HIGH-SPEED
HEALING

HIGH-SPEED HEALING

The Fastest, Safest and Most Effective Shortcuts to Lasting Relief

By the Editors of **PREVENTION** Magazine
Health Books

Edited by William LeGro

RODALE PRESS, EMMAUS, PENNSYLVANIA

Book Designer: Debbie Sfetsios
Cover Designer: Stan Green
Copy Editor: Mary Green

If you have any questions or comments concerning this book, please write:

Rodale Press
Book Reader Service
33 East Minor Street
Emmaus, PA 18098

Library of Congress Cataloging-in-Publication Data

High-speed healing : the fastest, safest and most effective shortcuts
   to lasting relief / by the editors of Prevention Magazine Health
   Books ; edited by William LeGro.
         p.   cm.
   Includes index.
   ISBN 0-87857-971-0   hardcover
   1. Medicine, Popular.   I. LeGro, William.   II. Prevention
Magazine Health Books.
RC81.H635   1991
613—dc20   91-7127
                                                              CIP

Distributed in the book trade by St. Martin's Press

   4 6 8 10 9 7 5 3   hardcover

CONTENTS

ALLERGIES

P ut a dust mite under a microscope and it looks like The Bug That Ate Buffalo. Actually, it's an unsightly, 3-millimeter-long relative of the spider and tick that is half of a Catch-22 situation for allergy and asthma sufferers. A dust mite lives in carpeting, furniture, and upholstery, feasting on dust—billions and billions of tiny pieces of residue from disintegrating life on this planet: the remains of carpets, draperies, blankets, furniture, toys, mattresses, insects, animal and people skin, hair, food, mold, and fungus—the whole allergen enchilada.

Without these mites, you'd be inhaling a lot more of these allergens. But as in all life, what goes in must come out: You (shudder!) inhale the dust mites' feces and body parts, along with everything they're eating. A British study has linked childhood exposure to high levels of dust-mite allergens to the development of asthma in later life.

Then there's mold—the fungus among us. Its spores are floating around looking for places to colonize. They land in our eyes and nose and lungs, which water and sneeze and sniffle and cough to get rid of them. An allergy is actually the body's own immune system fighting off a foreign invader.

You don't have to be a victim of the war going on inside your body. You can take the offensive and eradicate the enemy. You'll discover that:

- In just 10 seconds you can relieve asthma, with a dose inhaler for asthma medication.
- In just 30 seconds—the time it takes to don a mouth-and-nose mask—you can dramatically reduce your

exposure to pollen and molds when you mow the lawn.
- In just 5 minutes you can wipe out the mold spewed forth by your window air conditioner.

SAYING "ADIOS" TO ALLERGENS

In your well-insulated, energy-efficient home, the allergic irritants can be floating all around you and colonizing all kinds of unsuspected frontiers. Yes, you can take antihistamines, but they have such side effects as drowsiness or wakefulness. Take a few quick, simple steps from this list and spend more time enjoying your home and less time sneezing and running for the tissues.

Diagnose yourself. Allergies have many symptoms in common with colds and flu. How can you tell the difference? Colds and flu come with a fever, sore throat, thick nasal discharge, aches, and chills. True allergies generally involve lots of sneezes (often in rapid succession); a thin watery discharge; itchy eyes, nose, or throat; postnasal drip; ears that pop or feel plugged; loss of smell; and sinus headaches. A cold or flu rarely lingers longer than a week. Allergy attacks don't end until the source—like pets or pollen—is gone.

Switch on the climate control. Optimum temperature is 70°F during the day and 65°F at night—setting an air conditioner on superfreeze may aggravate allergy symptoms. Optimum humidity is 40 to 50 percent.

Turn off the fan. The greater the air disturbance, the more chance there is for allergens to circulate.

Card your vacuum cleaner. Unless you have a dust-free vacuum, vacuuming your carpet is actually one of the worst things you can do to remove dust. Instead of capturing dust particles, most vacuums suck them up and spit them into the air, where they can float up your nose. To test your vacuum for its dust spreadability, get a 3 × 5 card and cover it with double-sided tape. Partially tape the card over the exhaust grille with the sticky side facing the machine; it should not cover the entire grille but should hang loosely. Pour a cup of dirt on the floor, run over it for minute with the vacuum, then check the card. If the card is dirty, you've got a dust-spreader.

Spray tannic acid on your carpet. Tannic acid is a compound found in tea, coffee, and cocoa. It's a common ingredient in astringents. But researchers have also found it can chemically alter dust, pollen, and dust-mite antigens so they don't cause allergic reactions. One research team sprayed a pale tea-colored tannic acid spray on carpet infested by cat allergens. The average amount of antigen level after treatment was only 6 percent of pretreatment levels. Even six days after the cats returned, antigen levels continued at less than half the pretreatment levels in the most heavily infested carpets. The best way to continue protection, of course, would be to not let the cats come back. (The only commercially available tannic acid is Allergy Control Solution, produced by Allergy Control Products, 96 Danbury Road, Ridgefield, CT 06877.)

Banish allergens from the bedroom. Another good place to start your drive toward an allergen-free environment is the bedroom—where we generally spend over a third of our lives.

- Sleep on a waterbed. Waterbeds may be good for most amorous couples, but not Mr. and Mrs. Mite. Without the dark recesses of a fabric mattress to cling to, they'll look for a more hospitable honeymoon haven.
- Damp mop the walls, including the closet walls.
- Use synthetic pillows and comforters. Hair and feathers have no allergic potential by themselves, but are always contaminated by animal dander. "Nearly everything in your bedroom should be either washable or contained in nonallergic encasements," says Michael Kaliner, M.D., head of the Allergic Disease Section of the National Institute of Allergy and Infectious Diseases in Bethesda, Maryland. That includes curtains, walls, window shades, blankets, and bedspreads.
- Wash your bedding and linens in *hot* water every week. Dust mites don't drown in the washer, and studies have shown that cool-water washes have no adverse affect on them.
- Bedroom carpeting should be removed or vacuumed thoroughly and frequently.

- Also throw out as many dust collectors as possible: stuffed toys, pennants, pictures, and knickknacks should be eliminated. Don't store items under the bed. Use shades instead of venetian blinds, and select furniture made of vinyls, plastic, and other synthetics. Encase box spring, mattress, and pillows in nonporous plastic or rubberized cloth. Even the zippers should be sealed with adhesive tape. Keep all clothes in closets, preferably outside the room, and keep the closets shut.

Walk on wood. Hardwood and linoleum floors rob dust mites and fungi of a place to grow, and help prevent dust accumulation. Studies have shown that removing carpeting, particularly from the basement and first floor, can help reduce allergic reactions. It will be worth your time and money to have someone rip out your carpeting while you spend the day away from the house.

Slim down your furniture. Overstuffed furniture may harbor cattle dander, goat hair, and burlap, which contains highly allergenic hemp and jute. Buy either hardwood or plastic furniture.

Dust with oil instead of feathers. Feather dusters often contain dander. Dusting with furniture oil or polish not only saves time, it saves your nose. Of course, the biggest time-saver would be to delegate the task. And avoid vigorous dusting; it kicks up the dust rather than catching it.

Rip down the wallpaper. Your walls should be smooth and painted. Fabric wall coverings and rough-textured wallpaper will aggravate your allergies. If pictures or paintings are necessary, they should be framed with narrow, smooth wood and covered with glass.

Dry up your basement. People with asthma should avoid basements as much as possible. However, it's still necessary to keep a cellar as dry and clean as possible. Plug in a strategically placed dehumidifier and it instantly begins to reduce mold and its trouble-making spores, Dr. Kaliner says.

Leave the motel light on for roaches. Roach motels effectively trap and kill the insects without the sometimes allergic and toxic effects of insecticides, says Mark Sneller, head of the Office of Pollen and Mold Control in

Pima County, Arizona. The traps are fast and simple to use, and the bugs don't go crawling around your house slowly dying from sprayed insecticide. A study conducted in southwest Chicago involving 100 asthmatics showed that 60 percent were allergic to cockroaches and their debris and were repeatedly hospitalized with asthma attacks despite religiously taking their medication.

Wipe mold out of its hiding places. Periodically, take a few minutes and a bucket of chlorine bleach mixed with water to clean bathrooms, basements, leaky windows, water vaporizers, humidifiers, and hot-air systems. The bleach instantly kills mold. Discard old, moldy, or mildewed books. Even so-called clean books should be kept in a glass-enclosed bookshelf, Dr. Kaliner says. And don't forget the drip pans under your frost-free refrigerator and freezer—another microbe hot spot. A 10 percent chlorine bleach wipedown, a good washing, and a fresh chlorine tablet in each pan should keep mold to a minimum.

Make sure there's a good venting system in the kitchen, clean and free of dampness. Keep the exhaust fan on while cooking. Replace filters in forced-air heaters and furnaces often.

Chlorinate your air conditioner. Drop a fresh chlorine tablet into the area where the water drains from your window air conditioner. Standing water is essentially a breeding pond for multiplication-minded mold and bacteria that can contaminate an entire unit. If your air conditioner's drainpipe stops dripping, you could be in for trouble.

Open the windows for mold. You may get more than cool air piped into your home the next time you turn on your air conditioner—the first short burst could be mold. Before you turn on your air conditioner in the summer, make sure the windows are open, close the door, and leave the room. After the first few minutes, the air coming out should be relatively uncontaminated.

Wash your hands. Eye symptoms in allergy sufferers can be reduced by washing hands after handling pets, foods, and other problem substances; invariably the hands touch the eyes.

Wash your hair with Head and Shoulders. Or Selsun Blue, or any good antidandruff shampoo, to control flaking. Researchers in Denmark found that people who had dandruff had almost four times as many dust mites in their home as those without similar skin conditions.

Tell your friends about your allergies. Make sure house guests know you're glad to have their company but that their cigarettes, perfume, scented cosmetics, and any other allergy-inducing items are unwelcome.

Bake your newspaper. You can eradicate irritants in fresh newsprint by simply putting new papers in an oven set on very low heat for 20 minutes.

Air-condition your car. If you can't afford to allergy-proof your car, roll down the windows, turn on the air conditioner, get out of the car, and let it run for 10 to 15 minutes. Your drive should be allergy-free.

Put the top up. If you suffer from allergies, convertibles give you a kind of air conditioning you don't want. A California doctor discovered that driving with the top down exposed the passengers to almost 50 times the amount of pollen as the passengers in a hardtop with the windows rolled up.

SURVIVING PET-HOOD

Heaven forbid that it could be little Fifi or big Rowf that's making you itch and sneeze, but facts are facts: Some allergy sufferers are troubled by proteins from their pet's urine, saliva, and dander that are spread throughout the house. By constantly flapping their wings, even small birds spread dust and dander throughout the house. If all else fails, you may have to give your pet away. But first try some of these quick antidotes to animal allergies.

Banish pets from the bedroom. People spend the largest part of their time at home in the bedroom. You can cut your exposure to your pet's allergens by preventing it from visiting you there or in any other room where you spend a lot of time, according to the American Academy of Allergy and Immunology.

Let your pet out. This will also reduce your exposure to your pet's allergens when you are in your home.

Brush up outside. Brushing your cat or dog outdoors helps remove pet hair and allergens before they get inside your home. You may want to have someone else do it.

Replace bedding and carpeting. If you removed your pet or banished it from a particular room, *replace* any fabrics or carpeting that may have been contaminated with dander. (Cleaning isn't recommended, because sometimes it can take years to remove dander from a fabric.)

Depollen your pet. Cats and dogs need exercise. But before Fluffy and Spike are allowed back into the house, they should be thoroughly cleaned. When they're sniffing all those trees and shrubs, they pick up pollen in their pelt. In some cases, people who think they're allergic to pet dander are actually reacting to petborne pollen.

Pet a snake. Animals without hair, like tropical fish, turtles, hermit crabs, and even snakes, are usually safe for those suffering from allergies. Cats seem to aggravate allergies more often than dogs, although it's not known why. In general, nearly 25 percent of the U.S. population is allergy sensitive to cats or dogs.

Decontaminate yourself after visiting a pet owner. If you've been to someone's house where there is a pet, remove and wash your clothing as soon as possible. The same goes for clothes worn while romping outdoors.

Get rid of pets. It may be an unhappy prospect, but giving your furry or feathered pet away will definitely reduce the number of allergens in your home. So widespread is the contamination that the allergen level may not go down to an acceptable level for some time after the offending pet is removed. In fact, during one Baltimore study of homes that had cats, researchers discovered that unless some "aggressive environmental control measures were undertaken"—like the complete removal of furniture and carpeting—allergen content lingered in the home for 24 weeks or more after the cat was removed.

Before you give your pet away, make sure it's the cause of your problem.

WEARING AN ALLERGEN-FREE WARDROBE

Could you be allergic to your clothes? It's possible, since clothes are made of fibers that not only catch dust but make it. And many fabrics are treated with all sorts of chemicals that make the clothes look and wear better but can make you sneeze and itch. You don't have to become a nudist; you can enjoy haute couture by following a few quick fashion fixes.

Strip off fashions treated with formaldehyde. A hypoallergenic wardrobe will not only make you *look* "mahvelous, dahling," as Billy Crystal's character Fernando says, but will make you *feel* mahvelous as well. Steer clear of fashions that are treated with formaldehyde —frequently a source of skin irritation—by buying 100 percent synthetics, silk, or linen, or fabrics that have been mercerized or Sanforized.

Slip into only good-quality wool. Spend a little time searching out clothes made with only good-quality domestic wool—it's processed to be dander-free. That's not the case with wool clothing produced in many Third World countries.

Dry your clothes indoors. Hanging clothes out to dry may make them smell fresh, but you've unknowingly created a trap that is perfectly suited for capturing airborne pollen. Use a clothes dryer instead. And be sure to keep the lint trap clean.

MOWING DOWN HAY FEVER

Now that you have made your house safe for your nose, it would be nice if you could just hide indoors all the time. Outside lurk trillions of evil little allergens just waiting for you to put one foot out the door. But it is such a nice day outside. Is it safe? It can be, with a few simple precautions.

Time your outdoor excursions. Most pollen takes flight between 5 A.M. and 10 A.M. Weeds, grasses, and trees are the big pollen spreaders, taking advantage of wind to spread from near and far to every corner of your yard.

The trick to beating hay fever is avoiding the aerial bombardment. You might even consider staying inside on days when the pollen count is high or the wind is strong.

Hire a yard service. Get someone else to mow your lawn and rake your leaves. Both stir up pollen, mold, and dust. And talk about saving time: *Think* of what you can do with the hours you'll have to spare.

Wear a mask. If you mow the lawn yourself, wear a mouth-and-nose mask. There are a variety of nuisance masks and respirators on the market that reduce particulate exposure dramatically, Dr. Kaliner says.

Go to the root of the problem. A few hours spent pulling, chopping, and otherwise eliminating plants you're allergic to can save even more hours of sneezing and sniffling. Ragweed is justifiably notorious, but there are hundreds of other sadistic pollen producers. Next to weeds in producing troublesome pollen are grasses, most notably timothy, redtop, Bermuda orchard, sweet vernal, rye, and some bluegrasses. The pollen of such trees as elm, birch, ash, hickory, poplar, sycamore, maple, cypress, and walnut is often the cause of early spring hay fever.

Evict some houseplants. Reduce the overall number of plants in your home—a flash point for allergy-causing mold. Dead leaves quickly become moldy. Again, you save time by not having to water, feed, and clean—let alone worry about—large numbers of plants.

Be pushy about property regulations. Unless routinely trimmed, an average vacant lot can produce almost 22 pounds of pollen in less than a week. If you have such a lot in your neighborhood, a quick call to city hall can get the owner to take care of it. Or push your local government to develop an Office of Mold and Pollen like the one in Pima County, Arizona, which enforces pollen control ordinances with the threat of strict fines.

Wash off the pollen. Even antihistamines won't help if you're still covered with pollen. Partially washing yourself down with a hose outside is even better—you won't drag the airborne pollen into the house. Make sure to shampoo your hair—it acts like a small net, capturing windblown pollen.

Take a vacation next pollen season. Once you discover the peak pollen season for your area—generally from March to September—pick a pollen-free place, perhaps near the sea, and plan to spend a week's vacation there. But don't just hastily relocate if you find relief; you can easily develop allergies in your new surroundings. Before picking your vacation spot you might also consider the area's temperature swings, humidity, industrial contaminants, road dusts, insect life, and local vegetation— all potential allergens. Desert areas are good because there's little pollen and the humidity is low.

BREATHING EASY WITH ASTHMA

Imagine what it would be like to be fine one minute, a normal, healthy person with a full breath of air in your lungs. Then, after an innocent whiff of the "wrong" flower or pet or perfume, you're suddenly fighting for your next breath, gasping for life-giving air as your chest feels like it's caught in a vise.

As many as 10 percent of Americans know this feeling. They're asthmatic. More than half the cases of asthma in children and young adults are allergic asthma. And most know the quickest relief comes from using their medication as directed, especially *during* an attack. But there are other ways to quickly control asthma.

Sippa cuppa hot soup. Actually, any *warm* liquid may lessen the severity of asthma attacks and quickly relieve them when they occur. "Cold liquids irritate bronchial tubes, while warm liquids have the opposite effect," says Eric J. Schenkel, M.D., an allergist and clinical immunologist practicing in Easton, Pennsylvania. "Even during an attack, warm drinks can soothe it in 5 to 60 minutes. During the day of an attack, I recommend drinking between six and eight glasses of warm water or another drink, continuing even after the attack ends. Every day you should have at least four to six glasses. The more liquids you consume, the less thick your mucus will be. And you don't want thick mucus."

Hava cuppa tea. That's regular tea, not herbal. Regular coffee will work, too. "The caffeine opens airways much like the inhalers used by asthmatics," says Henry Gong, M.D., an associate professor of medicine and researcher at the UCLA Medical Center's Pulmonary Division. "The relief the caffeine brings isn't as quick as that from an inhaler, but it's just as effective—and a good thing to know if you have asthma and you forget to bring your inhaler." Cola will do in a pinch, although if it's cold it can irritate bronchial tubes.

Get a flu shot. "Viruses are one of the key factors that trigger asthma attacks," Dr. Schenkel adds. "So get a flu shot every year."

Take time to acclimate to temperature changes. "Any extreme of weather can trigger an attack, so take

5 minutes or so to try to acclimate," Dr. Schenkel advises. "If you're coming from one extreme outside to another inside, stand in the foyer—or another place cooler than the rest of the building—for a few minutes to get your body used to the difference. And when it's cold, take an extra minute or so to put mask or scarf over your face and cover your neck."

Evacuate during house cleanings. If you have asthma, leave the house while it's being cleaned. And when the house is being painted, plan to take a full week's vacation.

Take your medicine before gardening. You don't have to give up gardening. Some asthmatics even report overcoming garden allergies altogether by faithfully pretreating.

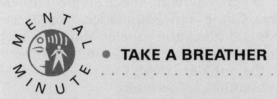

• TAKE A BREATHER

These exercises can make breathing less strenuous for asthma sufferers by helping them learn to control and coordinate the rate of breathing, increase the air supply, and maximize the function of the diaphragm.

- Lie flat on your back with your head lower than your body. (Use pillows if the bed can't be adjusted.)
- Place your left hand on your upper chest and your right hand on your abdomen. Inhale deeply through your nose, pushing out your stomach so your right hand can feel the abdomen rise. Use your left hand to make sure that you're not inhaling with your chest. Purse your lips and exhale slowly for as long as you can, pushing your stomach inward and upward with your right hand.
- Now sit up, leaning back slightly in a completely relaxed position. Repeat the same breathing technique described above.

Once you've mastered the breathing technique, you can practice using it when standing, then walking, and ultimately even when climbing trees.

Free breathing at once. If you have an asthmatic child who's unable to breathe, lightly pound him *on the back,* using a cupped hand. This series of gentle blows can dislodge mucus that accumulates in the trachea and obstructs breathing. To boost this treatment's effectiveness, make sure the child's head is below his waist, Dr. Kaliner says.

Uncork mucus with a hearty morning cough. The cough reflex shuts down during sleep, but a hearty morning cough uncorks much of the mucus that can accumulate overnight in the bronchial tree.

Use your inhaler properly. Between 20 and 75 percent of people who use metered-dose inhalers to relieve their asthma are using them incorrectly, notes James T. C. Li, M.D., Ph.D., a consultant in the Allergic Disease Clinic at the Mayo Clinic and Foundation, Rochester, Minnesota. You should place the inhaler about an inch and a half away from your mouth and begin breathing in before activating the inhaler. Hold your breath for 10 seconds and then breathe out normally.

Encourage kids to drink lots of liquids. Use a shot glass to trick kids into drinking more liquids than they might want. Children can be fooled into drinking the right amount of fluids by giving them a shot of liquid every 10 to 15 minutes.

Have a wheezing baby checked immediately. Don't wait—run to your doctor if you hear your baby wheezing. Breathing problems in an infant can become critical in a matter of hours. A pregnant woman with asthma symptoms should call a doctor also; if she can't breathe, neither can her baby.

Stick with methodical sports. Some exercise can trigger an asthmatic reaction that starts 6 or 7 minutes after exercise begins. But sports such as baseball, doubles in tennis, and golf are okay: They don't require the constant prolonged movement that can cause an asthma attack.

Think positively to breathe positively. "Asthma, like other chronic diseases such as migraines and pain syndromes associated with cancer, *can* be treated with biofeedback, self-hypnosis, and other relaxation techniques," says William T. Kniker, M.D., professor of pediatrics, microbiology, and internal medicine at the University of Texas Health Science Center at San Antonio. "And that can be done in about 25 minutes a day." Dr. Kniker and his colleague William Braud, Ph.D., a psychologist, are currently studying the effects relaxation and imagery have on preventing asthma attacks.

Meanwhile, a study from England showed that asthmatics who regularly practice yoga breathing exercises significantly improved their condition.

"It's the old business of mind over matter," Dr. Kniker adds. "The mind and body are highly connected, and thinking good thoughts and practicing positive imagery can improve some physical conditions. In past studies, we have found that some children who have learned self-hypnosis improved their asthma significantly. In a matter of a few days, you can learn self-hypnosis well enough to do the same."

Dr. Schenkel adds, "Short of medication, what I often recommend for asthma is relaxation. What happens with asthma is you're hungry for air so you panic and the panic tends to make asthma worse. Simply relaxing the way you usually relax is one of the best treatments you can give yourself—and relaxation can help soothe an asthma attack in about 15 to 20 minutes."

CHAPTER 2

ANEMIA

. . . .

The stairs. You're halfway up one flight and feel like you need to pitch camp for the night. Each step . . . feels heavy . . . as if the grocery bag in your arms . . . were 50 pounds . . . of potatoes. . . . Where's the top?

Iron-deficiency anemia. Just saying it brings to mind other words — like weakness, fatigue, tiredness, poor health.

In fact, anemia *is* poor health — iron-poor health. It means your body isn't producing enough hemoglobin, the substance in red blood cells that's responsible for carrying oxygen through your bloodstream. It takes iron to build hemoglobin. Without iron, hemoglobin can't do its job. Your blood gets starved for oxygen. You feel weak, fatigued, tired. Even slight iron-deficiency anemia can leave you dragging.

There are many types of anemia, but iron-deficiency anemia is by far the most common. And it's most common among women. Normally, as your body takes iron in, it uses only what it needs and stores the rest, retrieving it on an as-needed basis. In theory, you'd figure you could do this by balancing the iron you lose each day with the iron you take in.

It seems simple, but it's not. It's hard to keep on top of the iron balancing act. And that's because your blood is kind of fussy when it comes to using iron. There are three main causes of low iron stores.

- Loss of blood through menstruation
- Lack of enough iron in the diet
- Inability to absorb iron, even if there's plenty in your diet

But you *can* bounce back. You can put iron back into your blood—quickly. For example, it takes:

- A few seconds to take a daily iron supplement, the best protection for those who eat a poor diet
- Five minutes to make *healthy* food choices at the grocery store
- Ten minutes to cook a piece of lean, red meat, the richest source of iron

THE HIGH-RISK PROFILE

You may *think* you're getting enough iron when actually you're not. How can you tell? Fatigue, pale skin, and cold hands are all symptoms of iron depletion. Severe anemia can result in poor coordination, impaired wound healing, the inability to concentrate, and a craving for ice or dirt.

Those most susceptible to iron deficiency include:

- Women in their reproductive years
- Vegetarians
- Female endurance athletes
- Children
- The elderly

Women of childbearing age are at risk because of iron lost with each period. Five to 15 percent of women of childbearing age and 30 percent of pregnant women are believed to be anemic. Pregnant women are susceptible because the fetus draws iron from the mother.

Vegetarians are at risk because they avoid red meat, a primary source of iron. The iron in grains, beans, fruits, and vegetables—called nonheme iron—is not absorbed by the body as readily as iron from meat sources. You have to eat large amounts of these foods to get your daily iron requirement, because your body can absorb only 2 to 10 percent of nonheme iron, compared with 25 percent of heme iron. Being a female vegetarian only compounds the problem. Also, vegetarians tend to eat lots of fiber, which binds some of the iron so the body can't absorb it.

Female athletes, especially distance runners, are at risk because in addition to monthly iron loss, they may also be breaking blood cells in their feet as a result of strenuous activity, says Edward Eichner, M.D., chief of hematology at the University of Oklahoma Health Sciences Center in Oklahoma City. Furthermore, both female and male endurance athletes can lose blood (about 1 teaspoon) from their gastrointestinal tract during a long event. Athletes develop lower hemoglobin concentrations as a natural adaptation to exercise, Dr. Eichner explains, and this can be misconstrued as anemia. Tell your doctor if you're an athlete so he can make allowances when reading your blood tests.

"By and large, the problem is that women these days are so obsessed with thinness, our culture being what it is, they often hold down on their total calories even though they're running 10 miles a day," Dr. Eichner says. "They sometimes switch toward vegetarian diets for health, and the problem is they're just not eating enough iron to keep up with menstrual losses."

Children, too, can develop iron-deficiency anemia because of inadequate iron in the diet. By the time they're 9 or 12 months old, infants run out of iron stores they were born with. Thus, they need iron-fortified formula or iron-enriched foods or cereals to keep enough iron in their system, says Gregory Landry, M.D., assistant professor in the Department of Pediatrics at the University of Wisconsin-Madison Medical School.

"When infants are fed cow's milk, parents need to pay attention to the iron content of other foods," Dr. Landry says. Cow's milk has only a trace of iron.

As people age, anemia is more common. Hemoglobin levels often drop in older persons, and they may have problems absorbing iron because they often have less stomach acid, says Paul Stander, M.D., associate director, internal medicine residency, Good Samaritan Regional Medical Center in Phoenix, Arizona. Iron-deficiency anemia in older persons is often caused by blood loss from peptic ulcers, hiatal hernias, gastritis, hemorrhoids, and colon cancer. Another common cause is poor nutrition.

"Iron-deficiency anemia is not different [in older persons], except that elderly people don't tolerate anemia as well," says Dr. Stander, who also is attending physician at the Kivel Geriatric Center in Phoenix. "The elderly can suffer more severe symptoms than younger people for the same amount of anemia."

So if you're at risk and you have symptoms of iron-deficiency anemia, it's important to get a doctor's checkup. If tests confirm your suspicions, it's time to start building up your iron reserves.

PUMPING IRON

Okay, it's painful advice, but you should have listened to your mother. Healthy eating is the best way to prevent iron-deficiency anemia.

"In general, the best nutritional advice is to eat a wide variety of foods in moderation," says registered dietitian Cindy Heiss, of Texas Women's University in Denton, Texas. "For iron, that's the case, too."

What was it Mom said about food groups? And wasn't there something special about eating green, leafy vegetables and garlic under a full moon? Your memory is faltering. To get things straight, here's a sampling of foods to keep you out of iron deficit. (See "Food Sources of Iron" on page 19 for a more complete list.)

Reach for lean red meats. Red meat is a rich source of the kind of iron—called heme iron—that the body can easily absorb and use. But meat is often high in fat. You can solve the high fat dilemma by selecting the leanest cuts, such as round or flank steak. A 3-ounce serving of most meats can provide 20 percent of the Recommended Dietary Allowance (RDA) for iron. If you eat a small portion of lean red meat three times a week, Heiss says— and be sure to eat other iron-rich foods—you'll probably get adequate amounts of iron and still keep fat under control.

Chow down a Cornish hen. Dark meat turkey and chicken breast without the skin can give you almost as much iron as red meat but with less fat. Cornish hen has an edge over its fowl cousins when it comes to iron content.

Deliver yourself from liver. Liver still reigns as king of the iron caste, but it has a high cholesterol content. Also, "the liver is a detoxifying organ, so if there are contaminants in any organ, they're concentrated in the liver," Heiss says. So eat liver only sparingly.

Dish out the meat, potatoes, and veggies. This is the MFP (meat-fish-poultry) factor. Combine nonheme iron foods (vegetables and grains) with heme iron foods (meat), Heiss says. There are certain substances in the meat that help you more readily absorb the iron in non-meat foods.

Pop open a can of tuna. You can still eat light at lunch and get your iron, too. While not as rich a source of heme iron as red meat or poultry, tuna is a rich seafood source. Place chunks of water-packed tuna on a bed of lettuce. Add chopped celery and onions and a dab of low-cal salad dressing. Other good sources of iron from the sea are clams, oysters, and shrimp.

Eat your beans. Kidney beans, limas, lentils, and soybeans are all iron-rich legumes. "Beans are one of the best iron sources for vegetarians," says registered dietitian Ruth Lahmayer of Atlanta.

Eat oatmeal in an instant. In the time it takes to boil water, you can prepare one packet of instant iron-fortified oatmeal and start out your day with almost 50 percent of the RDA. But any whole-grain fortified cereal, especially Most, Product 19, and Total, is a good iron source.

Slap together a peanut butter sandwich. Just 2 tablespoons of peanut butter between two pieces of whole-grain bread can give you up to a quarter of your RDA for iron.

Don't forget your peas. Snow peas top the list when it comes to green vegetables with iron. They're one of the few green vegetables with ample amounts of iron. Collard greens, spinach, and kale are also excellent sources.

Pop a potato in the oven. Eat your peas with a medium baked potato and you can get a third of your daily need for iron. Potatoes are another rich vegetable source of iron.

Snack on figs and nuts. Dried apricots, dried figs, raisins, and prunes are among the few fruits with moderate amounts of iron. Sunflower seeds, cashews, and peanuts are also iron-rich snacks.

Chug-a-lug some orange juice. Nonheme iron sources — vegetables, grains, fruits, nuts, and beans — are absorbed better if vitamin C is consumed at the same time. So drink a glass of C-rich juice — such as orange, grapefruit, or tomato juice — especially with your morning cereal.

The RDA for vitamin C is 60 milligrams a day. Even

if you think that's low, you don't need supplements: An orange gives you 70 milligrams; a cup of broccoli 98; a cup of strawberries 85; a potato 26; a cup of red cabbage 40.

FOOD SOURCES OF IRON

Here's a list of foods that are good sources of iron. Remember, it's important to eat a variety of healthy foods to get enough iron to keep you going.

FOOD	SERVING	IRON (mg)
Clams, canned	3 oz.	23.80
Cereal, iron-fortified, breakfast	1 cup	21.00
Cream of Wheat, regular, cooked	1 cup	10.30
Tofu, raw	¼ block	6.22
Chicken liver, cooked	½ cup	5.93
Oysters, canned	3 oz.	5.70
Beef liver, fried	3 oz.	5.30
Soybeans, boiled	½ cup	4.40
Apricots, dried, sulfured, uncooked	½ cup	3.79
Lentils, cooked	½ cup	3.30
Spinach, boiled	½ cup	3.21
Potato, baked with skin	1 medium	2.80
Tuna	3 oz.	2.72
Sunflower seeds, dried	¼ cup	2.44
Beans, lima, large, boiled	½ cup	2.30
Beans, navy, cooked	½ cup	2.25
Beef, lean, broiled	3 oz.	2.15
Cashews, dry roasted	¼ cup	2.10
Beef, ground, extra lean, broiled	3 oz.	2.00
Swiss chard, cooked	½ cup	2.00
Spaghetti, cooked	1 cup	1.96
Chicken breast, roasted	1	1.78
Raisins, seedless, packed	½ cup	1.70
Beet greens, cooked	½ cup	1.40
Turkey breast, roasted	3 slices	1.33
Wheat germ	2 tbsp.	1.30
Peanuts, dried	¼ cup	1.20
Prunes, dried, cooked	½ cup	1.20
Broccoli, cooked	½ cup	0.89

Drink your coffee or tea alone. Both can hinder iron absorption, Dr. Eichner cautions. The tannins bind with iron and hinder absorption. If you wait 1 or 2 hours after a meal, the beverage should not have any effect.

Cook in an iron pan. Cooking foods in iron cookware increases your iron absorption, because some of the iron actually leaches out of the pan and into the food, Dr. Eichner says. Acidic foods like tomato sauce will draw out the most iron.

Ask your doctor about iron supplements. If you've already been diagnosed as anemic (a diagnosis, by the way, that should be made only by your doctor), you're probably already on iron supplements.

If you suspect you do not get enough iron in your diet, discuss it with your doctor. He may recommend supplements.

"For some women, especially vegetarians with heavy periods, I'd consider iron pills," Dr. Eichner says. "You can get them over the counter. Some women will need that extra boost of iron to keep up with their menstrual losses. They might consider taking one pill a day for two non-consecutive months every year—June and December, say—or two pills a week year-round."

Remember, balance and moderation are the keys—to eating enough iron, eating healthfully, and enjoying life.

. . . .

HOW MUCH IRON DO YOU NEED?

Here are the Recommended Dietary Allowances (RDAs) for iron. (The U.S. Recommended Daily Allowance is 15 milligrams.)

- Infants: 0 to 5 months—6 milligrams; 6 months to 1 year—10 milligrams
- Children: 1 to 10 years—10 milligrams
- Boys and men: 11 to 18 years—12 milligrams; 19 and older—10 milligrams
- Girls and women: 11 to 50—15 milligrams; 51 and older—10 milligrams; pregnant women—30 milligrams; breast-feeding women—15 milligrams

. . . .

ARM AND SHOULDER PAIN

Maybe you painted a ceiling all day without stopping, and now you know how Michelangelo must have felt when he was do-it-yourselfing around the Sistine Chapel. Or you stayed out in the garden an hour too long because you just *had* to get those tomatoes in, and now you're grumbling about Mr. Burpee and his abundance of seeds. Your shoulder feels as if it's on backward and your elbow feels upside down.

If our arms and shoulders could talk, they'd probably tell us we pay too much attention to our hands. "After all," your right arm says, "what do you think gets your hands to where you need them?" "Yeah," your left arm chimes in. "And what about watches and bracelets and blood pressure cuffs and walking arm-in-arm?"

Okay! Okay! You get their point. An arm has essential muscles hooked up to essential tendons that move essential joints, which are held together by essential ligaments and lubricated by essential bursae. The whole system has to endure a lot of stress and strain, and sometimes the parts hurt. But all your arms and shoulders want is a little attention, and you can give it to them quickly and easily. For example:

- You can completely chill out your aching elbow in 5 minutes.
- In 10 minutes, sound waves can wash away muscle pain.
- A new form of surgery cuts recovery time so much that you have to be careful to remember that you really *did* undergo surgery.

You may still have "the weight of the world on your shoulders," but today's medical knowledge can banish any pain in those arms and shoulders almost as fast as you can say "ouch!"

LEAPING LIGAMENTS! TESTY TENDONS! BLAZING BURSAE!

After your first tennis game in six years, your shoulder ligaments are feeling lousy, your biceps' tendons are throwing a tantrum, and your elbow's bursa is being downright beastly. The clue that it's these connective tissues and not your muscles? "With an inflammatory problem like tendinitis or bursitis, you'll feel a chronic, dull, throbbing pain that radiates out from the joint," says physical therapist Scott Hasson, Ed.D., an assistant professor at the University of Texas. Here's how to quickly take the "-itis" out of your tendons and bursae.

Act fast! "For those people who have overworked their elbow or shoulder and inflamed the joint, the first 48 hours afterward are critical," says William D. Stanish, M.D., an associate professor of surgery at Dalhousie University in Halifax and director of the Orthopedic and Sports Medicine Clinic in Nova Scotia. "Almost everyone may achieve relief in those first two days." Okay, you're going to act. But how?

Rub it away. Mommy was right. Rubbing the pain can make it go away. It's a pain-control technique with solid scientific backing. "It's something that you can begin to do instantly to reduce the sensation of pain from something like a stiff shoulder, tendinitis, or bursitis," says Edward Resnick, M.D., professor of orthopedic surgery and director of the Pain Control Center at Temple University Hospital in Philadelphia.

"Pain has to travel a fair distance from the injured area for us to perceive it," he explains. "When you rub the area that's injured, you're generating other impulses that will travel along the same pathways. These nonpainful impulses often interfere with the painful ones."

Freeze the flame with ice. Ice's cold competes with pain better than any other nondrug method, says Ronald Melzack, Ph.D., of McGill University, past president of the International Association for the Study of Pain. Freeze ice in a paper cup—that makes the ice a handy size to use. "The most effective technique is to slowly rub the ice in circles on the spot that hurts. Within about 5 to 7 minutes, that spot will feel numb and your sensation of any pain will be greatly diminished. The intense stimulation that ice provides is an excellent way to 'close the gate' to the spinal pathway and inhibit painful information from reaching your brain." Use ice massage three or four times daily until you're fully recovered. If you don't improve, or if the pain gets worse, see a doctor.

Put the squeeze on pain. It's called compression. You may find that wrapping the aching area in an elastic bandage will reduce swelling and thus ease pain. Make sure the bandage is snug, but not so tight or applied for so long that it's uncomfortable or blocks the flow of healing blood. Watch for any swelling or discoloration anywhere on your arm. Take the bandage off when you give yourself an ice massage, and don't sleep with the bandage on.

Boost it up. Arms tend to hang down whenever they get the chance. They swing back and forth and blood can pool, both of which cause pain. Keeping the hurt area raised above the level of the heart, or in a sling to restrict motion, helps control swelling and pain.

Rest . . . kind of. Dr. Stanish advises that you avoid the offending activity for a full week. That doesn't mean become a couch potato. Do things that don't aggravate the injured arm or shoulder. If it hurts to raise your arm over your head, then don't, but use that arm below shoulder level.

Swing your baby. After two days, when the pain is mostly gone, begin performing gentle "range-of-motion" exercises that put the joint through all its moves. The exercises help to prevent things from stiffening up and make sure that the injured area receives adequate blood flow in order for it to heal properly. Lean over and grasp the back of a chair with your uninjured arm, letting your tender arm hang down. Start swinging it slowly back and forth and side to side, until you get it going in circles. Do this for no more than 2 minutes at a time, several times a day; stop if it hurts too much.

Brace yourself. "When someone has no choice but to 'work through' the pain, a splint will give temporary relief," Dr. Stanish says. One common example of such a splint is "a forearm band" that greatly relieves the pain of forearm tendinitis—the correct term for what most people call "tennis elbow"—almost instantly. "The splint spreads the stress around instead of allowing it to concentrate in the joint," Dr. Stanish explains. It's often the only way to control the occupational tendinitis that people have—mail sorters or ice cream scoopers, for example, or others who have to make many repetitive motions in their job.

Pop the right pill. Aspirin and ibuprofen (Advil, Nuprin, Motrin, or the much cheaper generic store brands) are highly effective painkillers. They work by reducing pain-causing inflammation. Take the dose recommended on the bottle or by your doctor. Both can cause stomach irritation, especially if taken for extended periods of time, so be sure to check with your doctor before taking either of them.

Forget about the popular aspirin substitute, acetaminophen (Tylenol and Anacin-3): It's *not* an anti-inflammatory drug.

MUSCLING OUT MUSCLE PAIN

Muscles are different from tendons and ligaments, and muscle pain needs different treatment than tendinitis. But how can you tell it's your muscles that hurt?

"Muscle pain is very specific to the area around the muscle itself," Dr. Hasson explains, "With an inflammatory problem like tendinitis or bursitis, you'll feel a chronic, dull, throbbing pain that radiates out from the joint."

Muscle pain, on the other hand, hurts only in the area of the muscle itself—especially when you try to use that muscle. It may commonly occur a day after you exert yourself. The pain is caused by a buildup of fluid in the muscle tissue, causing pressure which in turn causes pain. Another sign of pain in a muscle is that it hurts when you press directly on it.

Here's what Dr. Hasson recommends to quickly relieve aching arm and shoulder muscles.

Milk your muscles. "Of everything we've tried, 'milking' your muscles is the fastest and best way to reduce muscular soreness," he says. "You need to repeat the motions that overworked your muscles the day before. Be gentle—don't extend your arm or shoulder too far or make abrupt movements—but keep moving the sore shoulder or arm pretty quickly. Repeat the motion 20 times, take a break and do it again. Repeat this for a total of six sets. This will keep that fluid moving and prevent it from building up."

Wash away the pain with sound waves. "Pulsed ultrasound—a treatment that most physical therapists can provide—uses sound waves that are much more powerful than the mild ones used to visualize internal organs in diagnostic ultrasound," Dr. Hasson explains. "We think they work by 'pushing' the extra fluid out of the muscle area, which decreases the pressure. A 10- to 20-minute session of ultrasound will provide almost complete relief. If the soreness returns the next day, one more treatment session should banish it completely."

STOPPING PAIN BEFORE IT STARTS

Now that you've recovered from that tennis match, you don't want to go through that pain and misery again. Your best long-term strategy, Dr. Stanish says, may be to "find a good physical therapist and 'marry' him or her. [A physical therapist] can teach you how to avoid the motions that are causing you pain and can help you build up and strengthen the muscles in that area. If you do that, you'll eventually be able to perform the same activity that previously troubled you without any discomfort." But for the short- and medium-term, pain experts have found several fast ways to prevent an elbow or shoulder from aching.

Stretch before you reach. "Warm up with some gentle stretching before you begin doing anything that requires a lot of overhead reaching," advises Tet-Sen Howe, M.D., a Singapore specialist and visiting Sports Fellow at the Cleveland Clinic.

Take a break. "Take frequent breaks if you have to do a lot of overhead work, like painting a ceiling or rearranging a top shelf," Dr. Howe adds.

Freeze pain after exercise but before it hurts. "After you've worked out, use ice, but don't wait until you get sore," says Joseph Estwanik, M.D., director of sports medicine at the Sports Science Center in Charlotte, North Carolina. "Apply ice *immediately* and keep it on for 12 to 15 minutes—however long it takes you to not be able to really feel the cold anymore. Then repeat the application every hour afterward for a few hours."

Lift light weights. Perform range-of-motion exercises to ensure a good supply of blood to your joints. And ask your physical therapist or health club instructor how to lift light weights to build up the muscles in that area, Dr. Howe says. If you're a menopausal woman or have osteoporosis, check with your doctor first.

Change your style. "The quickest way to get rid of a nagging soreness in the upper body is to learn how to modify the activity that caused the soreness so that it doesn't constantly inflame the joint," Dr. Stanish says. "So if you have tennis elbow from playing tennis, take lessons from a good professional and become a better tennis player! Tennis elbow is *not* a condition that you see commonly in professional tennis players. And that's because they have refined their form to the point where they just don't do anything awkward that puts undue stress on their elbows."

HIGH TECH

THE AMAZING ART OF ARTHROSCOPIC SURGERY

Sometimes the problem in your arm or shoulder isn't just inflammation. There could be loose stuff (physicians call it "foreign bodies") floating around inside the joint. Maybe the tendon has a small tear. Or a big one. Or there could be a structural problem limiting your range of motion.

Surgery might be the only way to find a long-term solution. How do you know what you need?

Get to a doctor. The sooner, the better. It may mean the difference between arthroscopic surgery

and the more traditional—and time-consuming and painful—open surgery. "Early on, when the tear is partial, we may be able to help with arthroscopic surgery," says Singapore specialist Dr. Tet-Sen Howe. "But if treatment is delayed and the tear worsens, there may be no choice besides open surgery."

Ask about an arthrogram. In this procedure, a needle is used to inject dye into the area to be examined, and an x-ray picture is taken. The dye makes the soft-tissue tendons and ligaments show up, and the doctor can then see exactly what the problem is.

Many of the more minor tendon and ligament injuries may heal on their own in a matter of weeks, Dr. Howe says. But one type of injury in particular can be stubborn. It's a rotator-cuff injury, one of the most common arm and shoulder injuries Dr. Howe sees in older people.

"Although the tear itself is up inside the shoulder, people generally perceive the pain from a rotator-cuff injury down the middle of their arm. The pain is usually increased when they're reaching up for something."

Now ask about arthroscopic surgery. If the doctor determines you have a rotator-cuff injury, and all conservative measures have failed, arthroscopic surgery may be the best way to heal it. "With arthroscopic surgery, recovery is usually short," Dr. Howe says. "You can be using that arm and shoulder for light tasks within just a few days. With conventional, open surgery, light activity would be restricted for at least 4 to 6 weeks."

If the problem is with your shoulder, you'll receive full anesthesia, and all the work is performed through two or three tiny holes, each about ¼ inch wide. Into one of the tiny holes goes a scope that allows the surgeon to see what's going on inside your joint. The other provides access for any equipment necessary during the procedure.

"The procedure involves removing pieces of torn rotator cuff, remaining spurs if present, and debris such as little pieces of cartilage that have come loose and are floating around inside the joint," says Dr. Ray Moyer of Temple University Hospital. "At the end of a month of physical therapy, you're likely to be fully recovered. With old-style, open surgery, the recovery is longer. That's because you actually have to cut through healthy tissue to get to the joint in open surgery. And besides recovery being faster, arthroscopic surgery has less risk of infection, scarring, and stiffness."

All arthroscopy is done on an outpatient basis. You're home the same day, as opposed to having a hospital stay with open surgery, Dr. Moyer says. "After an arthroscopic procedure you're usually back at a sedentary job in a week. You may have your arm in a sling for a little while for support. Ten years ago, when only open surgery was available, that same person might have been out of work for a month."

Sometimes the results of this futuristic fix are a little too spectacular. Some people feel so good afterward, Dr. Moyer warns, that they kind of forget that they just had surgery.

"Although recovery time from arthroscopic surgery will vary from person to person," he says, "you'll recover faster and more completely if you take your time, don't overuse the injured area, and follow a good physical therapy program."

WHEN THE DOCTOR KNOWS BEST

Sometimes the pain in your arm or shoulder can be so intense, or so incapacitating, that you want a doctor's help. Your doctor may advise you to try the remedies already discussed, but you can also ask what other treatments he has in his arsenal. There are two that are truly fast pain-relievers. Both involve injections of medication.

Lean on lidocaine. It's a local anesthetic. "The pain relief this provides is pretty dramatic," Dr. Howe explains. "If the injection is given in the right place, the results are almost instantaneous. By the time the needle comes out, the medication is already taking effect."

Count on cortisone. It's a steroid hormone famous for its long-term anti-inflammatory action. A local injection of cortisone will have calmed down the pain-causing inflammation by the time the more immediate "deadening" effect of the anesthetic wears off.

And the staying power of the steroid portion of such an injection is truly amazing. "If it's given in the correct area, the shot should relieve the inflammation for at least a month," says Ray Moyer, M.D., director of the Sports Medicine Center at Temple University Hospital in Philadelphia. If it doesn't last that long or is ineffective, Dr. Moyer says, it's a good indication that the problem isn't where the physician thought. Injections into other areas are then used to determine the real location of the problem, making injections a diagnostic as well as a painkilling technique.

This careful use of cortisone has few side effects, but if overused it may lead to deterioration of the connective tissue you're trying to treat. That's why strengthening and proper form, as well as less radical treatments like ice, heat, aspirin, or ibuprofen are the mainstays in handling arm and shoulder pain.

ARTHRITIS

. . . .

I f you suffer from arthritis, take some comfort in the knowledge that you are not alone. In fact, about 14 percent of all Americans have some form of the disease —and suffer enough to seek medical care.

Arthritis is not a simple disease. There are more than 100 different forms of it. The two main types are osteoarthritis, which is the most common and causes a mechanical breakdown of joint cartilage, and rheumatoid arthritis, which attacks and inflames the linings of the joints. Both types cause pain and stiffness in affected joints. The inflammation of rheumatoid arthritis adds swelling and heat to the list of symptoms. Gout is also a fairly common manifestation of arthritis.

Arthritis can be a discouraging disease because there is no real cure for it. Fortunately, there are lots and lots of speedy ways to relieve pain and release stiff joints.

You can, for example:

- Protect your gouty toe instantly with a bedtime accessory.
- Use moist heat to chase away pain in a matter of minutes.
- Ease pain, unlock joints, and improve your mood by taking a half-hour walk.

ACT NOW FOR FAST RELIEF

Sometimes the best moves against arthritis are just that— *moves*. Modest exercise doesn't cost anything, works to relieve arthritis symptoms, and gives prompt results.

Take a walk. "Walking can greatly improve a person's attitude and fight the vicious circle of depression and pain," says rheumatologist Sam Schatten, M.D., of Atlanta, Georgia. Walking provides a natural tranquilizing and mood-elevating effect, and it can help ease arthritis pain.

Kate Lorig, Dr.P.H., of the Stanford University Arthritis Center, coauthor of *The Arthritis Helpbook,* also endorses walking. At the Stanford Center, she encourages patients to use their common sense. "I tell people to start slowly, walking as far as they can without feeling more pain than before they started. If that means walking across the room, fine. One block or two blocks? That's a good start," she says.

Dr. Lorig also advises these walkers to listen to their body for signs of overuse or misuse. "Although arthritics may experience some pain with any movement, if the pain worsens when they begin to walk, they may be damaging their joints. Strengthening or stretching exercises—or perhaps some medication—may be needed. It's very important to work with your physician," she advises.

If you're afraid that you might be stranded by incapacitating pain on a long walk, Dr. Lorig advises that you can walk 5 miles and never be more than a half block from your front door—if you just walk up and down the street.

Walk on water. Sound too hard? Well, try walking *in* water. It's a treatment that all physicians agree will work. The water supports most of your body weight, taking the stress off your back, hips, knees, ankles, and feet. Once you're free to disobey the Law of Gravity, you'll discover that you can move with relative ease.

You don't need any fancy aerobic dance steps. Just head for the deep end of a pool, stand in chest-deep water, wave your arms, bend your knees and—walk in water!

TRY HEAT, COLD, AND OTHER HANDY HELPERS

Here are some quick tips for relief of pain and stiffness, plus some ways to make everyday chores easier.

Use moist heat to chase pain away fast. Moist heat can quickly chase away pain and stiffness from both rheumatoid arthritis and osteoarthritis, according to Donna King, a massage instructor at the Atlanta School of Massage.

King recommends that you rub Eucalypta-Mint ointment on the painful joint and wrap the joint in plastic wrap. Then apply heat with warm, damp towels, or soak the joint in warm water.

Chill out the pain. "Cooling treatments can soothe some inflamed joints," says Charles Jones, D.P.M., dean and vice president of academic affairs at the Dr. William Scholl College of Podiatric Medicine. "But make sure you keep a layer of cloth between the cold pack and your body to avoid skin damage, and avoid too much cold if your circulation is poor."

Toast your clothes. "Most arthritic pain responds to heat," Dr. Jones says. "Heat reduces the stiffness, too." During the winter, as Dr. Jones advises his patients, you can warm up your clothes in the dryer for a few minutes before dressing. The warmth will help loosen stiff morning joints.

Wash away stiffness with a warm shower. Another short cut to loosening up stiff morning joints is to take a warm shower or bath first thing upon arising, Dr. Jones says. Some people get a head start on the process by wearing socks or leg warmers to bed. They find this helps keep the pain away at night, too.

Get a gadget. "The best quick fixes for arthritis are the ones you can do around the house or on the job to make life easier," says Valery Lanyi, M.D., clinical associate professor of rehabilitation medicine at New York University Medical Center. "There are dozens of techniques and easy-to-use, inexpensive devices to help you conserve energy and save wear and tear on the joints. Thousands of gadgets and widgets can make your life easier," Dr. Lanyi says. "Some you can make yourself." For example:

- Opening and closing things: Looping a cloth through the refrigerator door handle saves wear and tear on the fingers. Smaller loops through zippers make dressing easier. And, Dr. Lanyi says, there are even gadgets that will open doors with the flip of a switch.
- Holding things: Wrapping foam rubber around the handles of eating utensils, razors, and hairbrushes makes them easier to grip and less stressful for sensitive, arthritic fingers. An extended mirror saves bending over while shaving, as can long-handled shoehorns and sock-pullers while dressing.

- In the bathroom: Install safety grips wherever necessary. A bar stool outfitted with suction cups to hold it securely to the shower or tub floor allows you to take a shower sitting down, Dr. Lanyi says.

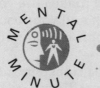 ● **WASH AWAY STIFFNESS**

While you were sleeping, did some loony laundress starch your body? Did the sandman drive a cement mixer up to the window and unload the whole 9 yards on your bed?

If you awake to morning stiffness, spend a mental minute loosening up.

First, be sure your blankets are snug and warm around you. Then close your eyes and visualize a scene that will help to unlock your joints and prepare you for a comfortable day.

Picture yourself resting on the bank of a gently flowing river. The sun is very warm. Feel it warm your body—warm your face . . . your neck . . . your chest . . . your belly . . . your thighs, knees, calves, ankles, and feet.

Your body is very warm, very soft, very comfortable.

The gentle river rises to flow over your feet. The water, too, is warm. It begins to flow inside your feet, warming them and washing away the stiffness. You can see strands of gray sand—the stiffness—stream away from your body, traveling down the river.

Your body is warm, and the warm river flows through your knees. Feel the sun's warmth, feel the warm water cleansing the stiffness from your knees. The gray strands of stiffness swirl into the river and flow away.

Send the river to any part of your body. Feel the sun's warmth. Allow the warm river to swirl and eddy through that place, catching up the gray bits of stiffness and sending them down the river.

Take your time. Enjoy the warmth.

Good morning.

PUT RELIEF ON THE SHELF

Stock your shelves with both natural and pharmaceutical treatments.

Try a lube job. Fish oil may provide fast relief from rheumatoid arthritis pain. There are good theoretical reasons why fish oil may help relieve arthritis symptoms, suggests Robert Zurier, M.D., professor of medicine and chief of rheumatology at the University of Pennsylvania: "[It] contains fatty acids that, in studies on animals and human cells in culture, have been shown to suppress the production of biochemicals that cause inflammation."

In an Australian study, 46 people undergoing long-term medical treatment for rheumatoid arthritis took 18 grams of fish oil every day. After three months, those taking the fish oil capsules had fewer sore joints and measurable improvement in grip strength, while a comparison group taking olive oil capsules showed no change. According to the researchers, fish oil brought relief by reducing levels of an inflammatory substance called leukotriene B4, and their results are strong enough to recommend adding fish oil capsules to the standard medical treatment for rheumatoid arthritis.

However, fish oil can have side effects: It can decrease the blood's clotting ability, raise vitamin A levels dangerously high, and interact with medications you may be taking. Consult your doctor before taking fish oil.

Try aspirin. The least expensive and most widely used antiarthritis drug is still aspirin, and most rheumatologists still recommend this ancient medicine as the first line of defense against pain and inflammation. According to arthritis expert James F. Fries, M.D., associate professor of medicine at Stanford University School of Medicine, the pain-relieving, or analgesic, effect of aspirin reaches its peak after two five-grain tablets and lasts about 4 hours. Dr. Fries says that "the anti-inflammatory activity," in which rheumatoid arthritis sufferers may be more interested, "requires high and sustained blood levels of the aspirin. A patient may need to take 12 to 24 five-grain tablets each day, and the process must be continued for weeks to obtain the full effect." This intense a regimen is standard for people with rheumatoid arthritis and requires medical supervision.

Block those betas. Rheumatologists know that stress causes arthritis to flare up. Would drugs that block the effects of stress also impede the inflammation of arthritis? Apparently so. Drugs called beta-2-blockers, which inhibit the effects of a stress-related hormone, norepinephrine, also apparently calm the fires of arthritis. "Other drugs currently used for the treatment of arthritis help reduce the pain and swelling, but beta-2-blockers have been shown to arrest further damage to the joint," says rheumatologist Jon Levine, M.D., of the University of California at San Francisco.

Dash for the sulfasalazine. According to recent research, a rapid treatment with this prescription drug at the onset of rheumatoid arthritis could put the brakes on joint damage. A study in the Netherlands found that the progression of joint damage was significantly reduced when sulfasalazine was given in the early stages of rheumatoid arthritis.

 HIGH TECH

ASK YOUR DOCTOR ABOUT RADIATION SYNOVECTOMY

Radiation synovectomy accomplishes the same effect as surgery for rheumatoid arthritis but does so faster. "A radioactive drug is injected into the joint," says Joseph Zuckerman, M.D., vice chairman of the Department of Orthopedic Surgery at the Hospital for Joint Diseases in New York City. The radiation destroys the inflamed joint lining, allowing less-inflamed lining to take its place. No incision or anesthesia is required, and recuperation is much quicker than for the comparable surgery. If symptoms return, the treatment can be repeated to provide several years of relief. And the radiation exposure is no more than that of a routine x-ray.

GIVE GOUT THE GATE

While rheumatoid arthritis and osteoarthritis generally develop slowly and stick around for a lifetime, gout strikes suddenly, with little warning, and may actually disappear after the first attack, never to return. In most cases, however, the potentially excruciating pain of gout does return.

Although any joint can be affected, the big toe appears to be the prime target.

In theory, anybody can suffer from gout. In reality, middle-aged men are the typical victims. Women don't seem to become vulnerable to gout until menopause.

Although it was once considered a royal disease, gout is actually very democratic, one caused by a chemical we all have in our bloodstream: uric acid. Some of us produce too much uric acid, and some of us produce more or less normal amounts but don't excrete enough. In either case, the excess uric acid crystallizes in the affected joints. And if you've ever seen photographs of crystals, you know they can have needle points and razor-sharp edges, which may explain why the pain of gout is so intense. "In some cases, the intensity is comparable to childbirth or a squashed testicle," says Charles Tourtellotte, M.D., chief of rheumatology at Temple University Hospital in Philadelphia.

An attack of gout is not a life sentence of pain, however. Gout can be treated quickly and effectively, and recurrence can be prevented.

First, get medical help. "There are conditions nearly as painful as gouty arthritis, but with different causes, so an accurate diagnosis is the first step in proper treatment," Dr. Tourtellotte says. "Pseudo-gout and infectious arthritis are all considerations. The treatment for these conditions will differ. An incorrect diagnosis will delay effective treatment."

Reach for the ibuprofen. Aspirin is the wrong choice for treating gout. It can actually make gout worse by slowing the elimination of uric acid. Ibuprofen, a nonsteroidal anti-inflammatory drug (NSAID), can reduce the tremendous inflammation that's causing the pain around the affected joint. "With NSAIDs like ibuprofen, you can be back on your feet within 24 hours," Dr. Tourtellotte says. "The effect is almost miraculous."

Take the pressure off. When the lightning bolts of pain start to hit, it's best to keep the affected joint elevated and at rest, according to Alabama pathologist Agatha Thrash, M.D., cofounder of the Uchee Pines Institute, a nonprofit health training center in Seale, Alabama. This advice will not be hard to follow, since the pain will be so intense. For most people, even the filmy weight of a bedsheet is like a crushing boxcar of pain on the tender joint. As a matter of fact, there is a product available to come to your rescue: a bar that attaches to the foot of the bed and supports the covers so they don't touch your feet. The bar is available for about $20 from Comfortably Yours, 52B West Hunter Avenue, Maywood, NJ 07607.

Tame the flame. John Abruzzo, M.D., director of the Division of Rheumatology at Thomas Jefferson University in Philadelphia, recommends applying an ice pack for about 10 minutes. The ice will soothe and numb the pain. If the pressure of the ice pack itself is painful, use a towel or sponge as a cushion.

Take a break from high-purine foods. Purine is a substance in food that can boost the body's level of uric acid, according to Robert Wortmann, M.D., associate professor of medicine and co-chief of the Rheumatology Division at the Medical College of Wisconsin. Some foods —anchovies, brains, consommé, gravy, herring, heart, kidneys, liver, meat extracts, meat-containing mincemeat, mussels, sardines, and sweetbreads—are so high in purine that they may actually bring on an attack of gout. Foods with lesser amounts of purine per serving may help bring on a gout attack, so don't eat more one serving per day. Asparagus, dried beans, cauliflower, lentils, mushrooms, oatmeal, dried peas, shellfish, spinach, whole-grain cereals and breads, yeast, fish, meat, and poultry fall into this category.

Go on the wagon. Alcohol not only increases uric acid production it also decreases the body's ability to excrete it. Beer may be a special offender because it not only contains alcohol, it also has more purine than other alcoholic beverages.

But don't give up drinking altogether. Be sure to drink plenty of *water* to flush excess uric acid out of your system.

BACK PAIN

F lat on your back. Again. Ask anyone who suffers from acute or chronic back pain what a back is for, and they'll probably answer, "Why, to be flat on, of course."

Actually, a back is good for much more than hurting. It's a place for arms and legs to attach. A good place to hang shirts and hide bouquets. There's walking, sitting, standing, swimming. There's running, jumping, riding, and dancing. Bending and straightening. Stiffening and relaxing and slouching. Twisting and turning. Itching and scratching. Rolling and tumbling and playing horsey.

With all those duties, almost any back can ache once in a while. Often it's a sprain, strain, or muscle pull. But sometimes it's a disk problem, or a symptom of some other serious condition. See a doctor when your back hurts suddenly for no apparent reason; when a backache is accompanied by fever, stomach cramps, chest pain, or difficulty breathing; when acute pain lasts more than two or three days, or chronic pain lasts more than two weeks; or the pain radiates down your leg.

But much of the time you can do something about back pain yourself; even if you see a doctor, he or she will often enlist you in the effort to relieve your own pain. The methods are fast ones. For example:

- In just 5 seconds, you can arrange pillows to relieve the pull of your hamstrings on your back.
- In just 10 minutes, and with two tennis balls, you can give yourself a pain-easing massage.
- In just 12 minutes, a back workout can wipe out pain.

Your back is hurting. It's saying, "Well, what are you waiting for?" Good question.

THE PRACTICE OF PAIN RELIEF

Generally, a strong back feels no pain. Exercise keeps it that way, and can also stop pain. That's why exercise and stretching are important parts of managing back pain. And the best thing is that you can relieve back pain remarkably quickly and easily, especially when you compare any of these remedies to hours of pain and immobility.

Hit the sack. The first and best thing you should do is go to bed. Depending on how severe the pain is, give your aching back up to two days of rest.

Get your back out of that bed, fast! Don't put down roots in your bedroom. Lounging in front of the tube watching another week's worth of game shows, soap operas, and Geraldo episodes may give your brain cells a well-deserved vacation, but studies show it's not going to do much good for your bad back. Bed rest helps, but only to a point. Back pain sufferers who stay in bed just two days miss 45 percent fewer days of work during the following three months than patients who are confined to bed for a full week. Your stomach and back muscles are growing weaker as they lie motionless for days on end.

Toss away that fear. There's another advantage to getting active as quickly as possible. The false security of prolonged bed rest can fuel fears that any movement will cause further damage. This mental paralysis essentially becomes paralysis of the body, trapping the sufferer into a cycle of periodic wellness—when cloistered in bed—and chronic suffering when forced to resume activity, says Wilbert E. Fordyce, Ph.D., professor emeritus of clinical psychology at the University of Washington School of Medicine.

Freeze pain with an ice massage. Icing your back for 5 minutes at a time over a couple of days can prevent swelling and soothe jangled nerves. Nicolas E. Walsh, M.D., of the University of Texas Health Science Center at San Antonio, recommends using water frozen in a paper or plastic cup to get at the point of pain. Lie down while your spouse or a friend slides the ice rapidly back and forth over the aching area. Spend no more than 30 to 60 seconds on each section of the area, and 5 minutes total on the massage.

Pump up the heat, pump out the pain. After two days of ice comes heat. Just 15 to 20 minutes of dry or moist heat widens arteries and veins, speeding the flow of blood to and from the muscles and flushing out wastes. A heating pad by itself is dry heat; putting a warm, damp cloth covered with plastic wrap between your skin and the pad creates moist heat. Set the pad at medium (or follow the pad's directions).

  HIGH TECH ● **TENS SAVES TIME**

Workouts without the sweat. That's the theory behind a device helping some back pain sufferers begin their reconditioning programs sooner.

Transcutaneous electrical nerve stimulation (TENS) electrically stimulates the muscles to relax and contract—like an isometric exercise —but without body movement. Electrodes from the battery-powered unit are attached to the skin and direct a low-level cur-rent to the appropriate muscle.

A study of 114 people with back injuries conducted at the Hospital for Joint Diseases Orthopedic Institute in New York City showed that electrical stimulation of the back muscles increased strength and endurance as much as isometric exercise.

Many medical supply stores across the country rent TENS units with a doctor's prescription.

Jump back and forth between hot and cold. Try the cold treatment for half an hour, then switch to heat for another half hour, then switch back again. This zigzagging has the benefits of both methods.

Stretch that spasm to a stop. In just a few minutes, a gentle stretch can work the painful kinks out of a back muscle spasm. As you lie on your back, bring your knees up to your chest and hug them with your arms. Hold the position until you feel like relaxing, then relax. Repeat until the spasm is gone.

Take 10 minutes, two tennis balls, and a rest. Massage therapist Ed Moore recommends this passive self-massage. Lie down on a firm surface—the floor is best. Slide two tennis balls (or billiard balls) under the small of your back, one on each side of your spine. Move them to the spot that hurts. Now take a deep breath and relax, allowing your weight to press down on the balls. The balls will stretch the sore muscles. You can vary the pressure by simply shifting your weight around. Rub your whole back for 10 minutes or spend 10 minutes in just one problem area. Don't continue massaging if the pain increases. This technique is not for disk or nerve problems.

Anti-inflammatories launch a blitzkrieg on back pain! Inflammation is a common companion of back pain, and both aspirin and ibuprofen decrease inflammation (acetaminophen isn't an anti-inflammatory). Aspirin and ibuprofen are famous as pain relievers for good reasons: They work rapidly, and with a minimum of side effects. For acute pain, follow the instructions on the bottle. For chronic pain, try one a day. A natural alternative to aspirin is white willow bark capsules, sold in health food stores.

A 12-minute workout wipes out pain. Physical therapist Robin McKenzie, author of *Treat Your Own Back,* and Vert Mooney, M.D., professor of orthopedic surgery at the University of California at Irvine, prescribe this easy exercise to help relieve the pain immediately. First lie face down. Relax your lower back, place your arms palms up beside your body, and turn your head to one side. Take a few deep breaths and relax for 4 or 5 minutes.

Next, place your elbows under your shoulders so that you're leaning on your forearms with your back arched and your head up. Stay in this position for no more than 5 minutes—less if it becomes comfortable sooner. Finally, place your hands under your shoulders, straighten your arms until your elbows are almost locked, and raise the upper half of your body as if you're doing push-ups. But keep your hips, pelvis, and legs relaxed and allow your lower back to sag. Repeat ten times, holding the sag for about 10 seconds.

If you don't feel better within a few days, try the exercise above but shift your hips away from the painful side—that is, while keeping both hips on the floor move the hip on the well side of your back higher (closer to your head) than the hip on the sore side—then complete the exercise. Often shifting your hip away from the bad side is enough to stop the pain, McKenzie says.

If the pain is so great that you can't do the exercise, you belong in bed resting your back. Try the exercise again the next day.

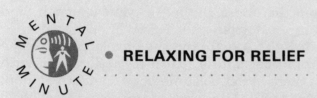

● RELAXING FOR RELIEF

Although there is still some debate over whether tension actually causes back problems, tension does contribute to pain, and there's little doubt that relaxation exercises can help ease back pain. At the very least, they can help keep your mind off the pain, even if for just a few moments. Try the progressive relaxation technique recommended on page 376.

THE PRACTICE OF PAIN PREVENTION

Just because you're able to get on your feet quickly is no guarantee, of course, that your back will stay healthy forever. The wrong movements will always have the potential to damage a weak back. But by following some of the fast-healing advice that follows, you may be able to help minimize the damage and speed relief. Better still, strengthening your back will vastly improve your odds against knocking it out of whack in the first place. As always, see your doctor before beginning any exercise program.

Cram a cushion into your curve. This is one of the quickest and easiest things you can do to prevent back pain when you're sitting. Just put a lumbar roll—a tube 4 to 5 inches in diameter available at most medical supply stores—behind the small of your back just above the belt line. A small, firm cushion also will do the job. These are especially good for driving.

Stand up straight. "Straighten up" Mom always told you—but did she mention the long-term consequences of slouching? Some doctors believe that poor posture is at the root of all back pain. Curves in our spine support our weight, but when the curves are rounded from slouching, the ligaments and soft tissues are stretched out of shape, McKenzie says.

The remedy is simple and takes only a few seconds, but needs practice to become natural. Stand as tall as you can, lifting up the chest, pulling in your stomach, and tightening your buttocks.

Sit up straight, too. To nip the development of low back pain from poor sitting, learn to sit correctly with these simple steps: First, assume your standard slouch. Then, says McKenzie, improve to the extreme of good sitting posture—back arched, neck straight, chest out—15 to 20 times, three times a day, morning, noon, and night. Soon your new sitting posture will become second nature, and your newly strengthened back muscles won't tire as easily.

Take a brief break. Taking breaks from sitting helps prevent "compression forces" from damaging your back, McKenzie says. Take frequent breaks from prolonged sitting by standing and bending backwards several times. Do the same when you have to stand in a bent-over position, as when you're vacuuming or working under the hood of your car.

Change chairs. A few minutes spent choosing a chair and adjusting it to fit you can help avoid a lifetime of back pain. Ideally, chairs should provide lumbar support and the seat should be the right height. How do you know how high to go? When your feet are on the ground, your thighs should remain horizontal, McKenzie says. Use a chair that has armrests to take some of the pressure off your back. Seats that change angle, like recliners and some power car seats, also help prevent back problems.

Ease behind the wheel. Throwing yourself into your car might save a second or two, but your back may nag you about it all day. Instead, go gently into that car: Sit down sideways, then swing your legs in. When you're in, make sure the seat is pulled forward enough so that your knees are comfortably bent to relieve back pressure.

A neat car seat. When shopping for a new car, remember to examine the driver's seat! "If the seat is not comfortable, all the gadgets and other options won't mean a thing," says Roger Minkow, M.D., founder and director of The Backworks in Petaluma, California. "The seat should be supportive, not too soft, and would be more comfortable if it had armrests and an adjustable lumbar support."

Dr. Minkow also recommends you rent a car like the one you want to buy, and take a long drive in it. "If the seat is uncomfortable, it won't take long to realize it," he says.

Lift with your legs, not your back. As strong as your back might be, it's not meant to bend over in a curve and pick up things, light or heavy. Always keep your back as straight and as upright as possible, bend your knees to stoop down, and use your legs to return to a standing position. When lifting several objects, interrupt the process a few times and bend backward, McKenzie says.

Cinch on a weight lifter's belt. Weight lifters and bodybuilders don't wear those wide leather belts just to look tough. The belts, available in any sporting goods store, actually provide heavy-duty low back support during workouts. You wouldn't want to wear one all the time, but it can help protect your back the next time you have to lift something heavy.

Drag that load. Whenever you can, push or pull heavy objects rather than lift them. This puts the strain where it belongs—on your arms and legs instead of your back.

Slip a piece of plywood under your mattress. A droopy mattress can sag in the middle, forcing your spine to match its shape, says Charles A. Fager, M.D., chairman emeritus of the neurology department, Lahey Clinic Medical Center, Burlington, Massachusetts. By placing a board between the mattress and box spring, you'll give your spine the support it needs—and save the time and cost of buying a new bed. Be sure to lift the mattress properly so the first thing you do after putting in the board isn't going to bed with a back strain.

Slip into a "lazy S" sleeping position. You've got to keep your back flat on the mattress to relieve pressure on the curve, and so here's the secret (takes all of 5 seconds):

Put one pillow under your knees and one under your head and neck. That relaxes the hamstring tendons, which then stop pulling down on your back.

Add a towel to your evening ensemble. Some sufferers experience low back pain only in bed, frequently caused by a poor lying position, says Robert Krotenberg, M.D., associate medical director of the Kessler Institute for Rehabilitation in East Orange, New Jersey. One way to correct that is to wear a rolled up towel around your waist fastened with a safety pin. When lying on your side, the roll should fill the natural hollow between your pelvis and rib cage. Putting on the towel shouldn't take much longer than threading a belt through loops and buckling it.

Sleep like a baby. The fetal position is a good one for chronic back pain. Stick a pillow between your knees to keep your upper leg from sliding up and twisting your hips, putting pressure on your back. Getting into this position is quick—so quick it takes you back in time.

Pick the perfect pillow. One of the least suspected villains of your back and neck pain could be your pillow. Think about it: You spend roughly one-third of your life with your head and shoulders propped up at an unnatural angle by a pillow. The good news is you don't have to sacrifice a pillow's sweet softness for support, according to Hugh Smythe, M.D., director of the Rheumatology Program at the University of Toronto and designer of The Shape of Sleep pillows. "Hardness is the enemy," Dr. Smythe says. A pillow need only be firm enough to keep its shape and to support the lower neck when you sleep on your side. Dr. Smythe's special pillows place a ridge between the shoulder and head, supporting the neck and allowing the shoulders and head to remain in more natural positions.

Drop a pair of innersole "cushions" into your shoes. When 382 back pain sufferers in one study switched to lightweight, flexible-soled shoes fitted with simple shock-absorbing viscoelastic cushions, something wonderfully soothing happened. Eighty percent of the patients reported rapid and significant pain relief. The doctors credit the fast relief to the special cushions' remarkable ability to soak up the pounding stresses that walking normally transmits to a weak back. The good results lasted as long as the patients remembered to wear their cushions on a regular basis. The cushions used in the study are not available commercially, but shoe stores carry a wide variety of similar shock-absorbing inserts.

EASY STRETCHING FOR BACK PAIN

Careful stretching takes only a few minutes and helps get muscles ready for exercise—particularly important for someone who suffers from muscular back pain. These stretches are recommended by orthopedic surgeon James Wheeler, M.D., former team physician for the U.S. Military Academy at West Point, and James Peterson, Ph.D., a former professor of physical education at West Point, in their book *The Goodbye Back Pain Handbook;* and by orthopedic surgeon Hamilton Hall, M.D., in his book *More Advice from the Back Doctor.* You can do these stretches to relieve pain; you *should* do them before you move on to the exercises in "Boot Camp for the Back" on page 46. But since stretching when your muscles are cold can also hurt your back, warm up first with a short, brisk walk or gently run in place. Do these stretches only if they feel good. Always do them slowly and smoothly. Stop if they hurt.

Knee-to-shoulder. Lie on your back on a mat or the floor. Pull your knees up toward your chest and clasp your hands behind your knees. Continue pulling your knees toward your shoulders as you feel a gentle stretch in your lower back. Hold for 15 seconds while breathing normally, then relax and repeat.

The chair slump. Sit on straight-backed chair and slump forward with your feet on the floor and legs slightly parted. Then slowly bend further forward at the waist while running your hands down your legs until they touch your ankles; by then your chest will be on your knees. Hold for a count of eight, gently straighten up, and repeat.

The shoe-tie. Stand with one foot on the floor and the other on a low stool directly in front of you, with most of your weight on the foot that's on the floor. Bend slowly forward until your chest touches the raised knee and your hands touch the raised foot. Slowly straighten up, and repeat five times. Then switch legs and repeat.

Brace yourself for the "achoo!" Try to lean backward while contracting your abdominal muscles when you cough or sneeze. "When most people sneeze or cough, there aren't going to be any problems," Dr. Krotenberg says. "But if you have a weakened disk, there could be some damage done."

Think before you drink. Rather than bending over a water fountain and straining your back, put one foot forward and bend your knees when drinking from it. Or simply collect the water in a paper cup. Here again, a few seconds can prevent hours of pain.

Stand up straight when brushing your teeth. Does your mouth lower itself into the sink to meet your toothbrush? Who's in charge here, your mouth or your toothbrush? Hovering over the sink may be a little neater, but why risk your back at the expense of a tiny spill? When you bend over like that the only thing that's preventing you from falling forward are your lower back muscles. Your lowly toothbrush should always rise to meet your mouth, giving your back the respect it's entitled to.

BOOT CAMP FOR THE BACK

For this treatment, all you need is an intense desire to overcome your pain. Hubert Rosomoff, M.D., director of the University of Miami's Comprehensive Pain and Rehabilitation Center, advocates comprehensive physical therapy so rigorous that it's been called a "boot camp for backs." But at the end of just four weeks, Dr. Rosomoff says, patients who've suffered debilitating pain for years are again active and healthy.

Back surgery used to be routine for Dr. Rosomoff. But the success of presurgery exercise in relieving his patients' pains has changed the way he practices medicine. Now he believes that imbalances and weaknesses in the muscles that support the spine and hips are the source of more than 90 percent of all back pain.

Treatment is more complicated than just strengthening muscles. Dr. Rosomoff's patients are caught up in a whirlwind of activity—massage, stretching, relaxation techniques, and workplace analysis. Patients are required to promise that they will work 8 hours a day at the center until the end of their program to meet their personal and work goals. The bottom line: Most of their pain can be alleviated at the center, and much of the rest will improve with continued activity at home.

But you don't have to check into the center to put some of their best back strengtheners to work for you. You can try them now, provided you've already been loosening up with exercises like those in "Easy Stretching for Back Pain" on page 45.

Pelvic tilts. Stand with your back and shoulders against a wall, your feet at shoulder width and your heels about 8 inches from the wall. Bend your knees slightly, then tighten your buttocks and pull in your stomach. Try to make the small of your back touch the wall. Hold for a count of six. Relax and repeat.

Arm and leg raises. Lie face down on a mat with two pillows stacked under your abdomen. Keep your arms at your sides. With your knees straight, lift your right leg off the floor until it is even with the top of the pillows. Hold 6 seconds, then lower your leg gently to the floor. Repeat with your left leg. Next, extend your left arm straight forward overhead. Simultaneously, lift your right leg, keeping your knee straight, until it is level with the pillows. Hold 6 seconds, then relax and repeat with your alternate arm and leg.

Curls. Lie on your back, bend both knees, and put your feet flat on the floor. Begin to exhale slowly while lifting first your head, then your shoulders, off the mat with your arms outstretched. Hold for 6 seconds.

Side-to-side sit-ups. Lie on your back with knees bent and feet on the floor. Touch your chin to your chest, stretch your arms forward and slowly curl up, reaching toward the right or left knee. Hold for 6 seconds. Alternate. Repeat as many times as you can.

Cat pose. Get down on your hands and knees with lower back relaxed. Drop your head, pull in your stomach muscles, and make your back as round as possible. Hold 6 seconds.

Butt-tucks. Lie on your back, knees bent and feet flat. Push your lower back toward the floor and lift your buttocks off the floor. Shoulders should remain on the mat. Hold 5 seconds, then slowly return to the floor.

Side-lying leg lifts. Lie on your right side, your bottom leg slightly bent, your top leg straight. Slowly lift your top leg up, keeping the kneecap facing forward and your body straight. Repeat several times. Alternate.

CHAPTER 6

BLADDER AND KIDNEY PROBLEMS

Bladder problems have no generation gap.

Urinary incontinence plagues half of all nursing home patients, while youngsters up to 16 know the frustration and fear associated with bed-wetting. Formation of kidney stones and urinary tract infections afflict people of all ages.

Whatever your bladder-related problems, here are some timesaving methods you can learn.

- A simple, seconds-long exercise to strengthen your bladder and stop urine leakage
- A way to get rid of painful kidney stones in just 1 hour
- A way for women to get rid of routine cystitis attacks in just one day

Keep in mind that serious bladder problems need to be seen by specialists, says urologist Kristene E. Whitmore, M.D., coauthor of *Overcoming Bladder Disorders* and director of the Incontinence Center at Graduate Hospital in Philadelphia. The good news is that many people could be cured or have their symptoms significantly relieved if they sought help. Two-thirds of elderly people could have incontinence stopped or significantly reduced, says Mark W. Zilkoski, M.D., assistant professor and associate director for geriatrics in the Department of Family Medicine at the Medical College of Ohio, Toledo.

TURNING OFF INCONTINENCE

The bladder is a storage bin for urine, which is produced in your kidneys. Your bladder walls stretch as more and more urine is collected. Nerve endings in your bladder tip you off that you have to go. Even if Pastor Brown's sermon or your friendly neighborhood rumormonger keeps you glued to one spot, your sphincter—a muscular ring around the bladder neck—keeps the bladder closed until you're ready.

But sometimes things get out of whack, and you find yourself voiding where prohibited. Such a condition is not only messy but also humiliating and hard on your feelings of self-worth.

Many incontinent people are so ashamed that they seldom let anyone know about their problem—including their own doctor. This is a mistake. With medical advice, you may fix what ails you—fast.

There are three common types of incontinence.

Stress incontinence. This is what you have when urine escapes from the bladder during such events as coughing and sneezing, laughing and jogging. It is associated with an increase in abdominal pressure.

Overflow incontinence. This occurs when the bladder becomes overloaded with urine because it isn't emptying properly due to an obstructed urethra, the passageway urine takes to make its exit. This can create a poor stream while urinating.

Urge incontinence. In this case, your irritable bladder doesn't allow you to hold your water when you begin to feel the normal urge to void. Accidents happen before you make it to the bathroom.

HELPING YOUR DOCTOR HELP YOU

Your doctor is the best judge of what type of incontinence you have. But there is something you can do to make the physician's job easier and to help him or her make a correct diagnosis.

Start recording your voiding. You can help your doctor make an informed judgment on the first visit by keeping a careful diary of every episode in which you eliminate urine (even a few drops) voluntarily and/or involuntarily.

Also log in your glug-glug-gluggin'. Keep a diary of all water and beverages that you drink. Doctors say some people's incontinence would let up if they didn't try to become a human Thermos. Let your doctor see if your body gets more swallows in a day than Capistrano gets in a year.

See if a drug is doing you dirty. When people visit Dr. Zilkoski with incontinence complaints, he figuratively rummages through their medicine chest. "I assume it's a medicine—if they're taking a medicine that could possibly do it—until proven otherwise," he says. Diuretics are the first suspects to be lined up, followed by any pill with "anti-" preceding its name—including opiates (anti-pain pills), anticholinergic medications, antipsychotics, antidepressants, antihistamines, antiarrhythmics, anti-diarrheal, and antiparkinsonian agents.

If you're taking any of these, consult your doctor. Your sprinkler system might be just fine—one or more of these drugs may have been turning it on prematurely. "Except for some long-term medicines, usually within 48 hours you should see a positive change—unless there's another participatory cause," Dr. Zilkoski says.

Get past any blockage. People who have constipation—from many causes, including taking opiates for pain—often suffer incontinence as a result, Dr. Zilkoski says. (See page 70 for advice on how to tackle your blocked bowel.)

STRENGTHEN YOUR RESOLVE, STRENGTHEN YOUR BODY

As with any health condition, diet, exercise, and habits play an important role in incontinence. Likewise, there are many truly quick and simple ways you can help yourself.

Head incontinence off at the pass. If stress incontinence is your bugaboo, you can strengthen your pelvic floor muscles with Kegel exercises (named after their inventor), Dr. Whitmore says. You can locate these muscles the next time you're on the toilet: First squeeze the muscles it takes to stop a bowel movement, then squeeze the muscles it takes to stop your urine in midstream. Hold each contraction for 3 to 5 seconds. These are the two stages of this complete Kegel exercise, and that's how you do them: Back to front, tighten the muscles, count to four, and release. Do this for 2 minutes, three times a day (at least 100 repetitions).

In short order, you'll be able to strengthen the muscles both while urinating and without urinating during several sessions daily. Placing yellow Post-It notes around the house can remind you to exercise. Build to an optimum of about 400 daily contractions, suggests Dr. Whitmore, and work up to holding each contraction for 10 seconds. You can do this while watching television or thumbing through your favorite magazine in three daily 20-minute sessions—although you can still get results in a much briefer session, she adds.

And, she says, this exercise has an added advantage: It can help improve your sexual response and you can achieve orgasm more readily.

Drop a few pounds. Men and women who are prone to stress incontinence exacerbate the problem by being overweight, Dr. Zilkoski says. "Couple weight loss with Kegeling, and you've got a great chance of getting a handle on your incontinence." Even dropping only a few pounds may be do the trick.

Jilt Mr. Coffee. "If you drink a diuretic such as coffee, you're going to be going to the bathroom even more," Dr. Zilkoski says. The caffeine in coffee, tea, and cola doesn't cause incontinence, he says, but it causes increased urine output and also irritates the bladder. According to Help for Incontinent People (HIP), when several of its members broke with coffee instead of taking coffee breaks, their dribbling ceased.

Stay away from alcohol. The drinks can be on you, but they shouldn't be *in* you, Dr. Zilkoski warns. Not only is alcohol a diuretic and bladder irritant but it makes you uninhibited and relaxed, so it's easier for bladder control to slip. Abstain.

Track down and eliminate other offenders. Many foods can cause incontinence in selected individuals, Dr. Whitmore says. Some of the more common culprits are chili peppers, spicy foods, tomatoes, and chocolate. She recommends keeping a food chart to see if there is a correlation between episodes of incontinence and what you eat. Eliminate one item at a time for three days to see if leakage stops.

Kick your butt. Nicotine irritates the surface of your bladder. Plus, if you have stress incontinence, your coughing fits can cause you leakage, Dr. Whitmore says.

Try an undercover solution. Adult underpants—equipped with special material to absorb fluid and control odors and elastic gathers to prevent leakage—should be absorbent enough to hold one void, Dr. Whitmore says. Absorbent inserts are available for adults who have less excessive leakage.

Make a stand, ladies. Women who need to use the nearest bathroom—no matter what its condition—or race behind bushes to relieve themselves can carry plastic funnels in their purse. Available in some camping supply stores, these funnels allow you to urinate like a man—standing up.

Take a toilet along. Since toilet facilities are often inadequate, Dr. Whitmore advises women to be creative. Keep a portable potty or a jug in your car.

Listen to some plane advice. Dr. Whitmore says that many incontinent people unnecessarily avoid traveling by plane because they fear a midair accident—although not the kind most travelers dread. She says that you can still take a flight if you restrict fluids before and after takeoff. Aboard the plane, sit on pillows to avoid vibration, wear absorbent pads, and choose an aisle seat so you can make a beeline for the toilet if the need arises. Alert the flight attendant about your potential need to go.

Make legislators privy to your needs. Write state and local politicians to demand that adequate numbers of public toilets be available to the incontinent. Let managers in stores, restaurants, and ballparks know you're dissatisfied with the facilities when they don't meet your needs. Give them a line if you're forced to stand in one.

"Seeing that many more women than men have bladder problems, it would only seem appropriate that there should be more female lavatory space," Dr. Whitmore says.

Get hip to HIP. HIP—Help for Incontinent People—offers assistance and advice. Send a stamped, self-addressed business-type envelope and an optional donation to HIP, P.O. Box 544, Union, SC 29379.

They also sell the *HIP Resource Guide of Continence Products and Services* for $10.

Become a two-timer. A technique called double void-ing helps you drain your bladder more efficiently. Dr. Whitmore suggests you stand up after you tinkle, and then try again, leaning your weight slightly forward on your knees until your pump is primed.

Excuse yourself. Good manners are important, but so is your emotional well-being. Ask to be excused from the dinner table when the urge to empty your bladder strikes you. Better to risk an incident with your host or hostess than risk an accident.

● MEET ELVIRA—YOUR BLADDER

If you have a painful form of incontinence and would like to feel in control of the pain, Dr. Kristene Whitmore, coauthor of *Overcoming Bladder Disorders,* has a visual-ization technique for you.

What you do is visualize your bladder as a person. "If you want to name it, that's fine," she says. One person with incontinence calls her bladder Elvira; others refer to their bladder by decidedly less complimentary names. Still others assign two names to the bladder—one to use on good days, one on bad.

It's a coping device that you can use each day to let that so-and-so inside you know "it's not going to get away with controlling your life," Dr. Whitmore says. "If your bladder hurts you, in order to accept it as part of you, you forgive it" by calling it a good name, she says. "But before forgiveness you have anger, so you call it a bad name."

By taking a minute to cope with your bladder on a person-to-person basis, you soon will feel more in control and can deal with old What's-Its-Face.

DEVELOP SOME CONDITIONED RESPONSES

The scientist Pavlov used to ring a bell when he fed his dogs. Eventually, when the dogs heard a bell, they salivated whether they were fed or not. What worked for Pavlov may work for you when it comes to overcoming incontinence. Here's how.

Learn to hold your water. Many people with urge incontinence have an involuntary bladder contraction when their bladder accumulates a certain amount of urine, explains Dr. Zilkowski. If you urinate before achieving that level, chances are you won't leak. How do you know what that "certain amount" is for you? Simply time the intervals between passages of water. Assuming that fluid intake is even during the day, Dr. Zilkoski says, most people can gradually increase urine retention to near-normal levels of 3 and even 4 hours.

Use an alarm. If you are consistently having a problem with urine leakage every 3 to 5 hours, outsmart the problem right now with a pocket alarm set to go off at appropriate times during the day and night, Dr. Whitmore says.

Certain diabetics should urinate every 4 hours. Some people who have diabetes lose the ability to sense when they have a full bladder, Dr. Zilkoski says. He recommends that these people go to the bathroom every 3 to 4 hours whether they think they need to or not. Otherwise, their bladder can fill to such an extent that they've destroyed certain muscle fibers that are necessary to urinate, and they end up with overflow incontinence.

TREATING INCONTINENCE MEDICALLY

Dr. Whitmore says that the vast majority of incontinent people—out of fear, ignorance, and embarrassment—fail to seek medical help for their condition. Others, Dr. Zilkoski warns, rush headlong into often-questionable surgical procedures—a drastic measure—when some other treatment might have worked as well or better. (Some women, for example, have a hysterectomy because of a tipped uterus putting pressure on the bladder.) Far too many people have ended up under the surgeon's knife before trying nonsurgical techniques. So when self-help measures have failed, see your doctor and get information about the following options.

See if there is a physical cause for the problem.

Eighty percent of women who go to incontinence clinics in England have atrophic vaginitis (a malady common in postmenopausal women because of an estrogen deficiency) as a contributing cause, Dr. Zilkoski says. And, he says, the percentage is probably just as high in the United States. If your doctor finds this is the cause, the cure is simple: treatment with estrogen creams three times a week, Dr. Zilkoski says. Results are noticeable in three or four weeks, the doctor says.

Give medication a try. Many prescription medications block the involuntary contractions that can lead to urge incontinence.

If all else fails, consider the surgical cure. Those with stress incontinence, particularly women, are frequently back to normal immediately following a surgical procedure. The operation for women is particularly quick —less than 45 minutes to insert two "stitches" that act as slings to support the urethra, notes Dr. Whitmore.

Incontinent men with sphincter problems often are helped by surgery, including such devices as an artificial urinary sphincter.

The latest surgical technique (not many have been performed) is done using a laparoscope, Dr. Whitmore says. This telescope-like device is put in a tube in the body cavity just below the navel. A second probe may be placed next to the bladder just above the pubic bone. *Voilà!* The repair is made instantly—ending incontinence —and you're on your way out the door to go home the same day (with a catheter in place).

Inject new hope in 30 minutes. Women who have had their urethra damaged from prior surgeries or childbirth may be treated "right away" by setting aside 30 minutes for injections of Teflon or collagen into the tissues surrounding the urethra, Dr. Whitmore says. Some people with severe damage may need repeat injections every couple of months until the damage is undone. There's a 75 percent success rate.

As a last resort only, accept a catheter or female collection device. A few people simply cannot empty their bladder because of disease or injury, Dr. Whitmore notes. If this is the case—and make certain you've gotten a second or third medical opinion first—an indwelling catheter can put a stop to incontinence. Be aware, however, that this invites bacteria into your system and promotes frequent urinary tract infections. Far too many nursing homes rely on catheters without exploring other alternatives, she says—up to 98 percent are unnecessary.

HIGH TECH ● PUTTING THE SQUEEZE ON INCONTINENCE

If you are a woman with severe incontinence, here's hope for you. A new device called the genisphere is now in the testing stages, and Dr. Kristene Whitmore, a member of the medical advisory board of Help for Incontinent People (HIP), believes it looks very promising.

The genisphere is a small inflat-able membrane containing silicone that's placed through a delivery instrument on each side of the urethra. The membrane is inflated, compressing the urethra tube to give it more resistance and thereby ending or greatly reducing incontinence. The device may be available sometime in the 1990s.

COMBATING URINARY TRACT INFECTIONS

An estimated 5 percent of American men and 20 percent of American women are troubled by urinary tract infections (UTIs). (The shorter female urethra is more prone to urinary infections. Consequently, women get infections 25 times more often than men.) UTIs in men and women seem to stem from different causes. Most infections in males are caused by prostate-related problems; in women, they appear mainly after sexual relations but most are not sexually transmitted. The most common UTI in women is cystitis—bladder infection. If the urethra is infected, it's called urethritis. A kidney infection is called pyelonephritis.

Some people show no symptoms. Others have cloudy, bloody, or foul-smelling urine. Some may have back pain below the ribs, frequent need to urinate (although only small amounts pass), and fever and/or chills.

If urinary tract infections are making you have a day not even Mister Rogers could love, here is some advice you may wish to heed.

Keep tabs on yourself. You can buy self-detection strips that measure the pH of your urine. High content will color the strip, which could indicate an infection. A cooperative doctor who knows you can then prescribe an antibiotic by phone to save you an office visit.

Have a cranberry cocktail. The on-again, off-again debate over whether cranberry juice is effective in treating urinary tract infections has attracted a new cheerleader. Researcher Itzhak Ofek, Ph.D., professor of microbiology at Tel Aviv University in Israel, says his work indicates cranberry juice has the "potential" to ward off UTIs. Dr. Ofek believes that both cranberries and blueberries may possess "antiadhesion effects" that keep nasty *E. coli* bacteria—the cause of most UTIs—from attaching themselves to the cells lining the bladder. Another study found that 4 to 6 ounces of cranberry juice cocktail (daily for seven weeks) may prevent UTIs in certain high-risk populations.

Create an unfriendly environment. The more acidic your urine, the more hostile it is to bacteria, Dr. Zilkoski says. He recommends drinking plenty of acidic fruit juices. "High-acid drinks help keep the bladder bacteria-free."

Take a quick dose of medication. Once upon a time, doctors routinely prescribed a seven- to ten-day course of antibiotics as treatment for cystitis. That's ancient history today—and overkill in most cases. Dr. Zilkoski says that the treatment of choice for routine cases in women is a one-day, single-dose treatment (two tablets) of a combination of the prescription drugs trimethoprim and sulfamethoxazole (Bactrim or Septra) or amoxicillin. (Some doctors instead prefer a three-day regimen, prescribing one tablet every 12 hours.)

Unfortunately, one- to three-day therapy is insufficient for the treatment of cystitis in men, Dr. Kilkoski says, nor is it recommended for women who are elderly, pregnant, or diabetic. In those cases, at least a ten-day course of therapy with the aforementioned drugs is usually prescribed. Ask your doctor about side effects—especially if you have allergies.

Fight recurrent UTIs with a new antibiotic. If your urinary tract infections keep coming back, you might ask your doctor about the prescription drug norfloxacin

(Noroxin). Research shows it may be a good choice to treat complicated cases. Treatment is 400 milligrams twice daily for 10 to 21 days. Call your doctor if the drug causes headache or nausea.

BEDROOM AND BATHROOM ADVICE TO HEED

A urinary tract infection, although usually not sexually transmitted, can be spread by engaging in sex and/or poor hygiene. Here is some prudent advice from doctors to keep from being the object of infection.

Play real hard to get. Women who have a urinary tract infection shouldn't have sex until it's cured. If symptoms persist—especially if you're pregnant—seek medical help before indulging again. Since bacteria can flourish in backed-up menstrual blood, if you're prone to UTIs, refrain from lovemaking while having your period.

Hit the sink before hitting the hay. To prevent urinary tract infections, both partners should wash their hands and genitals before lovemaking commences. Those prone to infections should use an antibacterial soap.

Make water your choice of beverage. Drinking plenty of water helps flush bacteria out of your system. Women in particular should drink a glass of water after lovemaking, then drink six to eight glasses daily to urinate frequently—thereby keeping the bladder free of bacteria.

Develop a routine. Women should cultivate a habit of urinating after sexual intercourse. One study found that the practice was "mildly protective" in preventing UTIs. One school of thought is that intercourse roughs up the membranes of your urethra, making you susceptible to bacteria already present in your body. It's still debatable whether urinating before having sex protects you, but it can't hurt.

Choose your method of contraception carefully. The most marked increase in urinary tract infections is seen in women who use diaphragms. Spermicides also were linked to recurrent UTIs in another study.

Wipe out cystitis. After each bowel movement, women should wipe their bottom with toilet paper from front to back. Good personal hygiene may keep you from infecting your bladder with bacteria from your fecal matter.

Get out of a bind. Women should choose a wardrobe that eliminates tight slacks and nylon panty hose. The latter trap moisture.

GIVING KIDNEY STONES THE HEAVE-HO

Midway through the 1990 baseball season, shortstop Kurt Stillwell of the Kansas City Royals had terrible back spasms for two weeks. One day the pain became so excruciating that Stillwell had to be carried from the team bus to his hotel.

Stillwell's problem had nothing to do with his back—even though one doctor mistakenly had diagnosed him as having a herniated disk. What he had was only an itty-bitty kidney stone, but the pain felt like he had ground glass flowing through his system. In a way he was lucky. Some stones (rarely, thank goodness!) can be the size of a golf ball.

Kidney stones tend to run in families, although men are more commonly affected than women, possibly because female hormones keep crystals from forming. The condition is sometimes found in people with high blood pressure.

Four-fifths of all stones are made up of stone-forming salts such as calcium oxalate. These seed crystals normally are swept out of the body in urine, but they solidify like rock candy in some people's kidneys—or in some cases move to the ureter or bladder.

Uric acid stones are granules formed in your body if your urine is consistently highly acidic and/or if your uric acid excretion is greater than normal.

Here are some ways to keep both types of stones from making themselves at home in your system.

WATCH YOUR DIET

Very simple dietary changes can go a long way toward preventing kidney stone formation. Here are some of the dos and don'ts.

Adopt a low-fat diet. If you have a fat malabsorption disorder, you can reduce your risk of developing oxalate stones by following a low-fat diet. You can greatly reduce your fat intake by drinking your coffee without cream and skipping desserts, junk food (pork rinds, potato chips, salted peanuts), and red meat, while limiting your intake of dairy products.

Resolve to dissolve. Drink lots of water daily to keep kidney stones from developing. Water dilutes urine, decreasing the concentration of the substances that form kidney stone crystals. It also flushes the kidneys, sweeping away crystals.

How much water is enough? People with a history of developing stones should consider drinking at least ten 8-ounce glasses of water daily. Be especially aware that hot weather tends to dehydrate you, raising the risk of kidney stones and requiring you to drink even more fluids than you normally do.

Negate the oxalate, mate. Doctors say you can minimize your chances of getting a calcium oxalate stone by avoiding or cutting down on your intake of oxalate-rich foods. These include baked beans; green, wax, and dry beans; beets; blackberries; blueberries; celery; chocolate and cocoa; eggplant; grapes; collard, mustard, and dandelion greens; kale; lemon peel; okra; parsley; green peppers; raspberries; soybean curd; spinach; strawberries; tangerines; tofu; tea; watercress; and wheat germ.

Chalk up the brocc. Broccoli is good for you, and George Bush would do well to cultivate a taste for it. Broccoli is rich in vitamin A, a nutrient that can help keep the urinary tract lining healthy and discourage the production of kidney stones. Vitamin-A-rich foods include dark green and yellow fruits and vegetables such as dried apricots, cantaloupe, carrots, brussels sprouts, and sweet potatoes.

Forgo that second cheeseburger. In those prone to stones, too much protein in the diet can lead to stone formation, says Brian L. Morgan, Ph.D., research scientist with the Institute of Human Nutrition at Columbia University College of Physicians and Surgeons in New York City. He suggests keeping protein intake in the low to adequate range. For example, lean meat, poultry, fish, and cheese are okay, but limit yourself to a total of 6 ounces of such foods daily.

Shake off the salt. Eating salt starts a chain reaction

that ends with more calcium being excreted. The result could be greater likelihood of kidney stones for people

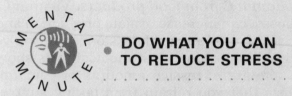

DO WHAT YOU CAN TO REDUCE STRESS

No, your kidney stones are not caused by stress, but tension can make things worse. What you can do to help yourself is imagine your stones vacating the premises. Do this exercise three times daily—in the early morning, at twilight, and at bedtime, says Gerald Epstein, M.D., author of *Healing Visualizations: Creating Health through Imagery.*

Sit on a chair with your feet flat on the floor, your hands and elbows resting comfortably on its arms, and your back straight. Do this for 1 to 2 minutes each time. Tell yourself that a flock of birds is going to eliminate your kidney stones for you (Yes, birds!).

Close your eyes and breathe in and out slowly three times. See, sense, and feel the presence of your kidney stone lodged in your kidney. (If you don't know what a kidney looks like, thumb through an anatomy book or encyclopedia until you find a drawing of one.) Investigate it from every angle.

Now breathe out once. Imagine a flock of golden birds with golden beaks descending into your kidney. See them pecking away at the stone and removing it. They chip away—you see and sense that—until it's completely eroded. Then they fly away.

Breathe in and out again. See, sense, and feel a light sunshower coming from above, washing through your body and flushing the kidney to take away any residue of the stone that remains. Sense the flow of urine—containing long strands of residue—going down through your urethra and out of your body, to be buried deep in the earth.

Know that your stones have been eliminated. Breathe in and out and open your eyes.

Do this for 21 days or until your stone disappears.

who are at risk, Dr. Morgan says. Table salt is out, as are high-salt luncheon meats, processed cheeses, snack foods, and foods packed in brine.

Get your vitamin C from food products. Vitamin C, taken in large doses, can increase oxalate production and increase the risk of calcium oxalate stones. If you've already had one kidney stone, or if medical tests show that you are excreting excessive amounts of calcium, research suggests that you refrain from taking supplemental vitamin C. Get your daily supply from citrus fruits, broccoli, and other foods.

Build B_6 to break down stones. Vitamin B_6 may help reduce the amount of oxalic acid in your urine that leads to calcium buildup, preventing new stones from occurring, according to researchers from India. The Indian researchers who conducted the study gave patients doses far above the U.S. Recommended Daily Allowance. Although no side effects were reported, be forewarned: B_6 can be harmful in large doses. Take this type of supplement *only* with the approval and supervision of your doctor. Better yet, enrich your diet with B_6 foods. Many foods are naturally high in B_6 including chicken, fish, and whole-grain cereals.

The rice bran cometh. From Japan comes a natural healing idea whose time has come. In one study, patients with a history of kidney stone problems were given two tablespoons of rice bran twice daily after meals. Of 61 patients, 52 had no recurrence. The researchers believe that a substance in rice bran seems to reduce the intestinal absorption of calcium, thereby reducing your chances of getting a kidney stone.

IF ALL ELSE FAILS, SUBMIT TO SURGERY

Thanks to surgery that uses shock waves to fragment stones (see "Smashing Kidney Stones" on the opposite page), the removal of kidney stones is hardly the dangerous, frightening affair that it was less than a decade ago. The method has decreased the need for conventional surgery to less than 5 percent. Doctors report that patients are back to work in two weeks.

● **SMASHING KIDNEY STONES**

If kidney or ureteral stones are causing you more pain and sorrow than the words to a sad country song, you may want to see a doctor about having them crushed with a machine called a lithotripter. No longer do patients dread the frustrating prospect of a long recovery period following surgery for stones.

The procedure crushes stones with shock waves. They disintegrate, but the kidneys and other organs are otherwise unaffected. The process takes about 1 hour. Most patients can be home the same evening or the next morning.

The only complication is the possibility that the stone will crumble into pebbles too large to pass through and will lodge in the ureter. Formerly, the only solution was to submit to surgery, but now there's an alternative. A long-tubed gadget called a ureteroscope—containing flexible optical fibers—coupled with a laser forms shock waves to break the ornery pieces into passable fragments. This, too, is a "hit it and git it" operation—in most cases, you'll be home from the hospital the same day as the procedure.

BRINGING BED-WETTING TO AN END

If both parents wet the bed as children, chances are about three in four that their boy or girl is a bed-wetter.

First, be certain that you're not rushing your child. Girls often attain control of urination before boys do. Doctors today say that the diagnosis of bed-wetting, therefore, should not be made until a girl is over five or a boy is over six.

In many cases, say doctors, the child simply has reduced bladder capacity, and the situation resolves itself nicely over time. Before any course of treatment, contact a doctor to conduct a thorough examination to determine if the youngster has a biological problem. There is no real evidence that methods such as restricting fluids and waking the child at night to urinate work. And reprimands and punishment are not only unnecessary but tend to exacerbate the problem. A child who wets the bed is not bound to become a failure as an adult.

There are many treatments for bed-wetting, but your child's pediatrician should be consulted, of course. There is no sure cure, but doctors report success with the following therapies.

"Stretch" your child's bladder. Rather than deprive your child of fluids, proponents of "bladder stretching" recommend giving extra fluids during the day to improve bladder capacity. Children then voluntarily hold off urination for as long as possible. In one study of 83 children over a six-month period, two-thirds of the bed-wetters who increased their bladder capacity had fewer episodes, including 30 percent who were cured or had only minimal bed-wetting. One problem with this method, however, is that it's often difficult to convince your child to do it.

Give your child a gold star. One treatment that doctors have found particularly successful involves encouraging the child to actively participate. The physician and parents do all they can to provide emotional support, and no punishment for bed-wetting is allowed. The child keeps a diary and puts a gold star on a calendar for each dry night. The treatment takes several months—longer than treatment with drugs—but it has no side effects and has a far lower relapse rate. In one study, 70 percent of patients treated this way improved significantly, wetting the bed only 20 percent as often as before. Experts estimated that one-quarter of the children stop wetting the bed entirely, and the relapse rate is only 5 percent.

Sound the alarm. In just three to five weeks, children can be taught to wake up on their own to urinate. Several safe and effective alarm systems are available, notes Barton D. Schmitt, M.D., a professor of pediatrics at the University of Colorado School of Medicine. Such devices consist of a small battery-operated alarm or buzzer that is attached to the wearer's pajama top, close to the ear. The youngster wears a moisture-sensor in a pair of tight-fitting underwear. Since only a drop or two of moisture sounds the alarm, the child wakes up before soaking the bed. The devices cost between $50 and $65. Beware of advertisers who offer to rent such devices for up to $1,000.

BOWEL HEALTH

While taking a cross-country vacation by car, Jerry Jeffers's body seized up. A stabbing pain drilled his left side. At a nearby hospital, a smiling nurse in the emergency room stopped smiling. In 10 minutes Jerry looked like the Clone of Frankenstein. His arms and chest contained enough wires to get cable, FM, and a hotline to Moscow.

The 43-year-old traveler waited for the results. An intern waltzed into the room. "Heart attack, Doc?" asked Jerry.

"Gas."

Jerry joked to hide his embarrassment. "I always stop for gas on long drives," he said.

Flatulence is but one gut-level problem that plagues us mere mortals. Some bowel problems are just socially painful, but others are deadly serious, requiring medical care. Jerry's flatulence is one of many difficulties with his plumbing that he has had over the years—including alternating bouts of constipation and diarrhea.

These internal matters can be frustrating, but happily, many commonsense or high-tech solutions can help you deal with them. With a little knowledge, Jerry—and you—can quickly control many bowel-related problems. For example:

- In just a few minutes, you can say *adios* to diarrhea.
- In one to three doctor's visits, you can banish hemorrhoids forever.
- In five weeks, you may be able to control the symptoms of irritable bowel syndrome.

DEFLATE FLATULENCE FAST

You like beans but they don't like you. You want the fiber that beans are rich in, but you're distracted by co-workers who wear clothespins on their noses when you're tooting upwind. Well, bean gene-splicers say that gasless beans won't be here until the year 2000. But in the meantime, here are some suggestions to hold down excessive intestinal gas, whether from beans or other natural gassers.

Go soak your bean. Much of the gas in beans can be eliminated by soaking them to break down the water-soluble starches your body can't break down.

Rinse 2 cups of beans until the water runs clear. Place them in a soup pot. Add 6 cups of cold water and boil for 2 minutes. Drain the water and replace with an equal amount of fresh water. Let the beans soak for at least 6 hours. Drain again and replace with fresh water. Boil then simmer these beans in a loosely covered pot until they are tender — 30 minutes to 2 hours. The process is a long one, so you may want to begin it the day before you plan to eat the beans.

Or take a tip from the Japanese. Buy kombu — a sea vegetable sold in Japanese gourmet shops and health food stores — and take the gas out of your beans. Simply add the kombu to the beans you cook, and discard it with the cooking water. You'll get the same effect you would have gotten by soaking the beans.

Try anasazi beans. Drop some anasazi beans in your shopping cart. They are the most user-friendly, gas-miserly legume known to man. To obtain more information on anasazi beans, call Adobe Milling Company at 1-800-54ADOBE (542-3623).

Be aware of other gassy foods. Every third-grader knows about the silent but deadly effects of starchy beans, but other foods that also produce gas include onions, celery, carrots, raisins, bananas, apricots, prune juice, bagels, pretzels, wheat germ, and brussels sprouts.

Give your vitamins the third degree. Some people find that supplements and vitamins — particularly vitamin C — can give them gas. Stop taking them for a day and see if that's the source of your gas. If your gas stops, start taking the supplements again, beginning with one, then adding another every two days until gas problems begin again. Then you've found the culprit.

Burst your bubbles, end your troubles. Simethicone is a nonprescription substance that does the job by breaking large gas bubbles into easily burst little bubbles in the small intestine. Simethicone is a common ingredient in over-the-counter preparations—for instance, Di-Gel, Mylanta, and Extra Strength Maalox Plus Tablets. The only dual-action OTC brand is Phazyme 95, which is long lasting enough to burst even Lawrence Welk's bubbles.

Get help with charcoal. You can relieve flatulence and bloating on the spot by taking two activated charcoal tablets before eating and two afterward. What happens is that activated charcoal effectively binds to either the gas itself or the foods that cause it. Caution: Because it binds to other substances as well, do not take it with supplements or medication (including birth control pills).

Try a little flour power. Some people just don't absorb wheat flour well, and the result is gas. If you've tried other ways to eliminate gas without success, you may want to try substituting rice flour for wheat flour.

DIARRHEA: COMMON PROBLEM, UNCOMMON DISCOMFORT

Diarrhea is an urge to purge that just won't quit. It can be nature's way of ridding the body of undesirable wastes. It can be a message from on low that you ate or drank something you shouldn't be eating or drinking. Then again, diarrhea may be the most visible sign of irritable bowel syndrome (IBS), a serious gastrointestinal disorder.

To be sure, an occasional case of the runs is hardly reason to race for help. Nonetheless, play it safe. See a doctor if you have diarrhea accompanied by fever, bloody stools, or vomiting lasting three days or more, or if you're awakened at night. In most cases, diarrhea does a disappearing act in a day or two. Here's how to help it along and how to prevent its appearance in the first place.

DEFEATING DIARRHEA

In isolated instances, over-the-counter medication is fine. But taking it daily is foolhardy. It can damage the bowel or mask the signs of serious disease. Frequent bouts of diarrhea need a doctor's attention. But for these isolated incidents, here are the main courses of action.

You ought to use ORT. Besides draining your body of water, diarrhea depletes such essential minerals as sodium and potassium. ORT, or oral rehydration therapy, saves the lives of thousands of diarrhea-stricken children in poor countries, and it can help you, too. Rehydrate with sugar water and a pinch of salt to correct a chemical imbalance caused by diarrhea, recommends Theodore Bayless, M.D., clinical director of the Meyeroff Digestive Disease Center in Baltimore. Or buy any one of the athletic drinks available in your supermarket to rehydrate your body. In any event, drink sufficient quantities of liquid to make you urinate every 3 hours and to cause your urine to turn pale in color. And remember, ORT becomes even more necessary if your runs turn into reruns.

Develop a yeast affection. An alternative to live-culture yogurt and acidophilus is a variety of yeast (*Saccharomyces boulardii*) prescribed in pill form in Europe that soon will be available in the United States. This pill stops the diarrhea that can develop when you're taking antibiotics.

You can overdo the bran power. Although a high-fiber diet is nearly always good for your bowels, occasionally you can have too much of a good thing, leading to cramps and diarrhea. If you suspect this may be the cause of your problem, try eating less fiber for two or three days. After all, eating fish is healthy, too, but scarfing a school of salmon in one meal would stretch your belly a mite.

Go bananas. Bananas banish diarrhea by soaking up water in your stool. They also are full of potassium, a mineral that diarrhea depletes in large quantities. Chiquita swears by them; so will you.

Counter it with over-the-counter products. Most diarrhea cases last only a day or two, but why not slam the door on them the way you would any other unwanted visitors? You can get immediate relief with remedies containing loperamide (Imodium). Imodium is not only quick acting but is also long lasting. It puts your intestine into low gear to slow down bowel action.

Get in the pink with Pepto-Bismol. Bismuth preparations (such as Pepto-Bismol) reduce cramps and also help relieve diarrhea symptoms by decreasing stool frequency and weight. Pepto-Bismol works in 24 hours or less.

STOP DIARRHEA BEFORE IT STARTS

When it comes to diarrhea, ignorance is far from bliss. Daily habits, what you eat, even an allergy can surprise you. Here are some quick tips to prevent your bowels from moving too fast in the first place, and keep them moving at a more reasonable speed.

Say no to beer and red wine. Some people have a problem when these two beverages go to their heads, but if you're prone to diarrhea they may send you to the head instead. Both are known to cause diarrhea. All alcoholic beverages, by the way, can lead to diarrhea when consumed in excess.

Choose an alternative to coffee or tea. An excess of either caffeinated beverage may not be good to the last drop. Coffee and tea speed up the digestive process—you need to slow it down.

Pass on eating sorbitol. "Sorbitol's not well absorbed by anybody," Dr. Bayless says, "and it can cause gas or diarrhea within a couple of hours." Sorbitol is a sweetener found in some brands of mints, candies, and gum. "We tell patients to check labels," Dr. Bayless says. So, if the chew gives you fits, put the gum on your bedpost, not in your mouth. Some people even have problems with apple juice or pear juice, both sorbitol-rich.

Round up all the other usual suspects. In addition to sorbitol, the sweeteners mannitol and fructose also can cause diarrhea.

Join the scrub team. Contagious intestinal bugs that cause diarrhea can be caught from toilet seats. Experts recommend avoiding public rest rooms if possible. If you can't avoid them, at least don't use stalls that are so soiled even flies shun them. You may also wish to use the less popular end stalls, use toilet seat protectors if available, and by all means wash your hands when you're finished. Clean your own toilet seat frequently when a family member comes down with an intestinal bug.

Have your diarrhea take a hike. If you're the outdoorsy

type, a few minutes of prevention may keep you from having to answer the real call of the wild. Before drinking water from streams, springs, or any untreated source, make sure that the liquid is rendered as pure as it looks. Guard against diarrhea-causing microbes by boiling your water vigorously for 1 minute, or inserting iodine tablets from your favorite outdoor shop.

Avoid pet peeves. Owning dogs and cats can be one of life's great pleasures. But if the wrong bacteria are present, affection may lead to infection. Thirty seconds of hand-washing after handling a pooper scooper can keep your pets from giving *you* a run. And, as your mother warned you—petting can get you in trouble. Wash your hands after stroking your Fido or Simba.

Limit your intake of antacids. If one of the ingredients in your antacid medicine happens to be milk of magnesia (a laxative), don't be surprised if you begin heeding nature's call more frequently than you'd like. Read the fine print on the label and do your bowels a favor. The laxative properties take effect in 30 minutes to 6 hours.

KEEPING YOUR BOWELS MOVING

Constipation may remind you of the silly riddles you asked back in junior high school. The question is: What goes in and never comes out? Unfortunately, you know the answer all too well.

It may make you feel better to know that one anal-retentive bloke was constipated for 368 days before finally achieving a bowel movement on June 21, 1901—a date that surely ought to be a national holiday somewhere. Surely there are easier feats to accomplish if you want to set a world's record. One of the most famous entertainers in the world—Elvis Presley—was plagued by constipation and lifelong laxative abuse. Instead of singing "I'm all shook up," the King could have lamented, "I'm all stopped up."

Constipation is more than an inconvenience. It tends to precede hemorrhoids and anal fissures. Sometimes it's a flag to alert your doctor that you might have a serious disease. Most of the time, though, it's a passing phenomenon that is quickly remedied.

ALL YA GOTTA DO IS ACT NATURALLY

The days are long past when so-called experts questioned the health of anyone who didn't have a daily bowel movement. In fact, studies show that many adults have but three bowel movements per week. The definition of normal defecation, like beauty, lies with the beholder.

Set aside a regular time. Research suggests that often all that is needed to put a stop to constipation is for you to set aside a time daily to use the toilet. A good time would be every day after a particular meal (such as breakfast) to take advantage of a gastrointestinal reflex that tells your body it's time to go.

When you gotta go, go. When nature calls, don't put her on hold. You can foul up your normal bowel cycle by trying to hold it in.

Stew some prunes. Stay away from commercial laxatives except under doctor's orders. They're unnecessary, habit-forming, and about as effective as Brazil's anti-inflation measures. You're better off trying to prevent constipation by making a lifetime practice of eating prunes, apricots, plums, and other natural laxatives. You can often beat constipation overnight by drinking prune juice or eating prunes before retiring.

Let nature take its course. Enemas once were as much a part of daily hygiene in enlightened circles as flossing is today. They went out of favor as doctors began realizing that healthy people didn't always need to move their bowels daily. Consequently, enemas today are used mainly by physicians for such purposes as cleaning out a colon for certain medical procedures. Even truly constipated people shouldn't have an enema more than once every three days. And enemas given at home should only be done under the guidance of your physician.

Brew some beans. Coffee beans, that is. A cup of coffee at day's beginning is a natural laxative.

LET FIBER KNOCK THE STUFFING OUT OF YOU

Studies have shown that fiber can reduce the transit time, the time it takes a meal to travel through your body, from 2 or 3 days to 1.6 days. The greater stool bulk produced by fiber decreases constipation. Here are some ways you can add fiber to your diet.

Munch muffins. Doctors recommend bran as a source of dietary fiber to combat constipation. You can easily reach your recommended ideal of 12 to 15 daily grams of fiber in your diet by eating a bran muffin or bran cereal. For best results, drink plenty of liquids to accompany the bran. Researchers recommend taking increasing amounts of fiber over weeks or even months to get all the benefits of bran without the drawbacks of flatulence and bloating.

Rice may suffice. You may see a dramatic improvement in your fight against constipation by using rice bran—instead of wheat—to increase the size and frequency of your stools. One European study says that rice beats the living chaff out of wheat when it comes to fecal output and frequency of bowel movements.

Bananas make constipation split. If constipation is your problem, eat a banana. The multitalented fruit can also help stop diarrhea, but when it comes to constipation, the fiber in the banana moves your stool through the bowel. In fact, nearly all raw fruits and vegetables are good fiber sources and so make good bowel buddies.

Psyllium will fill ya. Psyllium (Metamucil) is an easy way to add bulk to your diet. It may need two or three days with one to three doses daily to take effect. Contented consumers say they never Metamucil they didn't like.

Work it on out. Constipation and a lack of exercise are often twin companions. Give your gastrointestinal tract a boost by firming up your overall body. Any exercise is useful. Try giving up the elevator in favor of the stairs. Start slowly and check with your doctor to come up with a sensible exercise plan for you.

PREVENTING AND TREATING HEMORRHOIDS

Hemorrhoids are rectal veins that have gotten too big for your britches. You probably didn't know you had them until you saw red—specifically, the symptom of bright blood at toilet time that scared you into seeing a doctor and rewriting your will. Or, if you're a pregnant woman, your ob-gyn probably spotted these bulging veins during a routine examination.

Internal hemorrhoids occur in your rectum; external —the itchy kind—end up on the skin around your anus. Straining at stool and undue abdominal pressure is what causes them, so hemorrhoids may be said to be a complication of constipation. The other symptoms of hemorrhoids, pain and inflammation, need no introduction to hemorrhoid sufferers. They once knocked Kansas City third baseman George Brett out of a World Series game.

Here are some treatments and preventive steps you can try at home. These won't *cure* your hemorrhoids, but you will gain some immediate pain relief.

Soften your stools. Drink at least three glasses of water daily and eat plenty of fiber-rich foods to produce soft stools, which keep you from straining. This regimen works in just one to three days.

Soothe them with a "sitz" bath. Take a 10-minute daily bath in warm water with Epsom salts to control inflammation, end itching, and reduce swelling. Immerse your hips and buttocks, then sitz until you feel better.

Anoint them with an OTC preparation. Spread good cheer fast with commercial hemorrhoid preparations. Ingredients known to relieve discomfort include witch hazel, zinc oxide, Peruvian balsam, ephedrine, and (for its anesthetic properties) tetracaine. Avoid prolonged use of treatments containing cortisone, which eases itching and inflammation but can cause more problems than it cures if you overdo it. Preparation H, the best-known ointment for hemorrhoids, should be applied three to five times daily—particularly at night and after bowel movements.

Try prescription steroids. Topical corticosteroid ointments, available by prescription, reduce inflammation. Apply a thin film two to four times daily. They work in two to three days. Caution: Corticosteroids weaken tissues with prolonged use.

Call time out. Take frequent short walks or rest breaks during the day. Sitting or standing too long aggravates hemorrhoids.

PREVENTING PILES

The good news about hemorrhoids is that they don't have to be a fact of life. They may be preventable. There are two basic strategies: adding bulk and stopping strain.

Bulk up. Hard stools are hard to move. That's why fiber is so important—it softens stools and escorts them to the door with dispatch. Bran, along with raw fruits and vegetables, is the best way to soften stools.

If you want to read, visit the library. Don't keep periodicals in the john. Sitting on the toilet more than 5 minutes at a stretch can put too much stress on anal blood vessels. Lord knows what might happen to your tush if you kept *War and Peace* in reach of the throne.

HIGH TECH ● THE BELLY BUTTON/HEMORRHOID CONNECTION

You can stop praying to St. Fiacre, the patron saint of hemorrhoid sufferers. Your prayers have been answered. Experts have come up with a new method to combat hemorrhoids. It can be an alternative to surgery in many cases, or a complement to surgery in more severe cases. It's safe, painless, and has no side effects.

The process, studied by René Lambert, M.D., of the Lyon School of Medicine in France, involves using a drug called Alphanon, whose active ingredient is 2-camphanone (camphor). Two drops nightly are dropped into your navel. The solution is absorbed by the skin and the bloodstream picks it up. Alphanon stops hemorrhoidal bleeding in over 50 percent of patients. Most people find their symptoms are improved in 3 to 14 days. Although success varies with each individual, many report that they have no more bleeding, discomfort, or inflammation. Results vary from slight improvement to complete regression of symptoms. However, since there's a slight possibility hemorrhoids will return, be sure to use preventive measures. Alphanon is in the final stages of testing for Food and Drug Administration approval.

WHEN YOU NEED TO SEE A DOCTOR

Sometimes hemorrhoids need medical care; two indications are severe pain and bleeding. But your doctor can treat them quickly with one of the methods described here.

Consider the "current" approach. When it comes to

removing hemorrhoids, the kindest cut may be no cut at all. A technique that directs electric current from a probe to the base of your hemorrhoids reportedly is up to 97 percent effective at zapping piles, according to Daniel Norman, M.D., clinical assistant professor of medicine at the University of Nevada, Reno. The treatment is painless, leaves no scar tissue, and requires only two or three treatments. There is virtually no recovery time with this procedure.

Once your pesky piles are gone, they may have vacated your premises for good. One follow-up study found that patients reported only 15 percent recurrence 3 years after treatment.

Submit to a taillight inspection. One small zap for man may mean one giant step for mankind. An instrument called an infrared probe coagulator uses infrared light to literally shoot down hemorrhoids by cutting off their blood supply. The device looks like a ray gun Flash Gordon might have used. The treatment leaves no scars. In many cases, one week after you're zapped, you're cured. The most stubborn cases could require two or three visits.

Have your doctor tie one on. Several hemorrhoids at once are tied off with elastic during a procedure called rubberband ligation. It takes only seven to ten days for your hemorrhoids to shrink and fall off. The treatment is repeated every three weeks until your hemorrhoids no longer are a problem.

If all else fails, try surgery. Hemorrhoid surgery will get you back on your feet. The drawbacks are that it's painful, recovery time is 10 to 14 days, and it's costly—up to $4,000 for the procedure.

PACIFYING AN IRRITABLE BOWEL

People, places, and occurrences that are a pain in the rear can cause problems in a part of your anatomy, too. The irritable bowel syndrome (IBS) is believed by some to be a symbol of today's high-paced, stress-laden existence. Thus far, it's one of the not-so-sweet mysteries of life. Physicians know it occurs, but they don't know why. Naturally, they can't cure it until they catch what causes it. Its

TEST YOURSELF FOR IBS

Want a quick fix on whether you may have irritable bowel syndrome? Here's a corny suggestion. Note how long it takes kernels of whole corn to pass through your body. Normally, the corn takes two to three days to appear in one's stools. If you see the corn in 36 hours or less, you may have IBS. See your doctor for diagnostic tests to rule out serious bowel diseases or giardiasis, a parasitic infection. If you don't have bowel disease or parasites, the kernels racing through your body like rapid transit trains may be a sign that you have IBS.

symptoms of abdominal pain, bloating, nausea, and alternating bouts of diarrhea and constipation continue to keep an army of specialists looking for answers. In general, if you've had the symptoms for many, many months or years, and your problem is hard to put into words, you likely have irritable bowel syndrome, say the experts. If you have serious bowel disease, you likely are experiencing very specific symptoms and would have been in a doctor's office before now. But see a doctor, of course, to be certain.

IBS is like a baseball game. It ain't over 'til it's over—meaning that once you get the syndrome you'll likely harbor it for life. The disease thus far is incurable and chronic and affects more women than it does men. It recurs whenever factors such as diet, stress, and environment (or a combination of the three) trigger symptoms.

The main comfort you can take if a cross bowel is yours to bear is that it's not a problem that can kill you—although some days you might feel it might. No one dies of IBS. Nor do doctors feel it automatically leads to more serious bowel diseases.

Like the rich, IBS sufferers may be different. It's suspected that their gastrointestinal tract and the smooth muscle tissue in their bowel are subtly abnormal compared with that of people without IBS. Some doctors theorize that hypersensitive nerves in the intestine may cause IBS.

The good news is that you can relieve the abdominal discomfort and alternating diarrhea and constipation that are the hallmarks of IBS. Your best chance of controlling the condition is not to allow it to control you. Here's how.

Scarf down fiber. Stock the fridge and cupboards with fiber-rich foods, which are thought to have therapeutic value. Researchers say the kind of fiber you eat is important. Wheat bran has a tendency to hold water better than, say, apples or carrots, thus helping prevent diarrhea.

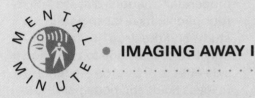

IMAGING AWAY IBS

In one study of the effect of hypnosis, self-hypnosis, and imagery on IBS, 20 out of 33 patients who tried it showed improvement in just seven weeks. Most impressive, 11 lost nearly all their symptoms.

As always, for imagery to work you need to relax. So first practice the progressive relaxation technique, which is similar to self-hypnosis, outlined on page 376. When you're relaxed, place a hand on your abdomen and focus on feeling all warm and relaxed in that area. Then envision a calm river and visualize your own gastrointestinal tract functioning smoothly and steadily like that river.

Or, follow the recommendation of psychologist Neil Fiore, Ph.D., author of *The Road Back to Health* and *The Now Habit: Overcoming Procrastination by Enjoying Guilt-Free Play:* Create an oasis of time for yourself by envisioning yourself turning your body over to the wise physician within you.

Dr. Fiore says, "Say to yourself, I will find a way to recover." Free your conscious mind from thinking about your irritated bowels and allow your body to be its own best doctor. Trust that your body possesses all the knowledge, talent, and tools it needs to calm your irritated bowels, heal the damage, and function properly. If your symptoms change or become worse, seek the advice of your physician, cautions Dr. Fiore.

• A GUTSY HIGH-TECH SOLUTION FOR IBS

People with serious bowel diseases have had "spectacular" success taking leuprolide acetate (Lupron), says John R. Mathias, M.D., a professor of medicine at the University of Texas Medical Branch. The injectable drug, usually used to treat prostate cancer, is given daily.

"The onset of improvement occurs usually about the fourth week," Dr. Mathias says. "It takes somewhere between four and six weeks to get a good therapeutic effect," although it takes somewhat longer in postmenopausal women and in women who have had their ovaries removed. All patients in one of Dr. Mathias's studies were symptom-free in three months.

Dr. Mathias says he's certain Lupron is going to be the treatment of choice for IBS sufferers "with moderate to serious disease." Sixty-four people have taken part in his study, and the drug has failed in only five cases—due to two known side effects of Lupron—edema (excess fluid) and bone pain. Your doctor will be familiar with Lupron. Ask him or her about trying it on your IBS.

Eat smart. Foods such as beans and cabbage that are known to cause gas may cause problems for IBS sufferers. Eating fat is also a problem because it prompts strong colonic contractions that make you run to eliminate what's inside you.

Eat slowly. If you're always first at your table to finish a meal, chances are you're also first in line to use the lavatory while the plates are being cleared away. Eating slowly may help you stop abnormal colon contractions from starting.

Put more stress on exercise. "I don't think that stress is what's causing the disorder," says Douglas A. Drossman, M.D., a gastroenterologist and psychiatrist at the University of North Carolina at Chapel Hill School of Medicine. "But it is one thing that causes it to flare up."

You can stop flareups with a program of regular intensive exercise, Drossman says. Once your doctor gives permission, start walking, swimming, biking, or some other activity. Build up gradually. Daily walks get your bowels moving, knocking out constipation—one of the troubling problems associated with IBS. Running is good also, but too much of a good thing can cause diarrhea.

Sit up and see if your colon takes notice. Hit the deck and reel off some situps for temporary relief. This exercise can stop your bowel spasms pronto and may start normal contractions in your intestine.

Stop the spasms. Antispasmodic agents have been found to be effective against the cramping and diarrhea of IBS. These prescriptions also quell your desperate need to use the john after meals—a normal urge that doesn't overwhelm people who don't have IBS. Some common antispasmodics include dicyclomine HCl (Bentyl), anisotropine methylbromide (Valpin 50), and glycopyrrolate (Robinul).

DIVERTING DIVERTICULOSIS

Refinement is a good thing on society hill, not in your diet. Since Americans started eating wimpy low-fiber foods made of refined sugar and flour late last century, a heretofore seldom-seen syndrome called diverticulosis has become a big-time problem. Today, more than half of all Americans have little hernias called diverticula—pouches or sacs that squeeze into the tiny passageways where blood vessels penetrate the colon's wall. The symptoms include cramps, gas, dyspepsia (severe indigestion), and—by turns—diarrhea and constipation when these pouches become inflamed.

Now that so many people choose to eat foods high in fiber, instances of diverticulosis ought to go down. This is one disease that may be preventable by smart eating.

A low-fiber diet requires the colon to squeeze like a python to move its load. All that unnatural pressure takes its toll on the colon.

In the worst-case scenario, you can develop a dreaded inflammatory disease called diverticulitis, which could be fatal because of severe internal bleeding or peritonitis, or could require surgery to remove a length of infected colon. Diverticulitis occurs in about 5 percent of cases of diverticulosis. But why not eat right instead of courting disaster?

Realize that physicians can spot the disease, but by

and large, you'll need to heal the symptoms yourself. Take these tips and you'll have your colon as long as you have life.

Feast on fiber. The good thing about this tip is that your body can stop damage overnight, and quite possibly stop the symptoms—although you're stuck with the pouches all your life. If you don't have colon hernias now, you may be able to prevent them by henceforth feeding on fiber. If you already have diverticulitis, skip this entry and read the next section. But if you have diverticula without complications, you don't have to eat a bland diet. Roughage from wheat bread, bran cereal, fruits, and vegetables provides the bulk you need.

Get a workout. Moderate exercise—daily walks, for instance—is a good treatment as well as a preventive because it helps keep you regular.

WHAT TO DO FOR DIVERTICULITIS

Diverticulitis needs a doctor's care and special attention to your daily diet. Here are the main guidelines for handling this serious complication of diverticulosis.

Eat with caution. Eat plenty of "soft" roughage in low-residue liquid form, including blender-crushed fruit and veggie soups—all without seeds. Seeds can catch in diverticula, causing inflammation and infection.

Get some serious sack time. Before resorting to surgery for diverticulitis, doctors recommend hospital bed rest accompanied by IV fluids to supply nutrients, because eating further irritates the colon when what it needs is to rest. The inflammation should subside in one to three days of bed rest, antibiotics, and fasting—plus acidophilus supplements to calm your throbbing gut.

Put your surgeon in charge. If diverticulitis persists despite these measures, the disease can be cured with surgical removal of the damaged bowel.

DOUSING THE FLAME OF IBD

Inflammatory bowel disease is a two-pronged devil's pitchfork. The two conditions that make up the disorder are called ulcerative colitis and Crohn's disease (also known as regional enteritis). Experts disagree on whether Crohn's disease and ulcerative colitis are one and the same. Both are inflammations of the digestive tract. At this time there is no cure for either one, nor do doctors know the cause of these afflictions that make you feel like Rambo's gone on the warpath inside you. But medical science in recent years has learned much about quieting the symptoms.

Fighting bowel problems—including serious bowel diseases—is not only a matter of treating symptoms, Dr. Bayless says. It's important that the patient take control of the disease. So here's what to do when IBD makes you feel like throwing in the bowel.

FIGHTING ULCERATIVE COLITIS

If a doctor has told you that you have "acute" colitis, you probably didn't blush and thank him. This inflammation of the colon's membranes is accompanied by abdominal pain, bleeding, and diarrhea. No miracle drugs are available to cure ulcerative colitis, but doctors have gotten positive results from some reliable medications.

Put out the fire down below. A drug called sulfasalazine (Azulfidine) works in three days to a week to reduce inflammation.

Take your medicine. An anti-inflammatory drug derived from sulfasalazine called 5-ASA (Pentasa, Rowasa, Asacol) is often effective in treating colitis attacks and causes fewer side effects than other drugs of choice. Taken orally or in enema or suppository form, it usually greatly reduces the number of rectal bleeding episodes and diarrhea attacks. Improvement is usually noticed in three to six weeks.

Steroids may help. Corticosteroids curtail inflammation, allowing the body time to heal. Prednisone works in two to four days.

Pack in the pectin. Some doctors who normally prescribe "bowel rest" for the ailment have had second thoughts ever since University of Pennsylvania researchers found that too much rest may make your colon atrophy. The alternative, say researchers, is to add pectin to your diet instead of typical fiber. This form of fiber is soluble—it "melts." Soluble fiber speeds bowel movement through the small intestine without taxing your colon, thereby helping you reduce the size of your feces. By reducing the fecal bulk this way, you get the same benefit as bowel rest without the most common problem related to bowel rest: atrophy. Although the medical jury is still out on pectin, some experts believe that it may keep your colon from weakening. Foods high in pectin are most fruits and vegetables, particularly apples, kiwis, brussels sprouts, and sweet potatoes.

Cyclosporine may prevent surgery. Until recently, removal of the diseased large intestine was the only remedy for the most severe cases of ulcerative colitis. Now, however, research at New York's Mount Sinai Medical Center finds that nearly half of patients tested benefited from treatment with cyclosporine (Sandimmune), a drug normally used to prevent organ rejection after transplant surgery.

The theory behind the drug's success is that this immunosuppressant curbs the tendency of ulcerative colitis patients' immune systems to misguidedly attack colon cells. Cyclosporine was given intravenously for up to two weeks, followed by six months of at-home medication with oral cyclosporine and steroids. And in just six months, five of the six patients who originally had responded to the drug were in total remission.

COMBATING CROHN'S DISEASE

Up to 10,000 Americans contract Crohn's disease every year. If you're one, surely you'd like nothing better than to return it to Mr. Crohn. "It's a very complicated disease," says N. H. Afdhal, M.D., a Boston-based specialist with the Department of Gastroenterology at City Hospital.

Crohn's is a painful inflammation of the gastrointestinal tract that can affect you anywhere from the mouth to the anus, although its usual stomping grounds are in the small intestine. This chronic illness is marked by diarrhea, cramping, fever, and weight loss. The diarrhea in Crohn's patients occasionally contains blood; seek medical help pronto if it occurs longer than a day or two. One frequent complication of Crohn's disease is partial intestinal obstruction — often accompanied by vomiting. Sometimes

Crohn's mimics appendicitis, causing pain and swelling on the right side of your abdomen. In worst-case scenarios, the best way to halt the vicious cycle of the disease is surgical removal of the diseased section of small intestine.

But there are several ways that you can help yourself without spending time in the operating room.

Stick to steroids. Since Crohn's disease is a serious ailment, you'll want to consult a specialist if you have not already done so. In most cases the best treatment is corticosteroids, which slowly begin to work in two to four days. "With corticosteroids you should see improvement in 4 to 6 weeks," Dr. Afdhal says. Stubborn cases, he cautions, may require medication for 12 weeks or longer — even "indefinitely." Corticosteroids curtail inflammation, allowing the body time to heal. Prednisone is the best steroid for Crohn's disease, but your doctor will watch for side effects.

Stash the smokes. Evidence has linked Crohn's to smoking. You'll need to can the tobacco, no butts about it, to be safe. Does smoking cause Crohn's? "No," says Don E. Brinberg, M.D., assistant professor of clinical medicine at Case Western Reserve School of Medicine in Cleveland. Can it exacerbate or make Crohn's worse? "Some evidence suggests yes," Dr. Brinberg says.

Eat to control your colon. Good nutrition is a primary goal in handling Crohn's, since you may often not feel like eating anything. So when your symptoms subside, be especially conscientious about loading up on calories, protein, vitamins, and minerals. In recent research, Dr. Afdhal found that Crohn's patients who were given nutritious diets to battle Crohn's-caused malnutrition were able to put their disease into remission. These patients had failed to respond to high doses of steroids and other drugs. Improvement was noted in just three weeks of tube feeding in the hospital. They then went home and for six months had regular meals that included potatoes, root vegetables, bread, and breakfast cereals, supplemented by liquid food. The amount was calculated on the basis of the patient's ideal weight, but all received three meals and three snacks. The patients were also given nutrients to supplement their diets. Patients were in remission on this diet for up to nine months.

Slow down your bowel movements. Dr. Brinberg recommends you limit your intake of fruits, vegetables, and high-fiber foods when your Crohn's disease flares up. Your aim is to slow down your diarrhea to make life more bearable at this time.

CELIAC DISEASE: UNDERCOVER OPERATION

Celiac disease—also known as sprue—is not one of the usual suspects that doctors round up when your bowels betray you. It is a relatively uncommon malabsorption syndrome in which gluten, a protein found in certain grains—such as wheat, oats, rye, and barley—causes a reaction in the small intestine. (It is gluten that gives dough made from these grains its tough, elastic consistency.)

This severe form of gluten intolerance is thought to be both hereditary and caused by a virus. The body's immune reaction to gluten destroys villi, the absorption sites of fluids and nutrients in the small intestine, resulting in a bad situation in which you starve after you eat—malnutrition is a common complication.

One sign of celiac disease is diarrhea which leaves a fatty oil slick on the surface of your toilet's water. Even solid stools are exceptionally fatty, frothy, and malodorous. Other signs are stomach cramps, emaciation and, in its worst forms, a distended belly.

The disease is bad but not hopeless. Here are some solutions to give you new hope.

Eat breadless meals and say nay to cereals. Although you'll need to seek your doctor's advice about celiac disease, a gluten-free diet is the standard treatment. So hold the wheat, rye, oats, and barley.

Switch to corn. Two common alternatives to gluten grains are corn and buckwheat. Use them often. Other safe bets are rice, millet, and gluten-free pastas.

Take vitamin and mineral supplements. When gluten no longer is part of your diet, your symptoms depart with your fatty stools. However, you're not home free. Because your villi need several months to recover, you'll have to ask your doctor to recommend supplements to build your body back up.

CANCER PREVENTION:
A Special Report

When it comes to preventing cancer, which is more important?

1. (*a*) Checking the radon level in your home or (*b*) eating the right kind of breakfast cereal?

2. (*a*) Losing weight or (*b*) banning food additives from your cupboard?

3. (*a*) Having a positive mental attitude or (*b*) shielding yourself from electromagnetic rays spewing from your home computer?

Tough questions, aren't they? Every day some new study is reported to have found another possible cancer-causer. You wonder if soon researchers will report that hot showers cause cancer. You have to sift through the confusion to get answers, to find out what's *really* important and what's not, so you can rationally set your own priorities to protect yourself and your family from cancer.

Well, here are some answers. (The answers to the questions above are 1:b, 2:a, 3:a.) They come from 200 leading cancer experts surveyed by Medical Consensus Surveys, a research arm of *Prevention* magazine, at the 44 National Cancer Institute-designated cancer centers around the United States. These physicians and researchers treat large numbers of patients and conduct full-scale tests of new cancer treatments. They have access to the most up-to-date information available on the causes and treatments of all types of cancer. Their work has helped establish the latest prevention and treatment guidelines.

Here they have prioritized 28 risk-reducing actions by checking one of five categories: Extremely Important, Very Important, Important, Not Important (But May Help), or Probably Worthless. Their responses were analyzed and statistically "weighted" on a scale of 1 to 100, with 100 being most important. Below is a priority list of the top 15 actions you can take right now to lower your risk of cancer.

THE TOP 15 PERSONAL CANCER PREVENTION MEASURES (ON A SCALE OF 100)

Don't smoke or chew tobacco—99
Get regular cancer screening tests—89
Perform breast/testicular exams—81
Limit exposure to sunlight—75
Avoid high alcohol intake—65
Avoid passive smoking—65
Reduce overall dietary fat—63
Eat more food fiber—62
Eat more fruits and vegetables—62
Eat more whole-grain/high-fiber cereals—60
Maintain normal weight—55
Avoid household toxins—54
Get regular exercise—53
Eat more cruciferous vegetables—51
Limit exposure to nitrites—51

Note: Avoiding workplace toxins was not included because the number of people at risk is relatively small.

Cancer is usually a slow disease, and preventing cancer is a lifelong process of awareness and self-care—it can't be called "high-speed." On the other hand, each of the many big and little steps in that process can be taken quickly, and most of them easily (stopping smoking is not easy, but it's the biggest and best step of all). And today half the experts surveyed agree that 50 to 70 percent of all cancers could be prevented if everybody were to follow the top-priority changes in lifestyle and diet outlined below. Add in the avoidance of environmental risk factors, and you can emerge from the confusion over cancer prevention feeling pretty confident that you're doing everything you can to reduce your risk, and doing it immediately.

TAKING CONTROL OF YOUR LIFESTYLE

It's a new buzzword—"lifestyle." When it comes to cancer, it means things like smoking, drinking, exercise, weight control, sun exposure, keeping track of your health—all things you have absolute control over, things you can change or avoid. You set the stage.

TAMING TOBACCO

As expected, tobacco use leads the list of risks: Nearly all of the experts surveyed say it's extremely important to avoid smoking or chewing tobacco. "If all the smokers in this country quit tomorrow, potentially 30 percent of all cancer deaths could be prevented," says Edward Trapido, Sc.D., chief of epidemiology at the University of Miami School of Medicine, Sylvester Comprehensive Cancer Center.

That's not just from lung cancer, either. Smoking causes cancers of the mouth, larynx, and esophagus, and it's linked to cancer in body parts that don't even have direct contact with smoke—notably the pancreas, cervix, and bladder. And it's no surprise at all that chewing tobacco causes oral cancers.

Tobacco has been a highly publicized risk for nearly 30 years, but all the warnings have been aimed at the smoker. Within the last ten years, so-called passive smoking—exposure to tobacco smoke from others in enclosed, poorly ventilated spaces (like airplanes)—has surfaced as a major concern. Over half of our respondents reflected that concern by saying that avoiding passive smoking was either very or extremely important.

"The latest information I've read says that a non-smoker's cancer risk increases 50 percent if he or she lives with a smoker," says William Shingleton, M.D., consultant and retired director of the cancer center at Duke University Medical School. Working 8 hours a day in a smoky environment can also raise your risk.

Bottom line for quitting smoking and chewing tobacco: Very High Priority—99 on a scale of 100.

Bottom line for avoiding secondhand smoke: High Priority—65 on a scale of 100.

BELTING BOOZE

High alcohol intake obviously isn't good for you, but is it a cancer risk, too? Most certainly: Nearly half the doctors rated avoiding high alcohol intake as very or extremely important. Alcohol in moderation seems to be a negligible risk. But the heavy drinker has a greatly increased risk of cancers of the mouth, throat, and liver. That's bad enough on its own, but it's a double whammy to the heavy drinker who smokes, too—an all-too-common combination.

Bottom line: High Priority—65 on a scale of 100.

SHUNNING SUN

In terms of the sheer number of cancer cases that could be prevented, however, avoiding excessive sun exposure is more important than both tobacco and alcohol. "Nearly all of the 500,000 cases of nonmelanoma skin cancer each year are caused by too much sun," says Paul F. Engstrom, M.D., vice president, population science at Fox Chase Cancer Center, in Philadelphia. "The good news is that nonmelanomas are highly treatable, so considerably fewer cancer *deaths* are attributable to sun exposure."

The bad news: Recent evidence links excessive sun exposure to those rarer-but-deadly melanomas. That's part of the reason over two-thirds of our respondents consider sunlight a very to extremely important risk factor. If you're outside during the period when ultraviolet rays are strongest (generally, 10 A.M. to 3 P.M.), use a good sunscreen lotion and wear protective clothing, a hat, and sunglasses.

Bottom line: Very High Priority—75 on a scale of 100.

GETTING THE JUMP ON CANCER

Regular cancer screening tests and self-exams are really methods of early detection rather than cancer prevention. But they're included here because early detection leads to a better chance of a cure—preventing *deaths* rather than the cancer itself. Getting regular checkups and self-exams garnered second and third places (right after smoking) on the "Top 15" list of cancer-preventing priorities.

The most important do-it-yourself tests are breast

self-exams for women and testicular self-exams for young men. It's also smart to keep an eye out for suspected skin cancers. The most important physician-performed screenings are the Pap test and pelvic exam, physical exam of the breast, mammogram, and colorectal cancer tests.

Bottom line: Very High Priority—89 on a scale of 100.

WATCHING YOUR WEIGHT

As recently as ten years ago, most doctors would have dismissed maintaining normal weight and getting regular exercise as unimportant to your cancer risk. But the experts think that these factors have at least a moderate effect on your cancer risk. So why the dramatic shift?

Studies over the past decade have linked obesity (defined by the American Cancer Society as being 40 percent or more overweight) with increased risk of colon, breast, prostate, gallbladder, and female reproductive system cancers.

Exercise is crucial in controlling obesity, and our experts rate regular exercise only slightly below maintaining normal weight. Direct links between exercise and cancer prevention are harder to establish, but some evidence exists. "Women who were involved in athletics during their teens and twenties seem to have a lower incidence of breast cancer," according to Silvana Martino, D.O., a breast-cancer specialist at The Harper Hospital in Detroit. Exercise isn't strictly for the ladies' benefit: "Studies suggest that people with desk jobs and sedentary lives are at higher risk of colorectal cancer. Exercise can help cut their risk, too," says Peter Greenwald, M.D., of the National Cancer Institute (NCI) headquarters in Bethesda, Maryland.

Bottom line for maintaining normal weight: High Priority—55 on a scale of 100.

Bottom line for regular exercise: High Priority—53 on a scale of 100.

MINDING YOUR MIND

Maintaining a positive mental attitude was rated "important" (or above) by 54 percent of the doctors in the survey, while 22 percent label it "probably worthless." A few years ago, those percentages would easily have been reversed. But today, mind/body interactions are accepted by many in the medical community. Recent studies show that stress-reducing techniques can cause measurable changes in the immune system. Whether these changes can help prevent cancer is still speculative at this point. "It's hard to prove scientifically that a positive outlook can help *prevent* cancer," Dr. Greenwald says. "But I think that people have a feeling that people with a positive attitude may smoke less and have better eating habits." Twenty-three percent of the survey respondents agree. They checked "Not important, but may help."

Bottom line: Moderate Priority — 42 on a scale of 100.

DOING RIGHT BY YOUR DIET

Twenty years ago, you'd be hard-pressed to find a doctor who'd say that diet had anything to do with preventing cancer. Things have changed dramatically, and the survey shows it. Most of the experts rated dietary habits "important," "very important," or "extremely important."

"Dietary factors probably account for up to 35 percent of all cancers," Dr. Trapido says. "That's according to a landmark NCI-sponsored report." And that's *higher* than the figure for smoking! (No surprise: Everybody eats; only a minority still smokes.)

EATING FOR PREVENTION

Cutting back on dietary fat is number one on the survey's cancer-prevention list. Eating more fiber and more fruits and vegetables are a close second, and right behind them is eating more whole-grain cereals. High levels of dietary fat have been linked to colon cancer, while fiber may help prevent this cancer. And fruits and vegetables, besides containing high levels of fiber, have nutrients that have been shown to be protective against cancer.

Bottom line for eating less fat: High Priority — 63 on a scale of 100.

Bottom line for eating more fiber: High Priority — 62 on a scale of 100.

Bottom line for eating more fruits and vegetables: High Priority—62 on a scale of 100.

Bottom line for eating more whole grains: High Priority—60 on a scale of 100.

DIETARY CHEMICAL RISKS

There are a number of items that can be termed "dietary chemical hazards." Like the environmental risk factors in the next section, most of these chemicals have a reputation far worse than their scores on this survey.

Nitrites, which are used to cure certain meats, are the dietary chemicals that head the list of concerns. Nitrites have indeed been associated with increased cancer risks. But the publicity surrounding that scare made most meat processors look for less-toxic substitutes.

Washing fruits and vegetables to remove chemical residues (and other contaminants) is a good health practice, but it counts as only a moderate risk reducer. "In general, the health risks of the currently approved chemicals have been overstated," J. John Cohen, M.D., Ph.D., of the University of Colorado School of Medicine, says. Food additives scored toward the bottom of the list in importance. As with other chemicals, frequency of exposure is the key to determining risk. Eating fresh fruits and veggies and avoiding high-fat prepared foods limits your contact with preservatives. Even eating grilled and blackened foods is okay, if done only on occasion.

Irradiated foods ranked as virtually a nonexistent risk. The irradiation kills bacteria and extends the shelf life of various foods. "It *does not* make food radioactive, although that idea circulated a few years ago," reports L. M. Glode, M.D., of the University of Colorado Cancer Center. "And there is no known cancer risk." With the exception of some spices, it's almost impossible to find food that's been irradiated.

Bottom line for avoiding nitrites: High Priority—51 on a scale of 100.

Bottom line for washing produce: Moderate Priority—44 on a scale of 100.

Bottom line for avoiding additives: Moderate Priority—32 on a scale of 100.

Bottom line for limiting grilled blackened foods: Moderate Priority—44 on a scale of 100.

Bottom line for avoiding irradiated foods: Low Priority—13 on a scale of 100.

YOUR ENVIRONMENT

Cars, trucks, and factories spewing out pollutants. Carpets and walls releasing formaldehyde fumes. Pesticides seeping into ground water. Toxic waste dumps in the neighborhood. You can't really control these things, except by taking political action, and that takes time. Thankfully, they rank surprisingly low in importance on the survey. While they are still considered risks, most of the experts think that these factors are not serious causes of concern. In some cases, it's because there hasn't been enough research; in others, plentiful research has failed to prove high risk, especially in comparison to known risks; and in still other cases, the risk is considerable but your chances of exposure are less compared with lifestyle factors.

MUCH ADO ABOUT MAGNETIC FIELDS

Thirty-three percent of our experts think it's ridiculous to worry about electromagnetic fields from high-tension wires, electric blankets, computer screens, and so on. In fact, the magnetic-field category was the second-lowest risk on the entire list! "It's a very, very, very rare cause of cancer compared with things like smoking and sun exposure. But people tend to overestimate the risk of outside factors they can't control," Dr. Engstrom explains.

Bottom line: Low Priority—24 on a scale of 100.

THE RADON WRAP-UP

Radon is a more controversial subject. The Environmental Protection Agency (EPA) maintains that radon is the second most important cause of lung cancer, right after smoking. The EPA's warning is based primarily on studies of miners exposed to radon far underground. Can we accurately relate those findings to the risk aboveground?

The majority opinion seems to be summed up by Dr.

Trapido: "None of us knows the real risk of radon in homes because there's just not enough studied about it." Yet probably because the American Cancer Society backs radon as a potential risk factor, 47 percent of the doctors surveyed say it's important to check the radon level in your home. The rest seem to be on the fence: Over 26 percent say it isn't important, but it may help. Very few of the experts picked the extreme responses.

Bottom line: Moderate Priority—45 on a scale of 100.

TOXINS AT WORK AND HOME

Industrial and agricultural toxins in the workplace scored quite high as risk factors. There is solid research linking certain industrial agents (such as nickel, chromate, asbestos, and vinyl chloride) to increased cancer risks in workers. Farm pesticides may also pose hazards to farmers. But the risks are limited. "I was surprised that industrial toxins would be up so high on the list," Dr. Trapido says.

Only a relatively small part of the population works with carcinogenic chemicals on a daily basis. (And even fewer people are exposed to toxic chemicals in their own homes on a continuous basis—hence the somewhat lower concern about this risk category.) EPA regulations and right-to-know laws make workers aware of the danger and help reduce some of the risks. Ironically, workers have more control than they think: Risks are higher for on-the-job smokers.

Bottom line for avoiding workplace toxins: High Priority—69 on a scale of 100.

Bottom line for avoiding household toxins: High Priority—54 on a scale of 100.

CHAPTER 9

CIRCULATION

Mel the plumber eats his favorite dinner—chicken-fried steak in brown grease gravy, french fries, and creamed corn, a little lettuce salad with half a cup of bacon bits, followed by apple pie à la mode—heavy on the mode. Then he falls asleep on the couch and, not surprisingly, drifts into a recurrent plumber's nightmare: He's trapped in a huge building with a 60,000-mile maze of pipes and tubes and valves. He's got to unplug the pipes, open the drains, stop up the leaks, weld the rusting walls, lower the pressure. *But he can't find his tools and he can move only in ver-r-r-y slo-o-o-w m-o-o-otion and his wife Tilly is yelling at him, "Mel, shape up or ship out!" and he knows the whole system is about to burst!*

Mel! Mel! Wake up! You're having a bad dream! It's not the building in your dream; it's your body. It's not plumbing; it's your circulatory system. *Your* pipes are narrowed, even plugged, with fat and cholesterol deposits called plaque. Your pipes are weakened by high blood pressure—they're about to spring a leak. In other words, you've got atherosclerosis and hypertension. You're risking a long, painful arterial breakdown into a real-life nightmare of strokes and heart attacks. That's what Tilly is trying to tell you: Shape up, or ship out before your time.

The good news is the tiny snippets of time it'll take for you to get your arteries shipshape. For starters, how about:

- An instant change in diet that can immediately begin scouring plaque from your artery walls?
- A 5-minute, twice-a-day routine that will end your cold hands forever?

- A 30-minute program, three times a week, to cut your risk of high blood pressure in half?

There's more good news. Although your doctor needs to treat and monitor your high blood pressure and atherosclerosis, you can help with a minimal amount of time and effort.

CHECKING UP BEFORE YOU CHECK OUT

Atherosclerosis is a fact of life: The older you get, the harder your arteries get. The harder they get, the stiffer they get. Stiffened arteries can't do a good job of moving blood.

And high blood pressure makes atherosclerosis even worse by putting excess stress on these now inflexible artery walls. The combination of high blood pressure and atherosclerosis increases your chances of having a stroke — when plaque or a blood clot blocks an artery leading to the brain, or when one of the brain's arteries leaks or ruptures under severe high blood pressure.

That's why your first goal should be to lower your blood pressure if it's high, or to keep it normal if it's already normal. (Your secondary goal should be to avoid speeding up the normal progress of atherosclerosis.)

Hypertension's sneakiest trick is that it's often without symptoms until it's done its damage. Headaches or flushing may be early symptoms; later symptoms include fatigue, dizziness, palpitations, rapid pulse, and nosebleeds. So it's important to have your blood pressure checked regularly.

What you're looking for on that blood pressure scale are numbers below 140 systolic and 90 diastolic — the first number shows the pressure in your blood vessels in the instant your heart beats, the second number measures the pressure when your heart is relaxing between beats. If your reading is below 140/90, you don't have high blood pressure. If either number is higher, you should discuss treatment with your doctor.

There are two main ways to check your blood pressure.

Have your doctor do it in a minute. It's fast, easy, and the logical place to start. Since blood pressure varies widely from situation to situation, one high reading in the doctor's office doesn't mean instant medication. But if repeated readings are high, you probably have hypertension.

Take your own for a day. You may have "white-coat hypertension": high blood pressure only when you visit the doctor. This can still be a good indicator of the heights your blood pressure is headed for in future years. But for your own peace of mind, you may want to get a blood pressure monitor and spend a normal day going about your daily business, periodically checking your blood pressure and recording it.

Then turn the record in to your doctor. It may reveal that you don't have hypertension at all. Or if you're already on medication, it can help your doctor fine-tune your dosage.

The best types of home monitoring devices are those with a mercury sphygmomanometer (these are the most accurate; one brand name is Baumanometer) or an aneroid sphygmomanometer (Tycos). As convenient as they are, the digital display models are not yet very reliable.

ATTAINING HEALTHY ARTERIES

There are three magic words that can cast a spell on your blood pressure and atherosclerosis and either cause or help prevent a stroke: diet, exercise, and lifestyle. Whether it's a good spell or a bad spell depends on you.

In a Northwestern University Medical School study, researchers found that 201 men and women at risk for hypertension halved their risk with a potent mix of a low-fat diet, reduced salt intake, limited alcohol, and regular exercise. You, too, can benefit from part or all of this kind of program. If you have only slight hypertension — your systolic pressure is between 140 and 159, or your diastolic is between 85 and 104 — you can lower your blood pressure without medication. If your numbers are higher, you can cut down on your drug dosage. And if you don't have hypertension, you can help prevent it.

And while you're at it, you can use the same strategies to slow the progress of atherosclerosis, hypertension's most intimate friend. If you have hypertension, you'll need your doctor's care, but there are many truly quick and simple ways you can help yourself.

A tiny new device called a rotablator can remove plaque blockage in your arteries in as little as a few minutes, and you can leave the hospital the very next day.

The rotablator, hooked to a spaghetti-thin catheter, sands down arterial plaque. The bloodstream then carries away the tiny grains. Because the rotablator leaves a smoother surface than other devices, scientists think the vessels will be less likely to catch more plaque, lowering the risk of reblockage.

The rotablator is only in limited use, and isn't the best thing for every kind of arterial plaque blockage, says Robert Ginsburg, M.D., director of the Center for Advanced Cardiovascular Therapy at Stanford University Medical Center. But it does seem to be the best bet among a variety of devices now being tested.

EATING FOR YOUR ARTERIES

When it comes to preventing or controlling high blood pressure and slowing atherosclerosis, *what* you eat is as important as *how much*. Fatty foods pack on the plaque and pile on the pounds. Other foods can scour your arteries clean, and some can help you shed fat. It should take you all of 5 minutes to scan these dietary recommendations, and seconds to put them to work.

Flatten that spare tire. You can eat and gain fat or you can eat and lose fat. Being too fat is linked to a number of health maladies, and hypertension tops the list. At least 60 percent of people with high blood pressure are too fat. The more overweight you are, the greater your risk. So eat to lose excess weight and you'll be gaining more control over your blood pressure.

Check the oil. Slice the fat in your diet to no more than 30 percent of your total daily calories, advises James J. Nora, M.D., author of *The New Whole Heart Book*. (One gram of fat churns out 9 calories.) That means you need a quick course in calorie-counting.

Squelch saturated fats. These fats are the kind that harden at room temperature — you can imagine what they do to your arteries! Cut the share of your total daily calories contributed by saturated fats to no more than 10 percent. You can do this quickly by reducing the amount of animal fat you eat. For instance, substitute polyunsaturated margarine for butter, skim milk for whole milk, take 10 seconds to rip the skin off that chicken, and restrict your beef entrées to only the super-lean cuts. Hydrogenated or partly hydrogenated vegetable oils are also thick with saturated fat, so eat natural peanut butter that you have to mix, and use liquid vegetable oils rather than solid vegetable shortening (but avoid palm and coconut oils, which are loaded with saturated fat).

Choke off the cholesterol. Keep the cholesterol in your diet to no more than 300 milligrams a day, and that may keep cholesterol from forming plaques that block and scar your arteries—atherosclerosis. You get 274 milligrams just in one egg, and 3 ounces of beef liver send you over the border. Only animal foods contain cholesterol: If you have hypertension and high cholesterol levels, the more you stick with plant foods the better. In fact, vegetarians have lower blood pressures than people who eat meat.

Cholesterol is a necessity of life: It's a type of alcohol made and used by the body to manufacture cell membranes and hormones. But your body makes all it needs. If you go on a low-cholesterol diet, that alone gives you a good chance of stopping the progress of atherosclerosis, and a small chance of even reversing it.

Change your oil. Whenever you can, use olive and canola oils. These contain high proportions of monounsaturated fat, which is actually good for your arteries. They can lower the level of artery-harming LDL cholesterol—the so-called "bad" cholesterol—while leaving the artery-cleaning HDL—"good"—cholesterol alone.

Polyunsaturated fats, found in vegetable oils such as safflower, soybean, and corn oil, lower both kinds of blood cholesterol. So the polyunsaturates have a "good" and "bad" effect.

Feast on the K-factor. Potassium-rich foods have been shown to lower blood pressure, and a deficiency of potassium—whose chemical symbol is K—has been linked to an increase in blood pressure. Fresh fruits and vegetables—especially bananas and potatoes—dry beans, and whole grains are rich in potassium, says potassium expert George Webb, Ph.D., an associate professor of physiology and biophysics at the University of Vermont Medical College. In one study, 859 people over a 12-year period reduced their risk of dying from stroke by 40 percent by eating just one extra serving of fresh fruits or vegetables a day. And the more of these potassium-rich foods they ate, the lower their risk.

When it comes to blood pressure, there seems to be a constant tug-of-war between potassium and sodium. Some doctors think that you need to maintain a 2:1 or 3:1 ratio of potassium to sodium in your diet. Thankfully, quick-to-fix-and-eat fruits and vegetables have large amounts of potassium and almost no sodium. A potato, for example has a potassium-sodium ratio of 130:1.

The only time you can't depend on food sources of potassium is when you're on a diuretic to reduce hypertension — the diuretic will leach potassium from your blood. That is the *only* reason to use a potassium supplement, and then *only* with your doctor's guidance.

Snuff out sodium. In some people with hypertension, sodium may elevate blood pressure or work against high blood pressure medication. If you're in this select group, a shaker full of herbs substitutes well for table salt. Even if your doctor says you aren't sensitive to sodium, for good health restrict yourself to a teaspoon or less per day. (Your minimum daily sodium requirement is a pinch.)

And remember that you can find sodium lurking in lots of places besides your saltshaker: aspirin, baking soda, diet soft drinks, canned foods, fast foods, frozen foods, condiments, pickles.

Eat it raw, steam it, bake it. Whatever you do, don't boil your veggies. Boiling leaches away much of their natural potassium. And your vegetables soak up the salt you may have added to the cooking water.

Go fishing. Fresh, frozen, baked, broiled, or poached — but never fried — choose fish for supper one or more times per week. Ten minutes of cooking brings you a delicious dish with multiple benefits.

- Fish contains little saturated fat.
- Fish, such as tuna, salmon, and rainbow trout, is packed with omega-3 fatty acids, a polyunsaturated fat that reduces cholesterol levels in the blood.

- Flounder, cod, haddock, and fresh salmon are good sources of potassium.
- Fish helps your arteries retain their flexibility. Researchers at Monash University in Melbourne, Australia, tested blood vessels in 53 people and found that people who ate one or more fish dishes a week had more flexible arteries, which means a healthier cardiovascular system, than those who ate no fish.

Get down to the C. In a study at Beltsville Nutrition Research Center in Maryland, 12 people supplemented their normal dietary vitamin C with a gram of C a day (nearly 17 times the RDA) for six weeks. The study showed that vitamin C may relieve mild hypertension for people of all ages by lowering blood levels of sodium and improving the ratio of potassium to sodium. Check with your doctor before adding any supplement to your diet; large amounts of C may give you diarrhea.

Breakfast on bran. If you're a typical American, you're eating only 12 to 15 grams of fiber a day. You can easily hike that to the recommended 25 to 35 grams just by eating more fresh fruits and vegetables, whole grains, and dried beans. One-third cup of oat bran, for example, has almost 8 grams of fiber and a potato with skin has 3 grams. Since doubling or tripling your fiber overnight can give you gas, take a few weeks or so to get your level up.

How does dietary fiber help your arteries?

- Soluble fiber, the kind found in apple and pear skins, oat bran, and beans binds to cholesterol, helping your body excrete it.
- Fiber also helps maintain a healthy potassium-sodium ratio in your diet, because fiber-rich foods like fruits and vegetables are also high in potassium and low in sodium.
- It can also help you lose fat, because fiber-rich foods fill you up and are low in fat.

LIVING THE ARTERIAL LIFE

The food you eat can make a big difference to your arteries, but you can undermine all your good eating efforts with a few bad habits. So spend the next few minutes reading how to supplement your good food with the good life, and then take a little time *doing* something about it.

Toss the tobacco. Smoking equals high cholesterol in the risk race. The study done at Northwestern University found almost 30 percent of smokers have high blood pressure, compared with only 11 percent of nonsmokers. Although it can't by itself *cause* hypertension, atherosclerosis, or stroke, cigarette smoking is still one of the most potent risk factors. How?

- The carbon dioxide in the smoke speeds up hardening of the arteries.
- Smoking constricts your arteries, which increases blood pressure.
- Nicotine raises blood pressure.
- Cigarette smoke changes the consistency of your blood, making it thicker, stickier, and faster to clot, according to Neil F. Gordon, M.D. and Larry W. Gibbons, M.D., coauthors of *The Cooper Clinic Cardiac Rehabilitation Program*. Fast-clotting blood puts you at greater risk for stroke.

So add tobacco to a host of other risk factors—diet, aging, lack of exercise, heredity—and it can put you over the edge.

Because nicotine is such an addictive drug, smokers often have to try a variety of ways to quit before they find the one that works for them. Once you do quit, however, your risk of dying from hypertension, atherosclerosis, and stroke drops each year that follows—and in five years you will have cut that risk to the same level as if you had never smoked at all.

Be moderate with martinis. A fast way to cut back on your drinking is to have just a single drink; then add water to it every time it drops to half-mast. If you drink more than an ounce of alcohol a day, cutting back to just an ounce—or stopping altogether—may lower your blood pressure. What's moderate? An ounce a day: That's one beer, or one glass of wine, or a shot of liquor. That much is safe even if you already have high blood pressure. Any more than that can raise your blood pressure, though by itself won't cause hypertension. And if you're a drinker and a smoker, then this combination is worse for your arteries than either alone.

Curb your caffeine. Caffeine is safe for most people, even those with hypertension. But if you do have high blood pressure, you are more sensitive to caffeine's effect, Dr. Gordon warns. He recommends you limit your daily dose of caffeine to no more than two cups of coffee, four cups of tea, or four soft drinks.

Go off the Pill. Birth control pills can actually *cause* high blood pressure in about 5 percent of women who take them. Women taking oral contraceptives have a six-times-greater risk of stroke than those who don't, because the Pill can cause abnormal blood clotting. If you smoke, too, the risk multiplies 20 times.

Getting off them is often the only thing you have to do. Sometimes it can take up to a year for blood pressure to return to normal, but it's a year well spent. Or you can try a pill with a low estrogen/progestogen content, which is less likely to raise your blood pressure.

Diet without pills. If you're taking diet pills to lose excess weight to control your high blood pressure, you're defeating the purpose and wasting time. If you're taking diet pills to lose excess weight, and you have your blood pressure checked, the reading will be inaccurate—another time-waster. That's because many diet pills contain a substance called phenylpropanolamine (PPA). This chemical is handy because it's believed to suppress your brain's appetite control center, but in some people it can raise blood pressure.

Ask about aspirin. As little aspirin as a quarter tablet a day offers some anticlotting effects, protecting against strokes caused by atherosclerosis. Check with your doctor before trying this remedy.

Cuddle your kitty. Some researchers say that interacting with a pet—dog, cat, or rabbit, any animal that's soft and cuddly—lowers your blood pressure on the spot. As soon as you start talking to and petting your pet, your blood pressure plunges and stays down until you're finished, according to Aline Halstead Kidd, Ph.D., professor of psychology at Mills College in Oakland, California. Why? A pet, she says, offers unconditional love—no demands, so no stress.

Look out! Develop a watching hobby and do it for 15 minutes, twice a day, advises Aaron Katcher, M.D., a psychiatrist at the University of Pennsylvania. If you're having hard times at work or at home, your blood pressure can go up temporarily. If the stress is constant, of course, your blood pressure can be too high too much of the time. But if you're spending energy looking and listening instead of worrying, you've found a natural blood pressure reducer, he says. You'll find there's more to fish than fatty acids—there's watching them glide and flip through an aquarium. Watch the birds in the backyard eat bugs and chase each other. Sit in front of the fireplace and gaze at the flames and let your mind wander.

Give yourself a belly laugh. Turn on the "I Love Lucy" reruns. Dig out the old home movies. Call a friend and share a joke—like the one Steven Wright tells about coming home from work one day and finding all his furniture stolen . . . but replaced with exact duplicates. A hearty 60-second chuckle causes a small, fleeting decrease in your blood pressure. It's also a good stress and anger reliever. Long-term effects of laughter are unknown, but there are no negative side-effects to laughter, so try it often.

Write in your diary. When you get a flat tire during rush hour, when you spend 2 hours looking for your car keys only to find them in your purse, when your next-door neighbor snubs you at a block party—take a few minutes to jot it down in an "anger diary." Tell this sympathetic listener what triggered your anger, what you did about it, and how you felt at the time. You may find this helps to defuse your anger. Suppressing your emotions if you have high blood pressure raises your risk of premature death five times, according to a study at the University of Michigan School of Public Health.

Sniff a slice of pie. Fragrance works in an instant. Merely catching the whiff of certain scents, particularly spiced apple, may nearly double any blood pressure benefits of quiet relaxation. One theory is that apple pie brings back memories of pleasant holidays. Research is too inconclusive to prove that one particular odor will give anybody's blood pressure a shove downhill, but test the notion by trying fragrances *you* find particularly appealing.

Tune in. Quiet, nonvocal, slow, predictable, rhythmic music may help lower blood pressure by helping you relax, according to music therapy experts.

Take a tip from nuns. Maybe you can't seek the cloister and veil as a way of relieving your hypertension. But take 10 minutes to jot down ways you might be able to arrange your environment for less stress and aggression with more meditation and quiet. Do you really *have* to be at your family's beck and call 24 hours a day—or can you give yourself a time-out? Do you really *have* to fight traffic every day—or can you take a bus or a cab or have something delivered? Do you really *need* shopping malls, credit cards, telephone sales calls, the very latest in this-that-or-the-other—or can you simplify your life?

Italian researchers studied nuns in a secluded order for 20 years and found they didn't develop high blood pressure as they aged. The scientists said these women had the ideal environment for normal blood pressure: silence, meditation, and isolation from society. They worked and prayed, free from economic and family tension, social stress, or anxiety about their earthly future.

GIVING YOUR ARTERIES A WORKOUT

Aerobic exercise is good for everyone, but it's essential for arterial health. A study of 3,000 men at the University of North Carolina found that those who exercised the least had an even greater risk of dying from stroke than did smokers. How does it work?

- Regular exercise can reduce and prevent high blood pressure.
- Exercise strengthens your heart, so that it can do the same amount of work with fewer beats—and that slows down atherosclerosis.
- Exercise helps prevent blood clots from forming. "Those who are the most physically fit may dissolve clots the fastest," says Edward R. Eichner, M.D., of the University of Oklahoma Health Sciences Center.
- Exercise speeds the loss of excess fat, which itself cuts your chances of developing hypertension and high cholesterol levels. The higher your level of fitness, the lower your level of cholesterol.

- Exercise works off stress—and constant unrelieved stress increases your risk of high blood pressure.

And best of all, a good exercise program will take a minuscule *1 percent* of your time—that's 2 hours out of a 168-hour week. Dr. Eichner's studies show that as little as *5 minutes* of strenuous exercise can give your bloodstream 90 minutes worth of "fibrinolysis," the body's own blood clot dissolver.

So what are you waiting for?

Get your doctor's okay. If you haven't had a physical exam in the last year, your doctor will probably want to give you one. He or she may also want you to take an exercise stress test. An hour or two in the doctor's office can help both of you determine the kind and intensity of exercise you need.

Start walking. It's probably the easiest, fastest, and cheapest form of exercise, and so it's the one you'll most likely stick with over time.

Start slowly. That is, begin with 15-minute walks three times a week. You want to condition yourself gradually —blisters and aching legs from starting off at too fast a pace can discourage you. Regular exercise may lower blood pressure four or five points, but if you quit exercising, your blood pressure will rise again. Your ultimate goal should be a 4-mile-per-hour pace—that's a "brisk" walk.

When you feel ready, increase your walking time to 30 minutes per workout. Then, add two more days of walking each week for a total of five days. At about your fifth or sixth week into walking, aim to cover 2 miles in your half hour by picking up the pace of your walking. Now you're walking briskly. Eventually try to increase your walks to 45 minutes or even 60 minutes a day.

Aerobicize. If walking isn't your thing, or if you'd like some variety, try cycling or aerobic dance for 30 to 60 minutes, three times a week.

REPELLING RAYNAUD'S DISEASE

Raynaud's disease is a mystery. No one knows what causes it or why, according to one study, up to 16 percent of women aged 18 to 59 have it. What is known is that the periodic attacks of Raynaud's cause the blood vessels in victims' hands and feet to constrict. The poor circulation makes fingers and toes first turn white, then blue with cold. It's often painful, and severe cases may even cause gangrene. Cold temperatures and emotional stress bring on the attacks, and warmth and relaxation beat them back.

Doctors can treat Raynaud's with drugs, and sometimes even with surgery, says John Abruzzo, M.D., director of the Division of Rheumatology at Thomas Jefferson University and professor of medicine at Thomas Jefferson University Medical College in Philadelphia. And here are some quick and simple ways you can help yourself.

Head South. Raynaud's is more common where the weather is cold. If Raynaud's is serious business for you, Dr. Abruzzo suggests you consider moving to a warmer climate. Or, a prolonged vacation during the snowy months is only a short plane ride away.

Get yourself into hot water. Place your hands in warm—not actually hot—water for 5 minutes twice daily. It will train your blood vessels to open up, allowing increased blood flow, and make them less sensitive to cold temperatures.

Electrify yourself. Carry a pocket-size hand warmer. Invest in a pair of sock warmers. Buy socks and gloves with battery-operated heat coils. Slip socks under fur-lined boots, gloves inside mittens, earmuffs under hats.

Button up your overcoat. "It's not just the hands and feet, it's the whole body that you have to protect," Dr. Abruzzo says. Your body automatically decreases blood flow to the extremities when your torso gets chilled.

Just say no. Avoid drugs such as decongestants, antihistamines, caffeine, and nicotine. They can increase the frequency and length of Raynaud's symptoms.

Eat something fishy. The omega-3 fatty acids in fish are good for vascular health. They also have been shown to improve cold tolerance and delay the symptoms of Raynaud's. A study at Albany Medical College in New York found that symptoms of Raynaud's stopped completely in 5 out of 11 people who took fish-oil capsules daily for 12 weeks. The other 6 people were able to extend by 50 percent the time they could keep their hands in cold water before their blood flow shut down. Consult with your doctor before taking fish oil supplements.

CHAPTER 10

COLDS AND FLU

o you think *you* have respiratory problems? Pity the poor schmoe with (take a deep breath now) *pneumonoultramicroscopicsilicovolcanoconiosis,* a lung disease caused by inhaling silicate dust. Not only is it reportedly the longest word in the English language, but just trying to *pronounce* it leaves both patient and doctor gasping for air.

Usually, though, it doesn't take a 45-letter disease name to leave you with respiratory problems. Whether caused by an isolated virus or a lifetime of smoking, many easier-to-pronounce ailments can leave you more breathless than a bull's-eye shot by Dan Cupid.

But in the time it takes to say *pneumonoultramicroscop* . . . (oh, you get the idea) you could be on your way to snuffing those sniffles, chilling that cold, decongesting that congestion, slowing that runny nose, and in general, breathing a sigh of relief from some of those ills.

- In just seconds—the time it takes to inhale deeply— you can unstuff a stuffy nose by either washing out your nose with a saltwater solution or snorting a lungful of steam.
- In just 1 minute, you can cut the congestion that comes with a cold, bronchitis, or allergies—*and* feed your appetite for spicy food at the same time.
- In just one day—if you're a man—you could start growing your own cold-virus filter.
- And in just one week, you could drastically cut your chances of getting many respiratory ills—and reduce the severity of some you may already have— just by stopping smoking.

So breathe easy—or at least, easier. Relief may be faster than you realize for a wide assortment of ills that can leave you short of breath, short of energy, and, until now, short of solutions.

FIGHTING THE COLD WAR

You think Mom's homemade chicken soup was hard to swallow when you were all stuffed up? Good thing you weren't in ancient Greece, where the recommended relief for the world's most common ailment—the all-too-common cold—was leech-induced bleeding. Meanwhile, the popular Roman remedy was to kiss a mouse on the mouth.

Throughout history, there has been no shortage of remedies. And, as you'll notice, no shortage of colds either. Today, Americans spend more than $1 billion each year on cold and cough remedies, and those sniffles and aches account for about $5 billion annually in lost wages —nothing to sneeze at.

"Sad to say, there really is no such thing as quick relief for the common cold," says Thomas Gossel, Ph.D., a professor and chairman of the Department of Pharmacology and Biomedical Sciences at Ohio Northern University. "Like the adage goes, you can suffer for a week, or take something and feel better after seven days. But no matter what you do, a cold is going to run its course— which lasts anywhere from a few days to a few weeks."

Of course, it doesn't take long to do a few things to help you *prevent* getting a cold in the first place.

Handle with care. Colds are infectious diseases caused by viruses, and these viruses are spread by human contact. Since avoiding other humans is impractical to most (unless your idea of home is an isolated mountaintop in Tibet), the best way to avoid cold viruses is to wash your hands frequently—every chance you get—especially when you come in frequent contact with cold sufferers. A 1- to 2-minute hand-washing removes many of the 200 or so different viruses that cause a cold, most of which can live several hours in the air, on clothing, on hard surfaces, or on hands after being spread from person to person.

"When you wash your hands frequently, you remove many of these viruses that cause colds," Dr. Gossel says.

"Even if you do wash several times a day, don't rub your eyes, and keep your hands out of your mouth."

Stay warm . . . "When you go outside and become cold and wet, what you actually are doing is lowering your resistance by raising your stress level," Dr. Gossel adds. "Before you may have been able to fight off the virus. But when your resistance is lowered, your body may not be able to do it." So take an extra minute or two to bundle up—especially when it's cold and damp.

. . . and chill out. Even if you stay toasty warm, stress can make you feel as stale as week-old bread, lowering your resistance and making you a prime victim for a cold. So take time from your daily routine to practice stress-reduction techniques—whether it's a few minutes of deep breathing or an hour of exercise or practicing your favorite hobby. "People under the most stress are the most susceptible to colds," Dr. Gossel says. "Trying to reduce the stress in your life can help keep up your defenses against colds."

Take your vitamins. Especially vitamins A and C, which help activate infection-fighting white blood cells and boost immunity (which, in turn, helps fight colds). These vitamins have been linked in several studies with protecting against respiratory ailments. It only takes a few minutes to eat winter squash, spinach, or sweet potatoes (which are high in vitamin A or beta-carotene); or citrus fruits, broccoli, or cantaloupe (good C sources).

Wet down the air. Ever wonder why the cold season is the *cold* season? Winter's chill has less to do with colds than the heated homes we run to in order to escape it. "In the wintertime, indoor air is very dry, and that lack of humidity is a great breeding ground for cold viruses," says Douglas Holsclaw, M.D., an associate professor of medicine and director of the Pediatric Pulmonary Division at Hahnemann University Hospital in Philadelphia. How dry is it? Typically, a heated room or classroom has only about 20 percent relative humidity—less than the Sahara Desert, which has 25 percent relative humidity. Add all those virus-carrying people *not* washing their hands who crowd into those heated rooms and breathe near each other, and you've got the makings of a regular sneezefest.

But in the time it takes to say *gesundheit,* you could be adding extra moisture to the air—ideally to about 45 percent relative humidity, according to the American Academy of Otolaryngology–Head and Neck Surgery. "The more moisture, the better for preventing colds," Dr. Holsclaw says. "To add moisture, leave bathroom doors open during showers, have a lot of houseplants (they add humidity), keep open pots of water around (especially near stoves and radiators). Or get a humidifier with a filter system so you don't get mold (which causes its own brand of respiratory ills); but if you go that route, you have to regularly clean it and change the water, which, unfortunately, many people don't do."

Go over-the-counter to get over the hump. Of course, the best-laid plans often go astray. In other words, the typical adult gets four colds a year (more if he or she is a parent), and kids usually get between six and eight—no matter what precautions are taken. When colds hit you, hit the medicine chest ASAP. "The best thing to do is take the recommended dose of aspirin or acetaminophen or ibuprofen and get plenty of rest," Dr. Gossel says. "The cold will continue to run its course, but you should start feeling better real soon, in about an hour or less. *Warning:* To protect against Reye's syndrome, don't give aspirin to those under 18, although the other pain relievers are okay.

30-MINUTE RELIEF FOR FEVER

A fever may be uncomfortable, but it's rarely dangerous. In fact, fever is a good thing. Turning up the heat is part of the body's normal defense mechanism against infection, injury, or inflammation. And yet, taking steps to lower a fever doesn't seem to interfere with recovery from illness. And you can bring down fever in as little as 30 minutes.

If an oral thermometer shows you have a fever of 100°F or higher, here's what to do.

Shed extra blankets and clothing. And lower the thermostat. Getting rid of unnecessary insulation speeds heat loss and lowers body temperature.

Take a comfortable bath. *Gentle* cooling is the goal here. Bathing or sponging the skin with cold water constricts your blood vessels, triggers shivering, and may actually *raise* your body temperature—to say nothing of the fact that a cold bath is downright uncomfortable if you're burning up. "Cool baths—and even lukewarm baths of about 80°—are torture to a person whose body temperature is 22 to 25 degrees warmer," say Thomas C. Rosenthal, M.D., and David A. Silverstein, M.D., in the journal *Postgraduate Medicine.*

Take aspirin, acetaminophen, or ibuprofen every 4 hours. And take it around the clock. These over-the-counter drugs lower fever. And although acetaminophen isn't as effective as the other two, it can help people whose stomach can't tolerate aspirin or ibuprofen.

Doctors have been using salicylates (that is, aspirin and aspirin-like drugs) to lower fever for more than 100 years. But "aspirin, acetaminophen, and ibuprofen are effective in reducing fever, [taking] effect in 30 to 45 minutes," say Dr. Rosenthal and Dr. Silverstein. (Don't take more than the recommended dosage, though. Your fever won't fall any faster, and more important, aspirin and acetaminophen are toxic when taken in massive amounts.)

Drink water, soup, and fruit juice. Liquids help prevent dehydration.

Call a doctor if fever lasts two or three days or longer. Fever usually subsides in a day or two, with or without treatment. If fever persists, or if it hits 103°F or higher, get medical advice. Also consult your doctor if fever is accompanied by shaking or chills, severe headaches, nausea and vomiting, change in alertness, or extreme sensitivity to light. These could be symptoms of serious illness.

Speaking of cautions, here's a list of "don'ts" for treating fever.

- Don't sponge with rubbing alcohol. Alcohol cools the skin surface too rapidly. As it evaporates, you'll start to shiver, and your body will react by generating heat.
- Don't take aspirin if you have chicken pox or influenza, if you have a peptic ulcer, or if you're allergic to aspirin.
- Don't take acetaminophen if you have liver disease.
- Don't give aspirin to a child or teenager who has a fever. The fever could be due to flu or chicken pox, and aspirin has been known to cause Reye's syndrome under these circumstances.

BITING THE FLU BUG BACK

Three things in life you *don't* want: a fight with a guy named Bubba; a ride on a horse named Lightning; and a bite by that bug named Influenza.

The first two you can avoid. The flu, however, is as predictable a winter ritual as a dead car battery—and leaves you with less energy. The flu starts innocently enough. A few aches and pains, maybe a sore throat or headache. Then, in a few hours' time, come the chills. The fever. The cough. The joint pains. The feeling as though you just had a fight with a guy named Bubba—and then rode Lightning.

This is one tough disease. There are 103 million cases of flu per year in the United States. Each year 72,000 people are hospitalized because of this disease, which along with pneumonia is the sixth leading cause of death in the United States; together, these diseases claim more than 69,000 lives annually. To keep from becoming one of these statistics:

Needle the bug before it needles you. "The best treatment for the flu is to avoid it in the first place, or lessen its severity, with a flu vaccine—and that doesn't take long at all," Dr. Holsclaw says. "I advise getting a flu shot each year—particularly if you're elderly or have asthma, bronchitis, heart disease, cystic fibrosis, or any other condition that involves the lungs." Since flu season usually strikes from December to February, he suggests getting vaccinated in October or November. "Usually, the vaccine isn't available until after October. If it's available *before* then, I'd be concerned about its effectiveness."

Make R&R your Rx... Even after getting stuck with a needle, some folks still get stuck with the flu. For them, as well as others infected with this bug, the quickest fix is getting plenty of rest and recuperation. Not that you'll feel like doing much else anyway. In fact, you probably will not be *able* to do much of anything else: Flu slows reaction time and actually impairs visual abilities, making driving, working, and most other chores difficult. In fact, a study at the University of Sussex in England found that drivers "under the influenza" had reaction times ten times *slower* than those driving under the influence of alcohol.

Suffice it to say, this is not the time to build that new addition or do your taxes.

... and drink plenty of fluids. "Stay in bed, eat small but frequent amounts of food, and ingest plenty of liquids, particularly juice, broth, and soup," Dr. Gossel advises. Besides providing your body with necessary fluids lost by a fever, nonalcoholic liquids—whether hot or cold—help fight germs in your body and provide you with needed nourishment. (Drinks with alcohol, however, further raise your already high body temperature.)

Give viruses a hot time in the old throat tonight. Hot liquids have the advantage of raising the temperature of the throat, which slows viral reproduction.

Give 'em the acid test, too. Meanwhile, the acidity of lemon tea, tomato juice, and orange juice is good, because viruses can't live in an acid environment.

And bore them to death with the cuisine. Foodwise, since the flu rarely brings out the gourmet in people, most prefer to stick with easy-to-chew, easy-to-digest foods like bananas and toast.

Drug that bug. "Tylenol, fluids, and rest," provide the quickest 1-2-3 punch for knocking out the flu, Dr. Holsclaw says—easing some of your pain in a few hours (although the flu will probably last several days). If you prefer generic drugs, aspirin is effective in easing the fever, headache, and body aches of flu, but as with colds, it *shouldn't* be given to those under 18. Acetaminophen or ibuprofen is also recommended—but stay away from most over-the-counter cold remedies because they can suppress symptoms and give you a false sense of recovery.

Hose down your hoarseness. Flu typically leaves your throat more pooped than a Pavarotti telethon. But those with a well-lubricated set of windpipes usually withstand the hoarseness and sore throat better when the flu hits—and you can do that in about 10 minutes a day (assuming it takes a minute to down a glass of water). "Drink ten glasses of water a day—with no ice," advises Robert J. Feder, M.D., an otolaryngologist and a professor of both drama/singing *and* ear, nose, and throat medicine at UCLA. "Ice water is too cold to protect your vocal cords as well as room-temperature water." Dr. Feder, who treats numerous singers, actors, and other entertainers, also advises against using mints or menthol candies to soothe your weary throat. "They're too drying. Stick with cough drops like Pine Brothers or hard candies."

Blow off that smoking gun. Gee, do we even have to mention it? Demon Weed is about the *worst* thing when you have flu. Besides draining the body of vitamin C and hurting your throat and lungs even *more,* smoke stuns the cilia, the tiny, hairlike projections whose job it is to keep airborne invaders from entering the lungs. Smoking slows recuperation time, keeps your immunity lower, and can lead to more serious respiratory woes.

A mere seven days is what it takes to totally rid your body of nicotine, the addictive substance in cigarettes. Get through that first week without cigarettes and you've made the greatest step toward a smoke-free and healthier life. "Want the quickest fix to *all* respiratory problems?" Dr. Holsclaw asks. "Just don't smoke. It's never too late to stop." (See chapter 20 for help with breaking the habit.)

SAYING "NO" TO PNEUMONIA

The usual symptoms are fever, headache, fatigue, chills, cough. . . . Hey, is this déjà vu or what? Sure, it could be a flu or a cold. But when you suffer through either of them and are *still* sick, the smart money says it's either viral or the more serious bacterial pneumonia. You may have a high temperature, shaking chills, painful, rapid breathing, abdominal pain, and coughing—first dry and then occasionally producing a rust-colored sputum. Quite simply, you have a lung inflammation in which air sacs are filled with fluid and debris instead of air. So what do you do?

See your doctor. You need immediate medical care. Pneumonia is nothing to fool around with. At times, it's difficult to clinically differentiate bacterial from viral pneumonia because they can share similar symptoms. But their treatments differ.

Take it easy—and take in liquids. Bacterial pneumonia is treated with antibiotics, which usually takes one to two weeks, but "you'll feel relief in a couple of days if they pick the right antibiotic," says Henry Gong, M.D., a professor of medicine and researcher at the UCLA Medical Center's Pulmonary Division. But since antibiotics are ineffective against viral pneumonia, at least 48 hours of bed rest is usually recommended.

"You won't feel like doing much else anyway," Dr. Gong adds. "The best thing to do is take it easy and drink plenty of liquids to get the mucus up that's in your airways." Of course, complete recovery can take up to eight weeks, since a possible complication of viral pneumonia is often bacterial pneumonia, in which antibiotics are needed.

Humid air helps. Again, your friendly neighborhood humidifier comes to the rescue. A cool-mist humidifier, or even moisture from the shower, helps thin mucus secretions and makes them easy to cough up. But be advised: Even after the infection clears, coughing may remain for several days or weeks.

BUSTING BRONCHITIS

Consider bronchitis the Mount St. Helens of respiratory ills: It starts with a few quiet rumblings—a tickle in your throat here, some discomfort there. Then the coughing gets louder. Deeper. More severe. Until . . . ERUPTION! Phlegm emerges from the depths of your lungs making you sound like a skid-row bum in need of an iron lung. In fact, sometimes the only way to distinguish bronchitis from pneumonia is with an X-ray. But if you do have bronchitis, here are the fastest ways to end the eruption.

Keep coughing. The cough may be ugly, but it's effective—and necessary. "The best way to treat bronchitis is to cough up the stuff that's down there [in your lungs]," Dr. Gong explains. "You don't want it to settle down there, because it can cause lung collapse or further bronchitis and you could develop pneumonia."

Liquefy the problem. From Mom's hot chicken soup to a cold glass of water or juice, drinking plenty of nonalcoholic fluids is one of the best and most time-efficient ways to thin out the secretions and bring up phlegm. "It doesn't matter what the temperature is," Dr. Holsclaw says. "The opinion that hot beverages are more effective at breaking up mucus and relieving congestion is nonsense. Whether they are 120° or 60°, *all* beverages are the same temperature inside your body. Just be sure to drink plenty of liquids."

It usually takes about two weeks to relieve acute bronchitis—but you could have a quicker fix by ingesting more than 10 glasses of fluids a day. "Water is the main thing in treating bronchitis," Dr. Gong says. "The more the better."

Reach for the red pepper. Congestion is to bronchitis as weddings are to Zsa Zsa Gabor. And one quick, inexpensive, and tasty remedy is to consume foods rich in capsaicin—the "hot" in hot peppers and other foods. "If it makes your eyes water, it's going to trigger the nose and lungs to water, too," says Irwin Ziment, M.D., chief of medicine and director of respiratory therapy at Olive View Medical Center in Sylmar, California, and a pioneer in the area of "hot" foods and their relation to respiratory health. "The 'hot' sensation from spicy foods like hot pepper or mustard, curry, or garlic stimulates a reflex in the tongue, throat, stomach, and most likely also in the lungs that causes mucus to lose its stickiness, making it more readily expectorated," he says. "Actually, these foods cause the very same reflex actions in the very same way as popular expectorants like Robitussin."

Best of all, he adds, this occurs immediately upon eating the food—hot or chili peppers, horseradish, Tabasco, or curry, to name a few. However, those with gastrointestinal problems should check with their physician before trying this remedy.

Get a checkup. Speaking of doctors, it's wise to speak with yours if you think you have bronchitis or pneumonia. True, most cases are caused by viral infections (like a cold or flu), so antibiotics don't do much good. But some cases of bronchitis are the result of a bacterial infection—and *are* relieved in about two weeks with antibiotics.

Bundle up. "Temperature changes may influence lung defense mechanisms that could affect bronchitis sufferers," Dr. Gong says. "We know that a sudden rush of cold air can cause asthma attacks in asthmatics. They learn to take a few extra minutes to put a scarf around their mouth and nose to better avoid a rush of cold air. I would advise those with bronchitis to do the same."

Most folks don't seem to mind spending the few minutes it takes to dress accordingly when leaving a nice warm house to face winter's cold wrath. But in the summertime? "People who go on cruises—where they're going from cool air conditioning to the hot weather frequently and suddenly, or vice versa—tend to develop upper respiratory infections; most frequently bronchitis," Dr. Gong adds. "So be careful in the summer, too."

Ban the butts. We said it before and we'll say it again: *Stop smoking now!* "The best thing you could do to either treat bronchitis or avoid it is not smoke," Dr. Gong adds. The vast majority of chronic bronchitis is *directly* caused by smoking. "If you have bronchitis now and you stop smoking, you'll still have it—especially if you've been smoking for decades. But your condition will improve."

SNUFFING THOSE NASAL NUISANCES

When sinuses act up, they inevitably either "drip" or "dry." Occasionally, they do both. Usually in the winter, the mucus dries out, and particles going through the nose get thick and sticky. The result: Postnasal drip. Here's how to get the drop on The Drip.

Use tissue tactics. "The fastest relief for a runny nose is blowing it," Dr. Holsclaw says. "It brings immediate relief and helps remove any irritants. The problem naturally tapers off, usually in a two-week period."

Wash relief in on a wave of salt water. "To stop the dripping, we use Ocean Mist," Dr. Holsclaw adds. (The generic equivalent would be a saline nasal spray or mist.) "It's a type of saltwater solution that helps cut thick mucus and dry out secretions. This brings immediate relief that lasts for about 20 minutes. You could also breathe in humidity or steam to get extra moisture in the nose that brings immediate, although short-lived, relief by helping to cut the stuffiness."

Do-it-yourselfers, take note: You can make your own saltwater solution by dissolving ½ teaspoon of salt (⅓ teaspoon if you have high blood pressure) in 8 ounces of warm water. Suck the water into a nasal aspirator and breathe in as you snort the water into your nostril while holding your nose straight back. Spit out the water and then blow your nose. And since the throat is connected to the nasal passages, gargle with salt water to help clear excess postnasal drainage.

Moisten the membranes. The very same type of saline solution used by contact lens wearers to relieve dry eyes does the trick a little lower. "Saline nose drops help thin out the dryness and stuffiness almost immediately," Dr. Holsclaw says. Other timely "thinners" include vaporizers, sipping steamy drinks such as hot tea, standing in the shower, and other methods described earlier to increase humidity and add moisture.

Beware of drug-containing nose sprays. It stands to reason: Your nose is stuffy, so unstuff it with a nasal spray, right? Wrong, say the experts. "Nose sprays can cause nasal congestion as well as relieve it," Dr. Gossel says. That's because using the sprays for more than three days can cause a "rebound" effect once you stop using them.

"In other words, you become dependent on the sprays," he explains. "Each time you use them, your nasal membranes do initially shrink—but then they swell up again (which can lead to blocked sinuses, blurred vision, and nasal infection). Nose sprays can help for a while, but your condition can become worse when you stop them." He, along with other experts including the American Academy of Otolaryngology–Head and Neck Surgery, strongly advises checking with your doctor before using the sprays.

DE-EMPHASIZING EMPHYSEMA

Sorry to report there is no quick fix to emphysema, which is characterized by loss of normal lung elasticity. Without this elasticity, the small airways collapse when you breathe out, making it impossible to fully exhale. Breathing becomes difficult, and simple chores—like walking across a room—can become nearly impossible.

There's no quick fix because this is no "quick" disease. Emphysema develops slowly—nearly always striking after age 50. It can be inherited; some people are born with "a deficiency in a protein that's usually there to sop up destructive enzymes," Dr. Holsclaw says. But emphysema usually hits longtime smokers or those long exposed to pollutants such as coal dust, industrial fumes, and other lung-busting substances.

And while there is no quick cure for this degenerative disease—which can lead to heart failure because emphysema interferes with the passage of blood through the lungs, making the heart work harder—you can take quick action to help prevent further damage and make the best of a bad situation.

Take C and see. "Vitamin C might reduce the amount of deterioration in the lungs caused by the processes that produce emphysema or other chronic respiratory illness," says Joel Schwartz, Ph.D., an epidemiologist and senior scientist at the Environmental Protection Agency in Washington, D.C. "It hasn't been proven, but preliminary research we have done indicates that those who consume high levels of vitamin C have less lung damage. In our study, those suffering from bronchitis and wheezing consumed lower amounts of vitamin C in their diet. If vitamin C is protective against these chronic lung diseases, it might be protective against emphysema.

"When your lungs are hit with foreign bodies—bacteria, particles, various irritants—a whole process of protective reactions occurs to get rid of that stuff. In the process, there's the release of basically toxic chemicals that kill these invading irritants, but they also do a number on your lung lining. And vitamin C helps repair that damage to the lung lining. It is also an antioxidant and may therefore directly protect the lungs." Vitamin C is a nontoxic, water-soluble vitamin, so you can't overdose on it; you eliminate excess amounts when you urinate. However, excess amounts can give you diarrhea, so look for a new form called Ester-C that's easier on your digestion.

And try E and A, too. Vitamin E and beta-carotene, a form of vitamin A, are also believed to have similar lung-aiding abilities, but Dr. Schwartz says they were not included in his study. So when you're doing your food shopping, spend a few extra minutes scanning the produce section for beta-carotene-rich butternut squash, carrots, cantaloupe, and sweet potatoes; and vitamin E-loaded almonds, figs, and sunflower seeds. Those looking to save even more time should note that vitamins A and E are toxic in large quantities and shouldn't be taken in supplement form without a doctor's approval.

Go easy on salt. "A high-salt diet is also a risk for respiratory illness, including, but not limited to, emphysema," adds Dr. Schwartz. "The reason is that sodium/potassium imbalances affect the nervous system, and respiratory inflammation is under the control mechanism of the nervous system. In other words, having too much salt may stimulate the nervous system to overreact, and this results in lung damage." *Advice:* If you eat a high-salt diet, counteract its potential damage by consuming equally high levels of potassium, found in bananas, orange juice, and potatoes.

Eat small meals. If you have emphysema, your lungs balloon with air, and that leaves your stomach unable to balloon with a large meal, making you feel bloated. You can avoid this by eating smaller, more frequent meals.

Give up tobacco. Sure, Demon Weed already did its damage by cursing you with this dreaded disease. And stopping now isn't going to reverse your condition (but then, nothing will). But quitting the habit *will* immediately help slow the deterioration of your already hurting lungs. Quit now and you'll also immediately help increase your capacity to exercise, a necessity to help boost lung power.

Use your head to use your lungs. Concentrating on your breathing—much as people with panic disorders are taught (see chapter 16)—results in more efficient inhaling and exhaling. And that means less energy is used, allowing you to actually breathe easier. Practice breathing from your diaphragm; also try to exhale twice as long as you inhale to help blow out trapped, stale air.

CUTS, BURNS, AND BRUISES

njuries aren't much fun, but if you must have one, you couldn't have picked a better decade in which to recover. Treatment techniques and technologies keep getting faster and better. And researchers keep making Baryshnikov-like leaps in their understanding of how the body heals from injury.

For example, in the not-too-distant future you may be able to buy a topical cream that contains growth factors, substances just like those the skin makes to repair itself and heal damaged blood vessels. Or you may find your doctor zapping a slow-healing wound with a low-energy laser or galvanic current to speed things up.

Of course, you don't always need high-tech solutions for speedy recovery.

- In just 3 seconds, you can douse burns of the mouth and tongue.
- In 5 seconds, you can protect a paper cut from further irritation.
- In just 1 minute, you can convert a common item in your freezer into a custom-fit sprain treatment.
- In just 5 minutes, you can peel away annoying microsplinters that are too small to reach with tweezers.

If you're ready for high-speed recovery, you're at the starting line.

PUT A QUICK STOP TO MINOR BLEEDING

When you damage a blood vessel, you bleed. If the damage is relatively minor, the bleeding will probably stop on its own within a few minutes. You can help nature along by following these tips.

Put on the pressure. The best way to stop bleeding when you've got a nick or cut is to put clean gauze over the area, then press down on it with your hand. Bleeding should stop in 3 to 5 minutes, says Judy Schmitt, R.N., of Allegheny General Hospital in Pittsburgh. You may have to apply a lot of pressure if you've sliced into the tip of a finger, where there are lots of small capillaries. Holding the finger higher than your heart can help.

If bleeding doesn't stop within 5 to 10 minutes of applying pressure, see your physician.

A tea bag on your tongue puts the bite on bleeding. Biting your tongue can cause it to bleed for quite a while, unless you take action. You can apply a compress and press firmly. But you'll get quicker results if you press a warm, wet tea bag against the wound. The tannin in the tea is believed to contain a coagulant that promotes rapid clotting.

Pinch here to stop nosebleed. If your nose is bleeding, sit down, lean forward, and hold both nostrils tightly shut for at least 15 minutes. (Obviously, you'll breathe through your mouth.)

Be sure to leave the scab in place, or you'll begin bleeding again.

SANE TREATMENT FOR PAIN OF SPRAINS AND STRAINS

If you want that muscle strain or ligament sprain to stop hurting and heal quickly, you've got to treat it right. Even though the injuries are different, basic care is the same, says Richard Parker, D.O., a staff physician with the San Diego Sports Medicine Center.

You get a *sprain* when you overstress a joint. Run, trip, and twist your ankle, and you're likely to sprain the supporting ligaments surrounding the ankle.

You get a *strain* when you overwork or overstretch a muscle. It's an injury common to anyone who's ever run too fast without properly warming up.

You can treat mild injuries yourself with the four-step RICE program: Rest, Ice, Compression, and Elevation (see the steps below). A mild injury should mend in a couple of days, Dr. Parker says. A more severe one can take four to six weeks.

But you'll need a physician's care if there's any looseness to the joint, or if you have difficulty walking. "There is no way to distinguish a sprained ankle from a fractured ankle without X-rays," says Dr. Parker, who is also team physician for the US men's and women's Olympic volleyball teams. "The fact that you can walk on it does not exclude the possibility of a fracture."

Aside from making sure you don't have a fracture, there are two additional good reasons why you shouldn't tough out anything more serious than a mild injury at home. A doctor can teach you how to stretch the strained muscle so that "the force of the stretch is applied along the length of the muscle fibers. You don't want a scar to form in a randomized way, crisscrossing the fibers," Dr. Parker says. Conversely, if you sprain a ligament, you may need a cast or brace to immobilize the joint so you don't stretch the adjacent ligaments, while allowing proper healing of the injured structure.

Now that you know what you can safely treat at home, try some healthy RICE.

Rest it. If you've injured a foot, ankle, calf, or thigh — parts of your body that help bear your weight — get off your feet immediately. Sit down, use crutches, do whatever it takes, Dr. Parker says. Rest for as long as it takes before you can walk in a relatively normal way. A significant limp can throw off your gait and lead to injuries in other areas of the body.

Ice it. After rest comes ice. You can use a bag of crushed ice, or if it's more convenient, use a bag of frozen peas or other small vegetables. Bang it on the counter to break the peas apart and it will conform to the contours of the injured area.

First place a thin, damp dish towel over the injured limb to protect your skin. Then put the ice on, make it conform to the body part, and leave it on for no more than 20 minutes at a time. (Longer than that can cause frostbite, Dr. Parker says.) You can help it conform by wrapping it with an elastic bandage. Ice the injury four to five times each day.

Ice can deaden the pain of a mild to moderate sprain,

reduce inflammation, and increase deep circulation, which will help get nutrients to the injured areas, Dr. Parker says.

Don't use the RICE technique at all if you have Raynaud's disease, peripheral vascular disease, or hypersensitivity to cold.

Compress it. Wrap on an elastic bandage to create 24-hour compression of the injured area, but don't make the bandage so tight that you've got a tourniquet.

You also want to make sure that the bandage has enough elasticity to it. If you've used one bandage to help hold the ice in place, use a fresh one to maintain compression after you take the ice off. And replace the bandage every couple of days, Dr. Parker says. He advises you to buy a good name brand like Ace. "Some of the off-brands are pretty flimsy."

Elevate it. Propping your twisted knee up on a footstool or putting your sprained wrist in a sling helps reduce inflammation and pain.

Rest and ice melt shoulder tendinitis. If you overdo any activity where you use your arms overhead—tennis or painting the ceiling, for instance—you can cause painful tears and inflammation in your shoulder. Rest the joint and apply an ice pack for about 15 to 20 minutes after you first experience pain.

Pop a pill. If the pain persists beyond the next two days or so, you can try an over-the-counter anti-inflammatory such as aspirin or ibuprofen or your doctor may prescribe an anti-inflammatory. (Acetaminophen—Tylenol—won't work because it's not an anti-inflammatory.)

Modify your workouts to eliminate the pain of muscle overuse. For pain that hits 24 to 48 hours after you've overdone a workout, take one day of rest. (Make your next workout shorter and lighter, repeating the one-day-off, one-day-easy sequence until all pain is gone.) Moderate exercise can alleviate pain from overused muscles faster than inactivity, though experts don't agree on why. But if the pain gets worse when you continue to exercise, stop and see your doctor, says Robert D. Willix, Jr., sports medicine specialist and director of the Willix Health Institute.

Take your vitamins. Vigorous exercise that strengthens your muscles works, in part, by damaging them. That's why you feel stiff and sore after a tough workout. A study at the University of California at Berkeley has turned up evidence that taking vitamins A, C, and E may limit muscle cell damage from exercise. Runners who ran downhill, then took 800 international units of vitamin E, 1,000 milligrams of C, and 10 milligrams of beta-carotene (which is converted by the body to vitamin A) daily for two months, showed fewer signs of muscle damage after a second downhill run. A word of caution: Such high dosages of vitamin E should be taken only with the approval and supervision of your doctor.

TAKE THE OUCH OUT OF THAT BANG OR BRUISE

There's no cut, but there is bleeding: You've damaged the blood vessels beneath the skin, and their bleeding causes a *bruise*. The leaked red blood cells appear blue under the skin at first, but can turn a lurid purple, then red, then yellow, or even green. Color changes in the skin reflect the activity of the blood's clean-up crew, made up of white blood cells. As the hungry little janitors gobble up and digest damaged red blood cells, the bruise goes through its chameleon changes and finally fades.

Here's how to get fast relief when you bang yourself.

RICE races to the rescue. The RICE technique — Rest, Ice, Compression, Elevation — is the best way to decrease internal bleeding and swelling and start that bruise on the road to healing. For the first 24 hours, cover the injured area with a towel, apply a bag of ice, and press firmly for up to 20 minutes at a time, alternating with 20-minute breaks. Elevate the bruise above the heart, if you can, and give it a rest, Schmitt says.

Plunge that bruise into cold water. For bruises to small parts like fingers or toes, this is the quickest way to reduce the trauma. The pain is reduced almost immediately. It also helps keep swelling down for less discomfort later.

BLOCK THAT BURN BEFORE IT GETS SERIOUS

What you do those first few minutes after you burn your-self can make all the difference in how well your skin heals. That's because your cells continue to fry even after you separate yourself from the heat source. The sooner you can bring down the temperature of the injured tissue, the sooner you call a halt to the destruction and the faster you'll heal. Cool the burn first, even before you take time out to call a doctor or drive to an emergency room.

Here's how to handle home care.

Plunge that minor burn into a container of cold water. And keep it there for up to 2 hours, or until there is no pain when you take it out. Use cold water only for superficial burns that cover a small area of unbroken skin.

Once you've cooled the area, wash with a mild soap to remove any opportunistic bacteria ready to make mischief now that the skin's barrier function has been compromised.

How quickly can you expect to heal? A first-degree burn, which affects the outermost layer of skin, usually heals in three to four days, the time it takes for the outer skin to peel off.

Pop some ice into a plastic sandwich bag to cool broken skin. If the skin is blistered or broken, try substituting ice encased in a plastic bag for cold water cooling. The plastic bag won't stick to broken skin the way cloth might, and will spare your skin direct—and *painful*—contact with the ice. Blistered skin "should heal within the week," says Linda Phillips, M.D., assistant professor in the Plastic Surgery Division of the University of Texas Medical Branch. A slightly deeper burn can take two weeks to heal.

Squeeze on some aloe. This cactus-like member of the lily family is full of a gel that has been found to promote healing of wounds, frostbite, and burns. In fact, aloe may help shorten the healing time of burns by up to 40 percent. In a study of 40 laboratory animals who had severe burns, those treated with aloe healed in an average of 30 days, compared with 50 days in a nonaloe group. After you've cooled the burn, snip off a bit of the aloe leaf and squeeze the gel onto the burn.

Reapply the aloe four to six times a day, Dr. Phillips says. You don't need to put on a Band-Aid or other dressing unless the burn is likely to rub against clothing or has blistered. Fresh aloe is safe to use on broken skin.

If you don't have an aloe plant handy, use a skin-softening lotion or cream that contains aloe. Choose one that doesn't have alcohol as its base, because the alcohol tends to neutralize the aloe, Dr. Phillips says. (Bottled aloe juice or gel may not contain the healing ingredients of fresh aloe or an emollient.)

You also may find that aloe can help with your pain. That's because it has a built-in mild anesthetic.

Dab on the Preparation H. This popular hemorrhoid treatment can shave 1 to 3 days off the typical 7-to-15-day healing time, according to Jerold Z. Kaplan, M.D., director of Alta Bates Hospital Burn Center in Berkeley. Preparation H contains a live yeast derivative, which has been found to speed wound healing, Dr. Kaplan says. Dab a little Preparation H on the burn and cover with a bandage or other sterile dressing, Dr. Kaplan advises. (The dressing helps seal in the ointment and keeps it off your clothes.) Change the dressing daily and check to make sure an infection doesn't develop.

Elevate the burn. One simple way to get the sting out of a fresh burn is to position yourself so the burn remains above the level of your heart. That helps prevent swelling, Dr. Phillips says.

Soothe away sunburn pain with an oatmeal soak. Fill the tub with cool or tepid water. Next add an oatmeal bath soak. You'll find several brands available in the drugstore; follow the directions on the package to see how long you need to soak. Don't use your breakfast oatmeal—the flakes are too large to do any good.

Sprinkle on sugar to cool that singed tongue. One of life's little annoyances is a burned tongue. You may be able to ease the pain somewhat by sprinkling sugar on the tongue.

Suck on a lozenge to relieve mouth burns. If food fresh from the microwave leaves you with a burned palate, over-the-counter cough lozenges containing benzocaine may lessen the pain. If they don't help, ask your doctor or dentist for a lidocaine anesthetic mouthwash.

Soak away hot pepper burn. If your hands burn after you've been cutting up hot peppers, soak them in vinegar for a few minutes—provided there are no open sores on your hands, of course.

HELP FOR SEVERE BURNS

A severe burn is one that fits one or more of these definitions.

- Large surface burns—more than 20 percent of an adult's body or 10 percent of a child's
- Burns that sear through all layers of skin, no matter how small the area
- Burns of the face, hands, or genital/anal area
- Burns caused by chemicals or electricity
- Burns that turn white, hard, black, or deep cherry red

All of these need immediate medical attention and probably hospitalization. If you've got severe nonchemical burns that (a) have nearly or entirely penetrated to the bone or (b) totally cover more than two of your limbs, don't cool with water or you could go into shock or hypothermia. Never immerse your entire body in ice water. That can be dangerous or even fatal.

Also see your doctor if your burn seems superficial but you find that the pain and redness increase two days or more after the incident, Dr. Phillips says. Do the same if you develop a fever, have difficulty moving your joints, or find a mild discharge at the burn site.

For chemical burns, remove contaminated clothing and flush the area with water for at least 15 to 30 minutes.

By working with your doctor, you can help hasten successful healing with these tips.

Ask the emergency room doctor about Biobrane. Several types of dressings are available to the doctor. One type is a premoistened gauze dressing which can dry out quickly and adhere to the burn. When you remove it, you may also strip off the new layer of skin. A second type is a sealed dressing. This type does *not* dry out. In fact, it will hold in the moisture that naturally drains from a burn, and that retained fluid may fuel an infection that also impedes healing.

A Biobrane bandage, however, eliminates both problems. (This brand of bandage is only available through your doctor.) The Biobrane bandage is a biosynthetic membrane dressing with pores which direct fluid up and into an absorbent gauze layer. The bandage itself substitutes for the missing skin and allows the underlying layers to heal. Within two days, the inner side of the dressing adheres to the surface of the burn and seals it. When you peel Biobrane away, the skin below will be healed, so it won't pull off the burn and it won't hurt!

The right nutrients will help you heal faster. Serious burn patients heal better and faster when given a special formula (either by tube or mouth) concocted at the Shriners Burn Institute in Cincinnati. Most formulas now in use are too high in the wrong kinds of fat and too low in protein, according to registered dietitian Michele M. Gottschlich, Ph.D., one of the formula's inventors. The Shriners' formula is high in protein, zinc, and vitamins A, C, and E. It's also enriched with omega-3 fatty acids (found in fish oil), but it's low in other types of fat.

The Shriners' formula has been tested against two commonly used formulas. The results of one small trial indicated that the Shriners' formula significantly reduced the length of time severe-burn patients stayed in the hospital. It also greatly decreased the incidence of infection.

The more severe the burn, the greater the reduction in healing time. On average, burns take one day to heal per percentage of body burned. So a person with burns covering 20 percent of his body would take 20 days to heal if he used the standard formula, or less than 17 days if he used the Shriners' formula. (The formula is currently available _only_ at the Cincinnati hospital—have your doctor call there for information.)

Check out cloned skin. Welcome to the option of laboratory-cloned skin. It's the latest lifesaver for patients burned over a large area of their bodies. Cloning is a process where a small section of your skin is removed, plopped in a special culture solution, and allowed to grow until it reaches the size needed to cover the burn. Then it's transplanted—grafted—onto the burn site. Regular skin grafting is slow. Patches of skin are surgically removed from one area of your body and transplanted to the burn site, and if the patch isn't big enough, doctors have to wait for the donor site to grow back, or find another place to take skin from. "Skin regenerates every 10 to 15 days, so you can't take a graft from an area faster than that," says Phil Walters, director of the skin bank at Shriners Burn Institute in Boston.

But cloning the skin can speed things up quite a bit, important because the skin is the body's first line of defense against infection. A relatively small section of unburned tissue can be cloned in a special culture medium to make an unlimited quantity of new skin—50 or even 100 times the surface area of the original. The average cloning period is about 18 to 20 days. When the cloned skin is grafted on, it 'takes' with no risk of rejection because it's essentially going back from where it came.

Consider artificial skin. In very serious burn cases, cloning (which replaces only the outer layer of skin or epidermis) may not be sufficient. To speed healing of deeper layers of skin, the use of artificial skin is the treatment of choice.

The best type of artificial skin was developed by Ioannis Yannas, Ph.D., professor of polymer science and engineering at the Massachusetts Institute of Technology, and John Burke, M.D., professor of surgery at Harvard Medical School. It includes an outer layer—an artificial epidermis—to seal out infection, plus a spongelike inner layer made of collagen, which replaces the skin's naturally thick, fibrous dermis. The collagen acts as a scaffold for new skin to grow into. The new skin eventually replaces the fake stuff completely as the collagen dissolves. When the process is complete, the artificial epidermis is peeled off and covered with cloned epidermal skin (see above) or replaced through other means.

SPEEDY RELIEF FOR CUTS AND SCRAPES

The right technique will help you combat inflammation, stave off harmful bacteria, and enhance healing. Here's how.

"Polish" that paper cut for irritant-free healing. First be sure the cut is scrupulously clean. Then daub on clear nail polish to protect the cut from irritants like air and soap, and leave it on until the cut heals.

Speed healing with antibiotic ointments. They can knock four days off the healing time of a cut or scrape. Unfortunately, many people still fall back on their grandma's favorite antiseptic remedy, such as iodine or peroxide. But doing that could be worse than doing nothing at all, according to one study.

Two different antibiotic ointments were tested against a variety of "traditional" antiseptic treatments, including iodine, hydrogen peroxide, and Mercurochrome. In the interests of science, 47 volunteers submitted to six minor wounds (three on each arm), which were later infected with a mild strain of staphylococcus. One wound out of every six was left untreated to act as a control.

Each untreated wound healed by itself in an average of 13 days. Both a dual antibiotic ointment (Polymyxin B-bacitracin) and a triple antibiotic (Neomycin-polymyxin B-bacitracin) healed wounds in an average of 9 days. That's more than 25 percent faster. None of the antiseptic preparations speeded wound healing. Some even slowed healing time down to an average of 16 days.

Why were multiple antibiotics better? Antiseptics kill bacteria, but they also kill innocent bystanders: the skin cells that are trying to regrow. Broad-spectrum antibiotic ointments kill bacteria without damaging the healing tissue.

Choose an airtight bandage. "Some people think that if you leave a cut exposed to air it will scab faster, but you should cover the cut, at least initially," Schmitt says. This is particularly true if the cut will be exposed to dirt.

So forget the old advice about "letting the air get at it." Keeping a cut moist with an occlusive (airtight) dressing can help it heal as much as 40 percent faster than using gauze or other bandages. Doctors aren't certain exactly why this speeds healing. One theory states that an airtight dressing keeps healing substances in body fluids from evaporating. But no matter what the mechanism, it works.

There are several types of airtight dressings made of polyurethane film. Each dressing is slightly different, but all have polyurethane exteriors with an interior layer of biocompatable material that "melts" into the wound. The best known of these are Duoderm and Spenco's 2nd Skin, available in drugstores.

Occlusive dressings are not ideal for chronic wounds such as diabetic sores. That's because there's an underlying problem in the skin's repair system that retards natural healing. But for most cuts, an occlusive dressing is best.

Change the bandage once a day. And never leave

on a wet bandage, no matter how many times you have to change it. It can increase your chances of infection, because even clean tap water breaks down the bandage's protective barrier and lets bacteria multiply and cause infection. If, despite your best efforts, you notice a red streaking in the area or any signs of infection, consult your physician.

Turn on the heat. Open wounds are likely to heal faster if they are heated slightly, reports John Rabkin, M.D., an instructor in surgery at the University of California at San Francisco.

In a review of several studies, Dr. Rabkin hypothesizes that heat dilates the blood vessels in the area of an injury, which increases blood flow and the influx of oxygen. Oxygen in turn is needed for the production of collagen, the protein building block of skin.

Clean the wound first, apply a sterile dressing, and then apply heat in the form of a heating pad, hot-water bottle, or warm, moist towel in a plastic bag for 15 to 30 minutes, four to six times a day.

Don't use heat therapy if you have an illness that has caused nerve damage—multiple sclerosis or diabetes, for example. You may not be able to feel if the heat you're applying is too extreme, and you could burn yourself.

PAIN-FREE REMOVAL OF SPLINTERS

Even the tiniest splinter can cause a whole lot of grief. Rather than dig around for it, wincing in pain—and everybody knows time seems to increase exponentially the more something hurts—try these fast, simple, and less painful remedies:

Sprinkle on a little vegetable oil. Just pat some on and wait a moment for it to seep around and into the puncture. Then gently remove the splinter with tweezers. The "lube job" should help it slide right out.

Dab a drop of glue on microsplinters. Splinters that are too small to get with tweezers can be removed with white glue or facial mask gel. Pour a thin layer of glue or gel over the skin and let it dry. Then peel the dried glue/mask off. The splinters go with it! The trick has worked for wood splinters, fiberglass fragments, and even cactus spines.

THE WONDERFUL NEW WORLD
OF GROWTH FACTORS

Three-fourths of a group of people who faced amputation because of nonhealing wounds avoided it after growth-factor therapy at the University of Minnesota Hospital and Clinic. Growth factors, hundreds of substances the human body makes to heal injuries, have always comprised our built-in repair kit. Now, through biotechnology, large quantities of these growth factors are being created in the laboratory. And research is under way around the country, testing their effectiveness in the treatment of cornea damage, burns, diabetic skin ulcers, and pressure sores. To date, over 850 Minnesota patients with sores that persisted for over two years despite conventional therapy were healed in about ten weeks by applications of growth factor.

Several growth-factor treatments have been approved by the Food and Drug Administration for preliminary testing. Where will it all lead? Perhaps to the development of ointments and creams that have these growth factors built into them, says Nelson Lee Novick, M.D., a New York dermatologist and author of *Super Skin: A Leading Dermatologist's Guide to the Latest Breakthroughs in Skin Care.* There could also be special growth-factor dressings, he says. "We might be seeing a magnificent set of products that do a really super job of healing."

SUGAR: SWEET SOLUTION FOR HARD-TO-HEAL WOUNDS

Modern research has proven the effectiveness of applying sugar to bedsores and other hard-to-heal wounds—a remedy that has been around since the seventeenth century. The treatment can dramatically speed the healing process in these more serious wounds. (It's not for minor cuts and scrapes.) By absorbing moisture from the wounds, the sugar forms a concentrated solution that creates an unfavorable environment for bacterial growth, says Alvin B. Segelman, Ph.D., professor of pharmacognosy at Rutgers University College of Pharmacy.

Sugar also acts as a kind of scavenger, picking up dead bacteria and white blood cells. This debris can then be easily flushed away when the wound is gently washed with warm salt water.

Because all serious wounds (including bedsores and diabetic ulcers) should be under the care of a physician, sugar treatments should be applied under medical supervision. The sugar treatment is not a home remedy, Dr. Segelman cautions.

HIGH TECH ● **LASERS: THE NEXT WAVE?**

The latest research into lasers shows that doctors may someday be healing our wounds with light.

Studies on animals and humans suggest that low-energy lasers stimulate the synthesis of collagen, one of the proteins responsible for the support and elasticity of skin. This may help explain why wounds and burns exposed to those low-energy lasers heal more quickly.

Intriguingly enough, a recent study at Tel Aviv Medical Center suggests that lasers can even speed healing on the untreated side of the body. A group of laboratory animals which had matching wounds on both sides of their bodies received laser treatment only on the right side of the body. But both wounds healed faster than a control group's. The researchers found the same to be true when they tested the laser on burns.

The next step for these laser researchers is to "hone in on which laser wavelengths are best for wound healing," says Dr. Nelson Lee Novick, New York dermatologist and author.

CHAPTER 12

DENTAL HEALTH

T he dull ache of one lonely cavity echoes through your whole mouth, leaving your head pounding. The tiny mound of a canker sore inside your cheek feels like a gaping gash at the awkward touch of your tongue, triggering fiery pangs. In the hyper-sensitive confines of your mouth, the most minor of problems can mean mega-pain. It hurts just to think about knocked-out teeth or chronic gum disease. You've spent hours on your back in a dentist's chair, hours that seemed like years. Is there a way to cut short all this aching and drilling, scraping and filling? Yes, by responding quickly when problems occur. Better yet, you can actually prevent many dental disorders, quickly and easily.

- In 1 minute, you can prevent tooth and gum disease by flossing.
- Ice a spot on your hand for 7 minutes and reduce the pain of a toothache.
- In 15 minutes of chewing gum, you can cut down on plaque.

Now, open wide!

COMBATING CAVITIES

So you've had a cavity or a few in your lifetime. Who hasn't? By the ripe old age of 2½, almost all American kids show some decay on the surfaces of their teeth. Adults, for whom dentures were almost inevitable not long ago, are keeping their own teeth more often, but those teeth are showing an increased incidence of root decay.

A cavity is your mouth's way of telling you that you have an active case of dental caries, a bacterial disease. Some 200 to 300 kinds of bacteria reside in your mouth, many providing worthwhile services like digesting food or producing vitamins. But others get their kicks ganging up in a sticky substance called plaque and looking for innocent teeth to beat up on. Usually invisible, plaque may briefly reveal itself as a slimy whitish film on your teeth first thing in the morning, because the glands that produce saliva, a natural mouthwash, are turned off while you sleep.

Plaque gobbles up sugars in the foods you eat and forms acids that attack your tooth enamel. Acid is produced within moments after you've ingested sugar and does its worst damage within 20 minutes' time. Your teeth are pretty tough, though: A year or two of recurrent acid attacks against a tooth can occur before the first signs of a cavity appear in the form of an opaque white or brown spot on the surface enamel. After that, the enamel's outer layers slowly break down, becoming rough and stained, and the bacteria invade the dentin underneath and spread, creating a large cavity.

Your cavity starts to cause pain as bacteria and acid seep inside your tooth down to the root through tiny tubes in the dentin. Worse yet, the bacteria dig into the pulp tissue near the center of your tooth. And then—talk about excruciating—the pulp becomes swollen, infection spreads, blood supplies are cut off, and the pulp can die. Then the pain subsides . . . until perhaps a few years later, when an abscess can form due to bacteria working their way from the root canal into the nearby bone and tissue, leaving them inflamed and infected.

Fortunately, cavities are anything but inevitable if you're careful about what you eat and how you care for your teeth.

Brush up. Proper cleaning of your teeth can virtually eliminate decay, says Chicago dentist Craig Millard, D.D.S. Forget the old "brush twice a day" rule. Brush your teeth after every meal and snack, he advises: "If you eat six times a day, brush your teeth six times."

No more than a minute or two is required for a good brushing, Dr. Millard says. Just make sure you're doing it properly. Use a soft toothbrush that effectively removes plaque without damaging tooth enamel or irritating gums.

Buy a fluoride toothpaste. It has been shown to reduce decay. Angle the brush at about 45 degrees against your gum line and move it up and down with a slight circular motion. Brush the fronts of your teeth, the backs, and the flat chewing surfaces. Then massage your gums with the bristles in a gentle circular motion to stimulate blood flow and eject plaque from beneath the gum line.

Brush your bacteria-laden tongue, too. You can buy a tongue-scraper at your drugstore for this exact purpose, but a toothbrush will do just fine in about 5 seconds.

Toss your old toothbrush. A toothbrush lasts for only three or four months, says Pennsylvania dentist Wistar Paist, Jr., D.M.D. "The bristles get worn out and stop doing a good job. Toss it and get a new one," he advises. You may want to replace it more often: Those old bristles are chock-full of food particles and water that provide the perfect breeding ground for germs, say researchers at the University of Oklahoma, who found that people with chronic sore throats or gum infections recovered sooner when they began replacing their toothbrush every two weeks.

Throw plaque a curve. Curved toothbrushes improve plaque removal by 63 percent compared with straight-bristle brushes, according to a study in the Journal of the American Dental Association. Choose your toothbrush on its ability to reach every one of your teeth. "A dentist uses angled instruments to get into your mouth," Dr. Paist says, "so why shouldn't you? Get whatever type of brush you feel most comfortable using, whatever you'll use most often."

Floss out plaque. Flossing can take as little as a minute, but remember, Dr. Millard says, that "you're not trying to remove food particles. You're trying to remove plaque from the surface of teeth. Just putting the floss between the teeth does not necessarily do the proper job." To do it right, break off about 18 inches of floss, waxed or unwaxed, wind it around your middle fingers, slide it between your teeth and curl it around them, scraping the sides of your teeth from the gum line.

Save money and time on mouthwashes. You've probably seen ads galore about mouthwashes that are supposed to fight plaque. But any such rinse is generally unnecessary—and time-consuming—Dr. Millard says, if you're doing a good job brushing and flossing. What's more, he says, the effectiveness of most of these so-called antiplaque rinses remains unproven. One exception is Peridex, a prescription-only plaque-loosening rinse approved by the American Dental Association. Dr. Millard often prescribes it for people whose poor eyesight or handgrip problems prevent them from cleaning their teeth well. Rinse at least twice a day for about 30 seconds, then brush and floss.

Check in for a checkup. The hour or so that you spend with your dentist twice a year in a checkup can save you from many a time-consuming dental problem in the future. Your dentist will examine your teeth and gums for cavities and disease. He may also take X-rays, but generally a full set of X-rays is needed no more often than every three years. He should also inquire, Dr. Paist says, about health problems you might have and medications you take, all of which can have an effect on your dental health.

Seal your mouth. An hour at your dentist's office can seal off your molars from bacteria. Plastic sealants, which go on in a liquid form and dry into an invisible but strong coating, have been shown to effectively prevent plaque formation and cut tooth decay in half. A single application of sealant can last up to several years.

Take the tablet test. Train yourself to get everything squeaky-clean, Dr. Millard advises, by occasionally testing yourself with disclosing tablets, available at any drugstore. After you brush and floss, dissolve one of these tablets in your mouth. Any leftover plaque will almost immediately turn a garish red. Brush and floss again to remove as much of the color as you can. Any remaining color will disappear in a day or so.

Have a piece of fruit. Plaque bacteria are like kids in a candy store: You can't give them everything they want. Instead, selectively satisfy their voracious appetite for sweets. Worst are sticky candy bars, raisins and other dried fruits, and lingering sweets like honey. Fibrous fresh fruits like apples, as well as raw vegetables, are actually good for your teeth, massaging your gums and stimulating the production of mouth-rinsing saliva.

Go ahead and eat dessert. Limit sweets to meals instead of between them. Plaque's acids start attacking your teeth only minutes after you ingest sugar and go on for at least 20 minutes. The fewer times you consume sugar, the fewer opportunities acids get to consume your teeth.

Say "cheese." Eating a piece of cheddar cheese after a meal seems to take the bite out of destructive acid. In a study conducted at the University of Toronto's Department of Preventive Dentistry, subjects who swished their teeth with a sugar solution showed significantly less tooth enamel damage if they chewed on one-half ounce of "extra-old" cheddar cheese for 1 minute immediately afterward.

Pop some gum. Chewing on gum made with xylitol can help bust bacteria. Subjects in one study showed reduced plaque buildup after chewing ten pieces of xylitol gum daily for two weeks. A natural sweetener found in fruits and vegetables, xylitol interferes with the growth of microorganisms that form plaque, says Kauko Makinen, Ph.D., who conducted the study at the University of Michigan School of Dentistry. You'll get best results, another study suggests, by popping sugarless gum into your mouth within 5 minutes after you've finished eating, and chewing it for at least 15 minutes. Check the label when you buy your next pack of sugarless gum to see that it contains xylitol.

DETECTING PERIODONTAL DISEASE

An infection of the gums and bones that hold your teeth in place, periodontal disease appears as early as puberty, and is very common among adults over 40. The culprit behind this is a now-familiar foe: plaque, this time doing its dirty work down between your teeth and gums.

Gingivitis is an early form of the disease. Usually striking in the teen years and hanging around in varying degrees of severity for a lifetime, it results when a buildup of plaque between the gums and teeth infects the gums. Signs of gingivitis are gums that are red and swollen and which bleed easily when touched or when you brush your teeth. It is usually painless.

Untreated gingivitis can lead to the more severe periodontitis, or pyorrhea, in which the continual buildup of plaque digs pockets between the teeth and gums. A vicious cycle takes hold as plaque collects inside these pockets, inaccessible to brushing and flossing. The plaque hardens into sharp splinters called calculus or tartar, which dig at the gums like a pickax. The gums start pulling away from the teeth, and more pockets open up. Eventually the whole structure can collapse, leaving you with no teeth.

Fortunately, Dr. Millard says, a vigilant program of proper oral hygiene can prevent and even reverse periodontal disease in its early stages.

Brush and floss. Just two or three days of proper brushing and flossing can clear up mild gum disease. More advanced cases may take a few weeks.

Irrigate your mouth. A water irrigation system like a Water Pik can be very helpful, Dr. Paist says. "Between each tooth and its surrounding gum there's a moat where water and plaque collect," he explains. "The normal, healthy depth of this moat is 1 to 3 millimeters—about $\frac{1}{100}$ of an inch. Periodontal disease deepens the moat, making it difficult to reach into with a toothbrush or dental floss without damaging the gums. That's where a water irrigation device comes in handy. What you're trying to do is change the water, flushing out all the bacteria that sits in there."

Go electric. An electric toothbrush can root out deep plaque, too. In one study, an electric brush with a rotating head was shown to be more effective than a human-powered brush in removing deeply-embedded plaque from the teeth of gum surgery patients whose molars' roots remained exposed.

Get plenty of vitamin C. This vitamin can help heal bleeding gums resulting from the early stages of gingivitis. Your gums need a constant supply of a protein called collagen that depends on vitamin C for its production.

Low intake of the vitamin may actually contribute to bleeding gums, according to a study conducted by Penelope Leggott, D.D.S., at the U.S. Department of Agriculture Western Nutrition Research Center in San Francisco. When a periodontist probed the gums of healthy subjects who received 600 milligrams of vitamin C daily (ten times the Recommended Dietary Allowance [RDA] of 60 milligrams for 25- to 50-year-olds), the number of bleeding gum sites was significantly lower than when the same subjects, at another time, took low amounts of vitamin C.

When it comes to bleeding gums, Dr. Leggott says, "the RDA of 60 milligrams daily may not be adequate." She recommends against swallowing megadoses, however. "If you have an orange, an apple, and a couple of green vegetables every day," she says, "you're almost sure to exceed the RDA."

Let your dentist clean up. Periodontal disease can persist despite your best efforts, so see your dentist at least twice a year for a half-hour professional cleanup.

THE FAST TRACK TO WHITER TEETH

Stains on the surfaces of your teeth are a common problem that result largely from foods, drinks, and other substances that you put into your mouth. Making matters worse is a buildup of plaque or tartar on your teeth, which can absorb bacteria that discolor your teeth. It's not a pretty sight. But a little prevention and prompt treatment can brighten things up.

Ban the offenders. Keep certain substances out of your mouth in the first place. In case you don't have enough other reasons not to smoke, consider that tobacco leaves a tarlike stain on your teeth—and consider the extra time the dentist has to spend cleaning those stains. Coffee and tea do a number on them, too. Switch to herbal teas—they won't stain. And don't go overboard with foods and beverages like citrus fruits and juices that contain citric acid. It can eat away at your enamel and thus give staining substances a foothold. Don't worry about drinking your morning juice, but a regular habit of sucking on lemons is sure to strip your enamel.

Have a water chaser. Protect your cosmetic dental work by taking a few seconds to rinse your mouth with water or brush your teeth immediately after drinking alcohol, which dulls the shine of bondings and crowns.

Brush around the clock. If you're particularly prone to stains, brush your teeth not only after meals but between them. And floss carefully, which prevents stains from getting started in niches and rough areas on your teeth.

Stick to toothpaste. Ordinary toothpaste is just fine for removing most stains. Steer clear of pastes and polishes that promise to whiten your teeth, as some contain bleaches that can irritate the soft tissues in your mouth. Others are abrasive polishes that can wear away enamel and roughen tooth surfaces, making them, ironically, even more vulnerable to stains.

Let your dentist do it. The professional cleaning your dentist does at least twice a year will give your grin extra polish. See him more often if your teeth are particularly stain-prone.

Whiten stains from the inside out. Your dentist can also help alleviate internal stains—those in which your teeth have actually changed color from the inside out. Among other causes, the antibiotic tetracycline can discolor the still-developing teeth of children (even while they're still in the womb if their mother takes the drug during pregnancy). Your dentist can bleach such stains, Dr. Paist says, by applying an oxidizing agent. Afterward, you sit for several minutes under a bright, heat-producing lamp to activate the bleach, which lightens the stain. Bleaching can take as few as three 1-hour treatments plus an annual touch-up. The results vary depending on the individual.

Do it yourself. You may have seen advertisements for "stain-removal systems." They're actually stain bleachers, not stain removers, says Dr. Paist, and are all basically the same. Although their "oxidating" or "oxygenating" bleaching agent is not as strong as the one your dentist uses, the procedure is simpler and cheaper than visiting your dentist, Dr. Paist says. The at-home treatment generally requires daily half-hour applications for four to six weeks. Just follow the instructions.

FAST-ACTING PAIN RELIEF

A pain in your mouth is nature's way of telling you to pay attention to it. Trouble is, it doesn't always speak very clearly. Sometimes pain can mean you've got a cavity or infected gums. Maybe a new wisdom tooth is drilling its way up to the surface. Or maybe you've got seeds from this morning's raspberry preserves jammed between your teeth. Whatever the source, there's no need to keep suffering. Cut pain short with these fast-acting techniques (but see your dentist if the pain recurs).

Release trapped food. Simply brush, floss, or rinse your mouth briskly with lukewarm water. One of these methods—or a combination—should dislodge it.

Change the temperature of a toothache. Hold a mouthful of very warm water for a couple of minutes or until the pain subsides, then spit it out and repeat if the pain comes back, Dr. Paist suggests. If heat doesn't work, try the same procedure with cold water. Or put ice directly on the aching tooth or on your cheek for 15 minutes three or four times a day, as needed.

Rub it down. Rub an ice cube into the V-shaped area where the bones of your thumb and forefinger meet in the hand on the same side as the toothache. Researchers at McGill University in Canada found that numbing the hand this way for about 7 minutes cuts the intensity of toothaches by about half, apparently by blocking the passage of toothache pain impulses along nerve pathways in your brain.

Swallow two aspirin. You've heard about placing aspirin directly on your aching tooth. Don't! This can cause an aspirin burn in your gums or cheek. But go ahead and take two aspirin every 4 to 6 hours as required to relieve pain. If you're sensitive to aspirin, try ibuprofen (Nuprin, Advil) or acetaminophen (Tylenol, Anacin-3).

Spice it up. Oil of clove has proven very effective in anesthetizing a toothache. Use a preparation available over-the-counter at drugstores, not pure clove oil, which can irreversibly damage nerves. Drop a small amount of the preparation directly onto the sore tooth, or dab some onto a cotton ball and place it over the tooth. A whole clove held against the tooth will work, too.

Make a breakthrough. Decrease the pain that accompanies the emergence of a new wisdom tooth by chewing something hard like pretzels. This may help the tooth break through your gums sooner. Unfortunately, this process can occur off and on unpredictably for a week or a lifetime, Dr. Paist says. Some wisdom teeth never come in completely, he says; if yours doesn't break through in a week or so, see your dentist.

Swig salt water for gum pain. Mix 1 teaspoon of salt in a glassful of very warm water. Swish a mouthful of the mixture around and between your teeth, spit it out, and repeat until you've used up all the water in the glass. This may reduce the pain for hours. If it doesn't, repeat the procedure every hour as necessary.

Desensitize your teeth. Some people's teeth are just plain oversensitive. Teeth whose roots are exposed due to gum disease or brushing too hard can become very sensitive. Hypersensitivity can also result from tiny cracks, broken fillings, or decay. Desensitizing toothpastes like Sensodyne, Promise, and Denquil can help. For 2 minutes, rub a cotton swab dabbed in the toothpaste along the gum line of the sensitive teeth. Repeat the procedure each morning and night for two weeks, then once or twice a week as the sensitivity diminishes. If it doesn't, see your dentist to check for deeper problems.

A dental technique called iontophoresis, involving the application of fluoride, can help, too. The procedure takes about 2 minutes per tooth. Sensitivity is usually alleviated after two or three treatments.

  HIGH
TECH ● **LASER DENTISTRY**

You won't be needing any anesthesia at your endodontist's office today. After all, he's just performing a root canal . . . on every one of your roots. But you won't be feeling much if any pain: He's using a dental laser. This space-age dentistry method is not only virtually pain-free but is quieter, more precise, cleaner, and ultimately more efficient than conventional dental equipment.

A dental laser emits concentrated energy in the form of an intense, pulsing light beam that vaporizes tooth and tissue with pinpoint accuracy, slicing out tiny sections of infected gum, closing off sensitive nerve endings exposed by gum disease, digging out cavities, and more. A laser seals blood vessels as it goes along, so the patient loses less blood and the dentist can more clearly see what he is doing. It causes less damage to surrounding tissue and presents less chance of infection, so most wounds heal better and with less pain. And when used carefully, a laser leaves little or no scarring.

Something else that a laser can do that nothing else can quite match is desensitize teeth. Very often if the gum has receded around a tooth, that tooth can be very sensitive to cold, touch, brushing, or even air. A dental laser seems to have an effect on the tubules in the dentin so that nerve endings are not exposed, reducing or eliminating sensitivity in as little as 10 minutes. "Nothing else I have seen is that dramatic in eliminating that source of pain," says Detroit periodontist Joseph Nemeth, D.D.S., who uses lasers to perform gum surgery.

Some dental procedures performed with a laser may actually take a few minutes longer than those performed with conventional equipment. In the long run, however, time may be saved by not having to give an anesthetic beforehand—meaning you don't unknowingly drool for hours afterwards, or feel like your lip is dragging on the ground. More time is saved in not needing to clean up bleeding or sew in stitches afterwards.

Laser dentistry can save countless hours of fear, loathing, and catch-up repair work for the millions of people who avoid dentists because they are terrified of pain, Dr. Nemeth says. Lasers cause little or no pain because their pulses come in bursts too short (10 to 30 times a second) to trigger nerve impulse transmission. "Many patients I have performed surgery on with lasers are remarkably comfortable without any anesthetic," says Dr. Nemeth. "Some have told me it's less uncomfortable than a cleaning."

While dental lasers are still relatively rare, having made their debut in gum surgery, the Food and Drug Administration's (FDA) pending approval of lasers for cutting out cavities could change all that. "This is the beginning of a new era in dentistry," says Dr. Nemeth. Already FDA-approved for gum surgery, lasers are now being used on cavities by some dentists. So don't be surprised to find yourself opening your mouth to a friendly laser during your next visit to your dentist's office.

BAN BAD BREATH

Periodontal disease is a major cause of bad breath due to the often odorous combination of bacteria, infection, and damaged tissue. The only remedy is conscientious care for your teeth and gums, starting with a visit to your dentist. Other diseases can also bring on bad breath, so if it persists despite your best efforts, see your doctor for a checkup. But often the cause of bad breath is simple, and the cure quick.

Brush away bacteria. Regular brushing and flossing help expel the bacteria that cause bad-smelling breath. Don't forget to also brush your tongue to remove bacteria that collects in its nooks and crannies.

Rinse your mouth. Protect your mouth from bacterial buildup for up to 3 hours with bacteria-fighting mouthwashes. Look for those containing the active ingredients thymol, eucalyptol, methyl salicylate, and menthol.

Cover up. You've just eaten Italian? Gee, except for the fact that your breath smells exactly like Giancarlo's Garlic-and-More-Garlic Surprise, we never would have guessed. Assuming you've brushed your teeth after your meal, this kind of bad breath doesn't originate in your mouth but in your lungs, Dr. Paist says. As you digest aromatic substances contained in garlic, they get into your bloodstream, circulate through your lungs, and greet your friends through your breath. In fact, the mere handling of lots of garlic can cause garlic breath because the smelly substances enter the bloodstream via the pores.

You can camouflage garlic and other potent-scented foods like onion and curry in minutes by chewing raw parsley, or peppermint or wintergreen gums and breath mints.

Drink away the stink of stress. Stress can reduce the flow of saliva in your mouth, giving odor-causing germs a chance to reproduce unchallenged. In seconds, a gulp of water or a breath mint can start things flowing again.

Soak your sinuses. The stuffy nose and postnasal drip of a sinus infection can give you bad breath. You'll probably need antibiotics to clear up the infection. While you're waiting for them to take effect, alleviate the smell by irrigating your nose with a few squirts of saline solution—½ teaspoon of salt to 1 cup of water—which washes away secretions and bacteria.

SOOTHING CANKER SORES QUICKLY

There you are, minding your own business, when—yeow! —out of nowhere this ugly sore erupts on your tongue or sprouts on the inside of your lip. A small, red wound at first, it quickly grows into a white, red-bordered, exquisitely painful ulcer that makes everything from eating to brushing your teeth an exercise in masochism. This troublemaker is a canker sore.

Medically known as aphthous ulcers, canker sores thrive inside your mouth on the wet tissues of your tongue and cheek. Nobody knows for sure what causes them although a predisposition for them may be hereditary. Sometimes biting your cheek or tongue or injuring them with a hard-bristled toothbrush or hard piece of food can get them started. They often seem to erupt during times of stress, such as after you've had a fever or a cold. There's some thought that they may be caused by a virus.

"There's not a whole lot you can do to speed up healing of canker sores," Dr. Paist says. "Usually I tell people that if I treat it, it'll be gone in two weeks. If I don't, it'll take 14 days." Although the pain can be so intense it seems to last forever, you will outlive canker sores: They tend to appear less and less the older you get. In the meantime, he says, you'll simply need to let the sore run its course. But you can do plenty to help it heal steadily and relieve the pain in the process.

Time to tingle. When you feel that first tingle of a canker sore, break open a vitamin E capsule and squeeze a little oil on the sore. And take 500 milligrams of vitamin C with bioflavonoids three times a day for the next three days to speed healing.

Nip it with a styptic pencil. This shaving-cut standby has been found by many canker sore sufferers to stop the development of a new, still-tiny ulcer into a big, painful one. The active ingredient is the astringent alum, which dries out the sore. The trick is to catch the canker sore early in its miserable little life. Take a few seconds dabbing it with a styptic pencil—it may save you a week or so of pain.

Peroxide it. Hydrogen peroxide and carbamide peroxide are antiseptics that kill germs and help canker sores heal. Both are available over-the-counter—carbamide peroxide sold as Gly-oxide liquid is often in the toothache-canker sore rack. If you catch a budding canker sore soon enough with these medications you may be able to prevent it from blossoming into a full-blown ulcer. Apply them several times a day—it's worth the few seconds it takes.

Warm salt water soothes. Mix a teaspoon of salt into a cup of warm water and slosh the solution around in your mouth for a minute. This cleans the tissue around your sore, helping it heal, and temporarily relieves pain. Water mixed with a little baking soda also works.

Numb it. Over-the-counter anesthetic gels containing benzocaine, phenol, camphor, or menthol can temporarily numb the pain. Since your saliva washes them away, just keep applying them as needed.

Paste it. Your drugstore also has an oral paste (Orabase) that sticks to the sore and acts like a protective bandage. Orabase-B has benzocaine added for a numbing effect. First gently dry the sore with a cotton swab; then apply the paste as directed. It takes less than a minute.

Take tea. Ordinary tea helps ease burning and itching. Soak a handkerchief or piece of gauze in cool tea and hold it to your sore for a few minutes until the discomfort subsides. Or use a cool, wet tea bag. Make sure it's regular tea, not herbal tea, because it's the astringent effect of black tea's tannic acid that does the trick.

Swish with milk. If eating becomes impossible because of canker pain, rinse your mouth with a bit of milk before eating, suggests David Burt, D.D.S, a Bethlehem, Pennsylvania, dentist. The milk will coat the sore and make supper possible.

Eat tastelessly. Bland, soft foods will help you feel better while healing. Avoid nuts and acidic fruit and hot, highly spiced foods, which can send you through the roof.

See your doctor. If the pain of a canker sore becomes very severe, it could be infected with bacteria. Your doctor or dentist can prescribe an antibiotic like tetracycline, which has been shown to reduce healing time, ulcer size, and pain in canker sores. He or she may also prescribe an oral paste-bandage that contains an antibiotic.

OVERCOMING INJURIES

Accidents happen. When they happen in the vicinity of your mouth—a tooth gets knocked out, a cap falls off, you take a bite out of your tongue—quick action can help prevent further problems and put you on the mend faster.

Stick that knocked-out tooth back in its place. You don't have to be a speed-skating, stick-swinging, puck-ducking professional hockey player to suffer the sudden loss of a tooth. You could be an everyday ordinary person who walks the wrong way into a swinging door or takes a fall on the sidewalk. But if you're a professional hockey player, you've got someone like Robert Duresa, D.D.S., busy dentist to the Chicago Blackhawks, on the sidelines to help treat tooth emergencies fast.

A quick response can save a knocked-out tooth, Dr. Duresa says. "The tooth has the best chance of healing if you rinse it off with contact lens saline solution or salt water and put it right back in," he says. When you rinse the tooth, make sure you don't wash away any roots or tissue attached. Do not clean it with any chemicals. Re-insert it with gentle finger pressure. Then get to the dentist right away.

Plop that tooth into milk. Getting a knocked-out tooth back in, and keeping it in until you get to the dentist, can sometimes be a problem, says Dr. Duresa, especially for kids, who might tend to swallow it. Another option is to clean the tooth as described above and keep it from drying out by putting it in a glass of milk or contact lens saline solution.

In their absence, plastic wrap provides good protection for about an hour. *Don't* store it in saliva, which contains harmful bacteria, or in tap water, which despite being wet can cause the surface of the root to die. Tow the tooth along with the toothless to a dentist immediately. "The shorter the period of time the tooth is out," Dr. Duresa says, "the better its chances of healing."

Put your cap back on. If the cap falls off your tooth, ruining your perfect smile, rinse the cap off with salt water or contact lens saline solution and immediately put the cap back in place, Dr. Duresa says. See if it will stay there by itself. If it doesn't, take it out and wrap it up in a piece of tissue or gauze, put it in an envelope, seal it, and mark it. Don't wrap it loosely in a piece of tissue tucked into a purse, he advises, or you could end up accidentally tossing it out.

Get to your dentist as soon as possible because, Dr. Duresa says, "the tooth now has nothing to keep it in place. Teeth aren't locked into place but are held in by fibrous material. There's always some movement, like a shock absorber. A tooth that's lost its cap can shift within just a day or two."

Compress your bleeding tongue. An accident to—or accidental bite of—your tongue can be awfully painful, not to mention frighteningly bloody. Try either of these fast remedies: Tightly press a wet handkerchief, face towel, or piece of sterile gauze over the injured spot. This will usually bring the bleeding under control without stitches or help from a doctor. Pressing a wet tea bag (regular tea, not herbal tea) against the wound may work even faster, thanks to the tannin in tea leaves, which helps blood clot more quickly. Firmly press a handkerchief or towel over the tea bag.

Get to your dentist pronto. It's the basic response to most other dental emergencies, from a tooth that's partially broken off to one that's pushed in or pulled out.

DEALING WITH DENTURES

Say, whose dentures are these, anyway? Godzilla's? Sometimes new dentures feel like they don't fit right when you're first adjusting to them. Instead of trudging back to the dentist right away, give yourself some time to get used to them—at least a couple of weeks. During this break-in period, and in the long run, there are fast and simple methods you can use to adjust to dentures and keep them—and your mouth—ready to take a good bite out of life.

Stick it to 'em. A soft denture adhesive paste temporarily "glues" your dentures to your gums. Once you're used to your new teeth, the paste should be unnecessary. See your dentist if the problem continues.

Soak up saliva. Your new dentures can be mouth-watering, and not because they taste good. Excess saliva is a common complaint among new denture-wearers, because your mouth thinks they're in there to be eaten. Simply suck on lozenges frequently for the first couple of days. This helps you rid yourself of the excess saliva by prompting you to swallow more frequently.

Soap 'em up. Avoid future trips to the dentist for new dentures by keeping the ones you already have in good shape. Remove them after every meal for a quick scrub with plain soap and lukewarm water, then rinse them and pop them back in.

BE GOOD TO YOUR GUMS

As important as your gums were before you got dentures, they're even more important now. Your gums are all you've got between — well, between chewing your food and gumming it, between speaking clearly and speaking unintelligibly. So you've got to take special care, and it takes little time.

Rinse them. Keep your gums clean by rinsing your mouth daily with a glass of warm water mixed with a teaspoon of salt.

Massage them. Give your gums a daily 1-minute massage to promote circulation and firmness. Take your gums between your thumb and index finger and rub gently back and forth and up and down. It feels wonderful, too.

Give them a break. And remember that your hardworking gums deserve some time off. When no one's looking, remove your dentures and let your gums do a whole lot of nothing for a few minutes. Avoid doing this all day, or for days at a time, though, because without your dentures your cheeks and lips will start to lose their shape.

BATTLING BRUXISM

Bruxism, the chronic, destructive habit of clenching and grinding your teeth (usually during sleep), can wear out more than tooth enamel. "If you wake up feeling tired, or with a headache or sore jaw muscles, you've probably been bruxing all night," says John Brown, D.D.S., former president of the Academy of General Dentistry. Other symptoms include increased sensitivity to hot or cold foods and drinks, pain while you're chewing, chipped fillings, and a spouse who's losing sleep because you're making noises like a squeaky door or a mortar and pestle.

Bruxism is often the result of teeth that don't properly fit together when your mouth is closed. Dentists themselves sometimes unknowingly cause it, Dr. Brown says, by installing a filling that's too high or a crown with a high spot in it. Your muscles attempt to correct the imperfection by grinding away. Physical or psychological stress can also set your teeth on edge.

If the surfaces of your teeth are soft, Dr. Brown says, bruxism will wear the enamel away. If you have tough teeth, bruxism can still do damage by rocking them away from supporting bones. At its worst, bruxism can lead to temporomandibular disorder, or TMD (see page 299). But the problem is usually correctable, sometimes quickly.

See your dentist. He or she can tell if your teeth themselves—or a crown or filling—are causing the problem. Correcting it may be as fast and simple as a little grinding to even things out or as easy as fitting a filling or crown properly.

Sleep with a guard. A cushiony plastic mouthguard or splint is one of the best ways to protect your enamel from nocturnal damage, Dr. Brown says. Designed by your dentist, it immediately reduces contact between your teeth while you sleep.

Change your position. Your lower jaw is hung in a sling of muscles that's not firmly attached anywhere. Sleeping in a different position, if you can manage it, can sometimes improve the way your teeth touch each other.

Squeeze a ball. "Some people don't realize it, but they 'doodle' with their teeth—clench, grind, slip, and slide them—just like they doodle with a pencil when they're on the phone or when feeling stressed," Dr. Brown says. If you're such a doodler, stress-management exercises like squeezing a tennis ball when you're feeling tense or exercising your head and neck muscles can help.

Have a ball. "In cases where severe stress is the cause of bruxism, the only way to deal with it is to change what's causing it, which in some cases means your job," Dr. Brown says. Whether they're anxiety-ridden New York cabbies or "professional volunteers," people who gnash their teeth need more fun and less stress. "Bruxism patients need to do everything possible to get rid of the stress in their lives," he says.

DIABETES

n the old days, Greek doctors dubbed it "diabetes," which means siphon or fountain, because people who suffered from this familiar disorder had to urinate copiously. They added "mellitus"—from the Latin word for honey—because the diabetics' urine smelled sweet from the large amounts of sugar it contained.

Those two observations have held up splendidly for the past 2,000 years. Taken together, they hint at diabetes' true, secret nature: a potentially fatal disorder of blood sugar utilization. Depending on the form of diabetes they have, people with diabetes either can't manufacture or can't properly use the hormone insulin, and that prevents the body from using glucose (blood sugar). Glucose is the body's main fuel, the kindling wood of all your cells. Without insulin, though, the sugar from digested food never gets properly burned; instead it just builds up in your blood. In a desperate effort to get rid of the stuff, your body dumps excess glucose into your urine. The result: lots of sweet-smelling urine.

What's wrong with that? Plenty. In the short term, blood sugar levels that are extremely high (hyperglycemia) or extremely low (hypoglycemia)—the opposite ends of the arc between which uncontrolled diabetes can swing —can lead to dizziness, "sugar shock" (mental confusion, unconsciousness), and even death. Over the long term, it can get worse: Of the 11 million Americans who suffer from diabetes, over 100,000 die from it each year, or from its various complications—heart disease, kidney failure, or nerve damage. Others go blind or develop gangrene, which may make it necessary to amputate a foot.

That's the bad news. But there's plenty of good news

to go around, too. For one thing, Type II or non-insulin-dependent diabetes (the kind we'll be talking about in this chapter), "is for many people a lifestyle disease," says Michael Stolar, Ph.D., of the American Diabetes Association. That means many Type II diabetics can control the disorder—even wipe it off the blackboard of their lives completely—simply by controlling their weight, diet, and exercise habits. (Type I or insulin-dependent diabetes requires daily injections, is much more severe, and can't be as readily controlled by the simple methods that follow.) Although Type II diabetes does tend to run in families, you inherit only the genetic tendency to become diabetic. By controlling your lifestyle, you can spit in the face of Fate and live a long, happy, crazy life just like everybody else. You may never have to find out whether you're "really" a diabetic at all.

. . . .

GIVE YOURSELF A TEST

Type II diabetics who take insulin need to frequently check their blood sugar levels. The doctor will use this information to optimize their insulin regimen. But most other Type IIs never do learn how. "It's not as important for Type II diabetics who don't take insulin to monitor their blood sugar levels daily," says the American Diabetes Association's Dr. Michael Stolar, "but self-monitoring data can be valuable—mainly because it shows you that you are really accomplishing something through diet and exercise." Nothing helps keep you motivated like knowing it's all worth it. And you can test your blood sugar in less than 5 minutes. Note: You'll have to suffer the indignity of a pinprick, but tests that measure glucose in blood, rather than urine, are much more accurate.

. . . .

Keeping your blood sugar levels under control doesn't have to take much time but does take a constant commitment. After all:

- In just seconds, you can add chromium to your daily diet to help control glucose tolerance.
- In 60 minutes a week, you can exercise your way to sugar metabolism management.

- You can save time, and slow down the rise in blood glucose levels, by eating your vegetables raw.

Diabetes doesn't have to take as much of your time as you thought, and these fast methods are ways to help you lead a healthier, more active life.

MAKING A 10-POUND DIFFERENCE

Approximately 80 percent of the people who find out they've got Type II diabetes are overweight. Why? Well, even diabetes specialists aren't exactly sure. But the bottom line is this: If you're diabetic and you're carrying around some excess baggage, weight loss is generally considered the single most effective treatment—the first step back toward a normal life.

"Many Type II diabetics are 30 to 60 pounds overweight," says Robert Henry, M.D., a diabetes weight-loss specialist in San Diego. "For some, there's no question that losing just 10 pounds can make a big difference."

And the sooner you peel off the lard, the better. "If weight is lost early in the course of Type II diabetes, the disease is often reversible," says Norman H. Ertel, M.D., of East Orange Veterans Administration Hospital in New Jersey. "In fact, non-insulin-dependent diabetes often disappears when people lose weight." But if you wait for ten years or longer, losing the weight will probably only lessen the severity, but not eliminate the disease.

To help take the weight off and keep it off, follow the guidelines in chapter 36 and add these special tips for diabetics.

Know thy sweet tooth. Some well-meaning people will turn up their noses at all sweets of any description, then later go on a sugar binge to beat the band. Nutritionists say it would be better for folks with diabetes to indulge themselves just a little each day than to follow up total deprivation with total degradation. Others do better cutting out all sweets. The key: Know thyself—and thy sweet tooth. If you're the kind of person who can live without sweets, do so; if not, be realistic yet responsible.

Eat a peach at teatime. Usually your natural insulin level peaks around four in the afternoon. And since insulin is a well-known appetite stimulant, that's your diet's most perilous moment. So try having a little snack around that time (or whenever your hungriest moment happens to be). But be sure you're stealing those calories from some other time in the day, not just adding them. Fresh fruit or raw vegetables, which come in bite-size, ready-to-eat packages are quick, convenient, safe, and nutritious snacks.

DESIGNING YOUR OWN DIABETES DIET

The key to successfully living with diabetes is avoiding extremes of blood sugar plus keeping cholesterol and blood pressure under control. And the key to doing that is sticking with the sort of lifestyle that's usually advised for everybody else: Keep your weight down, exercise regularly, and eat a low-fat, high-fiber diet rich in complex carbohydrates. You could consider this fact the Diabetes Silver Lining Award: Having diabetes just means that you're doubly motivated to do what you ought to be doing anyway.

As far as diet goes, one thing that so far appears not to help Type II diabetes is that otherwise-wonderful stuff, fish oil. The omega-3 fatty acids in fish oil have been shown to work a variety of metabolic wonders, like reducing cholesterol and triglycerides in people prone to heart disease. But when high doses of fish oil were given to a group with diabetes, it actually raised their fasting glucose levels. So for now, it's fine to eat fish, but stay away from fish-oil pills.

So now that you know how to lose weight, and how to manage your special daily dietetic quirks, it's time to learn how to meet your nutritional needs over the long haul.

Consume your cauliflower in the raw. In general, raw, unpeeled foods raise blood glucose levels more slowly than foods that have been peeled, mashed, beaten, cooked, fooled with, and otherwise trounced into submission. By cutting down on cooking, you can also save time.

Have two breakfasts, two lunches, and two dinners. It's easier to avoid blood glucose highs or lows if you space your meals throughout the day, instead of gorging yourself in one or two big blowouts. For example, try eating two small breakfasts, one at 7:00 and one at 9:30 A.M.; a small lunch at noon and another at 2:30 P.M.; a small dinner at 6:00 and another at 8:00.

Have a slice of whole-grain bread. Bread made from whole flour is good, but bread made from whole, unmilled kernels is better for diabetics. The reason: The more of those crunchy little unmilled kernels in your bread, the slower the stuff digests, the more gradually your blood sugar levels rise. And it only takes a few more munches to swallow a slice of whole-grain bread.

Chrome(ium)-plate your diet. This obscure trace mineral acts as a sort of booster rocket for insulin, at least in people whose insulin needs a little oomph, like people with glucose intolerance—an early sign of Type II diabetes. In one study conducted by the U.S. Department of Agriculture, eight people with mild glucose intolerance spent four weeks on a low-chromium diet (typical of the diet about 25 percent of Americans consume). An hour after chugging a glucose solution, their blood sugar soared to 170 mg/dl. But after five weeks on a chromium-loaded diet, their after-meal glucose readings averaged only 130—a 50 percent decrease. By boosting the effectiveness of insulin, chromium apparently reversed their glucose intolerance.

Where do you find chromium? There's not much in the typical American refined-food diet—only 50 micrograms a day. But unprocessed fruits, vegetables, grains—especially corn and wheat—and chicken are good sources. There is no Recommended Dietary Allowance (RDA) for chromium, but the Committee on Dietary Allowances says up to one 200-microgram supplement daily is safe. Just ½ cup of apples, plums, or peanuts will supply more than 100 micrograms.

Plop a dollop of olive oil into your salad dressing. It used to be thought that saturated fats were uniformly bad, unsaturated fats were good, and monunsaturated fats, such as those in olive oil and canola oil, were more or less neutral. But the latest wave of research has begun to demonstrate that monos have a wealth of benefits to bestow, particularly upon diabetics. In one recent study, patients on diets generously garnished with olive oil brought down their blood sugar levels. As a free bonus, their triglycerides also went down, and their HDL cholesterol went up, all signs pointing in the direction of better cardiovascular health. Replace saturated and polyunsaturated fats with monounsaturates whenever you can, but don't exceed 30 percent of calories from fat.

Take a taste of tabbouleh. This tasty Middle Eastern bulgur salad is rich in soluble fiber, the right kind of fiber for your diabetes. It's well known that all that hard-to-digest roughage slows the absorption of sugar through intestinal walls and thus moderates your after-dinner blood sugar high. Other foods high in soluble fiber are barley, beans, baked (not deep-fried) falafel, cracked wheat, fruits containing pectin (like apples), oat bran, parboiled rice, peas, pumpernickel bread, rye bread, and whole-grain pasta. On the other hand, foods rich in insoluble fiber — like the bran part of wheat and the cellulose in most vegetables — will have relatively little effect on your diabetes.

Eat an orange. Making sure your diet is rich in vitamin C, that sweet inner sunshine, may help protect you against two problems commonly associated with diabetes: gum disease (gingivitis), and slow-healing wounds. Both of these disorders are caused by defects in the production of collagen, a protein essential to the manufacture of tough, strong tissue. Studies at the University of Southern California (USC) have shown that diabetic mice fed large doses of vitamin C were able to overcome this inborn deficiency and produce more, higher-quality collagen. The reason: Blood sugar and vitamin C both compete for entry into the cells. The higher your blood sugar levels, the less vitamin C can enter the cells, and so the poorer the collagen quality.

A diet bathed in the sunshine of vitamin C may be able to help. Although these studies in mice have so far not been duplicated in humans, many other studies seem to point in the same direction, and "these things are all starting to add up," says USC biochemist Michael Schneir, Ph.D. Like mice, humans cannot store or make vitamin C in their body, so a good daily dose is needed. Citrus fruits (and especially their juices), cantaloupe, mangoes, and bell peppers are good natural sources.

Check out a C supplement. Nerve disorders and cataracts are two more potentially serious ailments in the dismal hit parade of diabetic side-effects. But vitamin C appears to slow the progression of both of these problems, too. Both are thought to be caused by an accumulation of sorbitol, a type of blood sugar, in cells. But according to studies at the University of Scranton, vitamin C can reduce the concentration of sorbitol in red blood cells, and in this way may protect against the awful possibility of diabetic neuropathy or blindness. Vitamin C has already been shown to slow the progression of galactose cataracts in rats (an animal model of human diabetic cataracts). The Scranton researchers went a step further and tested it in humans. Result: At a level of 500 milligrams a day, vitamin C (in the form of a citrus fruit extract dissolved in juice) reduced sorbitol in red blood cells of diabetic volunteers by 27 percent. At a level of 2,000 milligrams a day (vastly more than the RDA), it reduced levels by almost half (an average of 44 percent). Although drugs that block the formation of sorbitol are now under development, no one knows what their long-term effects might be. A vitamin C supplement is safer and quicker, but check with your doctor first: High blood levels of C can affect urine sugar tests.

Get a dietitian to design a diabetes diet. You may run into problems designing your own diet—it's a complex assignment. So you should try getting a professional dietitian to help you custom-design a diet that accommodates all your little food fancies and fetishes, along with your typical workday and exercise times. Your doctor or local American Diabetes Association office may be able to refer you to a qualified local dietitian.

WORKING OUT DIABETES

Inactive older people are three times more likely to develop diabetes than those who exercise regularly. But even if you've already developed diabetes, exercise can help you keep it under control in a variety of ways. It helps you maintain your weight. It improves your insulin sensitivity and may improve your glucose tolerance. It reduces your risk of heart disease. It reduces the clumping of blood platelets, which can lead to strokes. If you're taking insulin or oral hypoglycemic drugs, it may help you reduce your dosage. And it improves your psychological health.

That's why regular workouts, in some form or fashion, should be a key part of your antidiabetes strategy. Before you embark on an exercise kick, however, get a physical exam to uncover any possible problems with your blood vessels or nerves. The American Diabetes Association also recommends you take a stress test if you're over 35.

Warm up and cool down. Low-intensity exercise before and after aerobic exercise prevents injury. First it gradually increases your heart rate and blood pressure, then gently decreases them, making your workout easier on vulnerable blood vessels.

Keep warm and keep cool. That is, avoid exercising in extreme cold or heat. Those vulnerable blood vessels are what keep your body temperature within normal ranges, so avoid stressing them too much.

Listen to your body. You may occasionally lose some control over your sugar-insulin balance. During these times you should avoid exercising.

Walk every day against diabetes. Aerobic exercise, like walking, jogging, biking, or swimming, is usually thought to be the best way to keep diabetics' sugar metabolism in working order. But the beneficial effect of exercise on blood sugar regulation is, alas, as fast-fading as a flower. That's why, in order for exercise to do you any good, you have to do it often. Pick something you can do three times a week for 20 to 45 minutes, like swimming or biking. Or, if you choose something less vigorous, like walking, do it even more often.

Take it easy. You may be the kind of person who likes intense workouts. Or, if you skip a workout or two, you may want to try to compensate by walking twice as fast, or twice as far, next time. Don't. Unusually intense exercise can actually boost blood sugar levels.

Pump iron. One study suggests that working out with weights may have almost as beneficial an effect as aerobic exercise on blood sugar metabolism. A three-times-a-week strength-training program would take only 3 hours or so.

Slip soft shoes on your athletic feet. Diabetics need to be especially careful of their feet, and diabetics who jog need to be extra-extra careful. That's because diabetes often leads to peripheral vascular disease, which reduces the blood supply to the feet and legs at the same time it also dulls the sensitivity of nerves (a condition called peripheral neuropathy). Taken together, these two problems are like some evil tag team: Reduced circulation increases the likelihood of infection at the same time neuropathy reduces your ability to feel it. As a result, the humble blister or callus on a diabetic jogger's heel can very quickly become a painfully infected sore. It may even lead to gangrene, which could require amputation.

To bypass that grisly possibility, diabetic exercisers should always wear comfortable running shoes. (Properly fitted running shoes can be so heavenly, in fact, that some doctors advise diabetics to wear running shoes all the time.) Try air-conditioned (mesh-vented) shoes and specially designed athletic socks to wick away sweat and help prevent blisters. Make foot inspection a daily ritual. Look over your tootsies for blisters, calluses, or cracks between the toes, and if you discover a nasty-looking sore, have a doctor take a look at it right away. A daily foot inspection only takes 5 minutes or so.

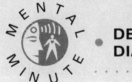

DE-STRESSING DE-SWEETENS DIABETES

Stress seems to have a negative effect on almost every metabolic pathway and process in the body, and sugar metabolism is no exception. Excess stress can boost a diabetic's blood sugar level as surely as a triple-decker sundae. But relax! Taking a minute to de-stress after meals may help. Researchers from Duke University Medical Center had 20 Type II diabetics try a relaxation technique called "progressive muscle relaxation" after meals, twice a day, for 24 weeks. Result: Their glucose tolerance improved by an average of 20 percent. (Relaxation does not seem to help Type I diabetics, however.)

So after meals, practice the progressive relaxation technique outlined on page 376.

CHAPTER 14

DIGESTION

f you think you've got digestive problems, be glad you're not a sperm whale. A sperm whale's ulcer might be the size of a turkey platter, its hiccup can swamp a cabin cruiser, its burp can launch a weather balloon, and its gastroesophageal reflux tastes (ugh!) like squid. Take pity on the poor whale that swallowed Geppetto and Pinocchio: They lit a fire in its tum-tum, probably causing a Guinness world-record case of heartburn.

Now that you've put your digestive ailments into perspective, you can relax. Some aren't terribly serious and respond readily to simple, quick, and easy remedies. Even the more serious cases can often be treated quickly and effectively.

For example:

- Wiggle your fingers for a few seconds and stop hiccups.
- Mix chocolate into your milk and forget about lactose intolerance.
- The latest gallbladder surgery can have you out of the operating room in 90 minutes and back on the dance floor in two weeks.
- New medication can heal your ulcer in a short time.

You'll save even more time by starting right now.

DEFEATING DYSPEPSIA

The feeling is universal: Yuck! The look is unmistakable: The lips curl up, the eyes register dismay, the forehead furrows, a hand caresses the abdomen.

You know it's only indigestion, but you hate it.

"I do not use the word 'indigestion,'" says gastroenterologist Paul Pickholtz, M.D. He favors "dyspepsia," but by any other name it would be as sour. There's nausea, regurgitation, vomiting, heartburn, bloating, and stomachache. It's painful, difficult, or disturbed digestion, and usually it's harmless, associated with overeating or eating the wrong foods.

Sometimes, though, dyspepsia may be a symptom of a serious illness—gastritis (stomach inflammation), peptic ulcer, stomach cancer, pancreatic disease, gallbladder disease, diseases of the lining of the small intestine, irritable bowel syndrome (the illness causing the majority of cases of chronic dyspepsia), and diabetes mellitus all can cause dyspepsia. When it's chronic, dyspepsia warrants a doctor's attention.

Blessedly, dyspepsia is usually short-lived. Still, there are ways to make its life span even shorter.

Just say no to food. "Your stomach should be able to handle anything," Dr. Pickholtz says. If your dyspepsia is from eating too much at a meal, it will go away quickly if you just stop eating. "Let your stomach rest," he says.

Drink ginger ale. If you want something to drink, ginger ale or herbal teas usually won't make your symptoms any worse. Beverages containing caffeine, however, produce more acid, Dr. Pickholtz says.

Slip your stomach into something more comfortable. When your stomach's irritated it puts out more acid, Dr. Pickholtz says, so you need a buffer between all that acid and your stomach. Antacids containing magnesium work well but can cause diarrhea, so if diarrhea is also a problem, take an antacid that contains aluminum hydroxide, like Gelusil.

Eat lite. A common cause of indigestion is fatty food. You may find that your dyspepsia vanishes when you cut back on meat and greasy foods in your diet. In fact, most of the time dyspepsia can be controlled by diet.

Be ready for "restaurant syndrome." This is a face-reality tip. There are all kinds of enticing dishes at the ethnic restaurants cropping up in our melting pot of a nation. But while your palate is experiencing the wide world of food and loving it, your American meat-and-potatoes stomach does the only thing it knows how to do in the presence of unaccustomed food: Pour on the acid. Be prepared when you eat ethnic: Keep a supply of antacids in the medicine chest.

GETTING A HANDLE ON HEARTBURN

Imagine: If your esophagus is the Mississippi River, the spot where it meets the stomach is the delta, and your stomach is the Gulf of Mexico. Pretend that gastroesophageal reflux is an especially high tide of salt water flooding the bayous, and heartburn is a very annoyed catfish.

Reflux and its symptom, heartburn, are the result of a muscle that either relaxed before it was supposed to or is weak to begin with. It's the lower esophageal sphincter (LES) muscle, and its function is to seal off the stomach and its bubbling, churning contents from the comparatively pristine esophagus.

Unfortunately, this little one-way valve occasionally goes both ways in 80 million Americans, and daily in 25 million. Twenty-five percent of pregnant women experience reflux and heartburn daily. "Open sesame!" Obese people are also prone to reflux and heartburn, says gastroenterologist Sidney Cohen, M.D., chairman of medicine at Temple University Medical School.

Chronic heartburn can be dangerous and needs a doctor's care. (See "When Your Heartburn Is Heavy" on the opposite page.) But when reflux and heartburn are temporary and mild, there are several quick and simple ways to handle it. At the top of the list are preventive measures, by their nature the fastest way to slam the door on reflux and heartburn.

Swallow ten times. Simple swallowing can wash away the reflux that has pushed stomach acid up into your esophagus.

Stomp out that ciggie. Cigarette smoking dramatically weakens the sphincter muscle.

Gobble turkey. High-protein, low-fat foods like skinless turkey or chicken breast, skim milk, fish, and dry beans actually reinforce the valve that guards your esophagus. High-fat foods weaken the LES muscle. Many people find this out right after eating chocolate, which

WHEN YOUR HEARTBURN IS HEAVY

Stomach acid is powerful stuff. If you have heartburn every day, see a doctor. Although it's the subject of humorous commercials, heartburn can be serious. "People think of heartburn in very simple terms, just an annoyance," says gastroenterologist Dr. Sidney Cohen. "But it can lead to inflammation, ulceration, narrowing of the esophagus, and precancerous changes in the lining of the esophagus. So it's more common than peptic ulcer and more difficult to manage. Because it's chronic and not well understood, it hasn't been treated properly, and so the inflammation often progresses."

When reflux and heartburn are chronic and don't respond to simpler measures—like dietary changes, antacids, or stopping medications known to cause heartburn—your doctor will first do "upper GI" (gastrointestinal) tests, including looking at your esophagus through an endoscope and perhaps taking a biopsy.

If there are signs of inflammation, he or she will probably prescribe the peptic ulcer medications Tagamet, Zantac, or Pepcid. All three cut the production of stomach acid, dousing the fires in your red-hot esophagus and letting it heal. "They work so well they're probably used more for esophagitis now than for stomach ulcers," Dr. Cohen says. If your reflux is particularly stubborn, you'll probably start taking Losec, which is an even stronger acid-beater approved just for esophagitis.

The great thing about these drugs is that they work almost instantly—within a half hour or 45 minutes they bank your acid fires. With Losec, the esophagus can heal in 4 weeks; with Tagamet and the other drugs, it may take 8 to 12 weeks. Side effects, if any, are remarkably few and mild.

---

contains a lot of fat. Other foods also relax the muscle, especially tomato products and caffeinated beverages. Heartburn sufferers can usually figure out which foods start the fire.

Eat five meals a day. Or even six. But make them small meals. A large meal is like a Mata Hari to your lonely GI Sphincter. It's very easy for Sentry Sphincter to be taken off guard by the insistent, seductive burble of stomach acid whispering, "Aw c'mon, lemme just loosen your tie a *little* bit."

Remain vigilant. Lying down after a meal is enticing, but it's also a sure way to let the enemy acid sneak past the flimsy sphincter gates and into sensitive territory. After meals it's better to sit upright, or even take an easy walk, until the acid retreats.

Strip off those pounds. When you have excess fat, especially in the abdominal region, something's got to give, and often it's the lower esophageal sphincter. Obese people with heartburn who drop below a certain weight often find their heartburn disappears. (See chapter 36 for tips on losing weight.)

Snap on suspenders. A tight belt can be like a big meal or 20 extra pounds, squishing up that which should go down.

Jack up your bed. Raising the head of your bed 6 inches puts gravity on the side of your sphincter, and so helps keep stomach acid in its place.

Douse the flames with antacids. "Antacids are the mainstay for heartburn," Dr. Cohen says. "Heartburn accounts for most of the sales of antacids like Gelusil, Rolaids, and Tums." They're effective in relieving symptoms of reflux, he says, but not for people who develop severe inflammation of the esophagus. And there are side effects from long-term use of antacids—diarrhea, problems with calcium metabolism, and too-high levels of magnesium in the body. If you have to use an antacid every day, take as directed and see your doctor.

GOING AFTER GALLSTONES

As a pearl is to an oyster, so a gallstone is to your gallbladder. A "seed" of sand becomes the center around which a pearl forms. In a similar way, gallstones grow: A cholesterol or bile pigment "seed" becomes the core of an unwelcome stone in your gallbladder.

There are significant differences, of course, between an oyster and your gallbladder. While an oyster shells out just one pearl at a time, your gallbladder can be a prodigious producer—up to several thousand tiny ones the size of grains of sand, many marble-size, or one or two egg-size boulders. These are the kind of pearls you can cast before swine with no regret, and you can pay a great price in pain and illness before you have them removed.

No one knows why some people form gallstones and others don't, but there seem to be definite sex and genetic factors: Women are three times more likely than men to get gallstones, and they run in families. High cholesterol levels, obesity, too-rapid weight loss, and high insulin levels also appear to play roles. Yet by the age of 60, almost 30 percent of all adults have gallstones. One third to one half of these people don't even know they have them—these stones are called "silent" because they don't produce symptoms, and it's considered best to leave them alone.

But in most cases they do cause pain—often intense—by lodging in the opening of the gallbladder's duct as the organ is squeezing its stored bile into the small intestine to aid in digestion. Nausea and vomiting may accompany the pain, until several hours later the stone drops back into the gallbladder. Sometimes a stone gets stuck in the duct itself. A stone can block the flow of bile from the gallbladder and from the liver, where it's made, or interfere with the flow of pancreatic fluids. The result of these blockages can be inflammation and severe damage of the gallbladder, liver, and/or pancreas—potentially fatal conditions.

So gallstones are nothing to fool around with. Thankfully, medication and surgery may treat them successfully and quickly. But you may even be able to prevent them.

PREVENTING GALLSTONES

If you were prone to gallstones—you're a woman, they run in your family, you're overweight—wouldn't not getting them in the first place be the fastest, easiest way to handle them? There's some evidence—controversial evidence—that diet can reduce your chances of forming them.

Start your diet today. Several studies have shown that obesity is a major risk factor for gallstones. It's a chain reaction: Cholesterol-rich bile is produced by the liver to aid digestion. Overweight people have more cholesterol in their bile because of their eating habits. But when there's too much cholesterol in bile, stones can form in the gallbladder, where bile is stored until it's needed.

It's also possible that insulin could be playing a role: It stimulates the body to make more cholesterol, and the fatter you are the more likely it is you have a higher-than-normal level of insulin.

So losing excess weight and keeping it off is a place to start (see chapter 36).

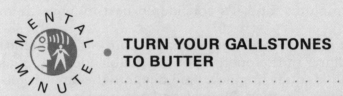

TURN YOUR GALLSTONES TO BUTTER

You can't expect to remove your gallstones by imagination, but you can visualize them dissolving, says Martin Rossman, M.D., clinical associate at the University of California Medical School in San Francisco, codirector of the Academy for Guided Imagery in Mill Valley, California, and author of *Healing Yourself: A Step-by-Step Program for Better Health through Imagery.*

Before trying the mental exercise that follows, first practice progressive relaxation, as outlined on page 376. Once you've relaxed, bring up a healing image in your mind. Gallstones are mostly cholesterol, "so imagine them dissolving like butter in a warm frying pan, into a liquid that can be excreted," Dr. Rossman suggests.

Since you should probably include a low-fat diet in your gallstone therapy, you can also incorporate that into your imagery. "As your body takes in less fat," he says, "it will look around to find discretionary fat that it can absorb because it's used to having more fat in the diet. One form of this discretionary fat—fat your body doesn't need to survive—is the fat and cholesterol in these gallstones. So you can visualize the body changing the chemistry of the gallbladder to melt down the stones, extract the fat it wants to satisfy its craving, and eliminate the rest."

• SCOPING OUT YOUR GALLBLADDER

The problem with treating gallstones is that they tend to recur. The way to prevent recurrence is to remove the gallbladder. The organ helps with digestion, but isn't necessary, since it's just a storage bin for bile. Without the gallbladder, bile flows directly from the liver to the small intestine. After surgery, no special diet or medication is needed, and you'll never have gallstones again.

More than 500,000 American gallbladders are extracted each year, the second most common surgery in the country and by far the most common and effective way to treat gallstones. And laparoscopy "is now the way to go," says Desmond Birkett, M.D., chief of the Section of Gastrointestinal Surgery at Boston University Medical Center.

Laparoscopic cholecystectomy has two stages. In the lithotripsy stage, a small incision is made and an endoscope is inserted. Through this thin tube the surgeon slides a wire probe into the gallbladder. An electrical charge is sent down the wire, creating a shock wave that shatters the stone. The fragments are scooped up in little wire baskets.

In the second stage, the surgeon slips tiny scalpels down the endoscope and snips out the gallbladder. Since the organ has to exit through the narrow tube, "it's easier to remove the gallbladder after the stones are out," Dr. Birkett says.

In the standard gallbladder operation "that's been done for the last 100 years," he says, a large incision was made. Recovery time included three to five days in the hospital, two to four weeks until you could return to work, and six to eight weeks to full activity.

Laparoscopic cholecystectomy takes the same 45 to 90 minutes in the operating room, but there the similarity ends: The incision is tiny; you spend only one or two nights in the hospital, go back to work two days later, and in a week dance the night away.

The procedure is so new that relatively few surgeons in the United States perform it, but Dr. Birkett predicts it will soon become standard operating procedure.

Drop weight gradually. And do it under your doctor's watchful eye. Obese people on rapid-weight-loss diets increase their risk of developing gallstones. When 51 obese men and women went on a diet for eight weeks in one study, their average weight loss was more than 35 pounds. That sounds good, but one-fourth of them developed gallstones, and three of those needed gallbladder surgery.

This is one case where slow could prove to be faster than fast.

PREVENTING AN ATTACK

When you have gallstones, and they're causing problems, a doctor will have to treat them. There are several choices of treatment, including surgery and medication. But although you can't get rid of them yourself, there is one major way you may help prevent an attack.

Eat a fish, an apple, and a slice of whole wheat bread. The aim here is to cut way back on fatty foods, which may play a role in making gallstones act up. Eating fatty foods stimulates the gallbladder to contract, shooting bile into the intestines to help digest the fat. If you have stones, it is thought that the contractions may squeeze them into the bile duct, bringing on an attack. So a low-fat diet can not only help you keep off unneeded pounds of fat; it may help prevent a gallstone attack. A low-fat diet would be one with 25 percent or less of the calories coming from fat (1 gram of fat equals 9 calories).

ATTACKING ULCERS

When people talk about ulcers they're usually talking about peptic ulcers. Peptic ulcers can occur in the esophagus, the stomach, and the duodenum (the upper part of the small intestine—when they occur here they're called duodenal ulcers).

Peptic ulcers are common, eating holes in the gastro-intestinal lining of 1 in every 10 Americans at some time in their lives. Surgeons operate 46,000 times a year on peptic ulcers, and ulcer complications kill 7,000 Americans each year—some bleed to death internally, others suffer a perforation, which allows food to spill into the abdominal cavity, causing abdominal inflammation called peritonitis.

The most common symptoms of a peptic ulcer are indigestion or heartburn. Other symptoms are nausea and vomiting, loss of appetite, or black, tarry stools. That's why it's important to see a doctor if you have these symptoms. Sometimes the main symptom of stomach cancer is a stomach ulcer, another important reason to see your doctor when you have chronic ulcer-type symptoms. Yet sometimes a stomach ulcer doesn't have any symptoms at all.

What causes ulcers? Heredity is a factor: If ulcers run in your family, your own chances of developing one are triple the norm. In people with duodenal ulcers, acid and pepsin can overwhelm the gastrointestinal lining. And that lining itself may be less resistant to the acid and enzyme.

Some stomach ulcers don't need excess stomach acid to form; they can be caused by aspirin and ibuprofen which can damage the stomach lining.

There are some things that don't cause ulcers, though a lot of people think they do. There's been a lot of research into possible dietary causes, for example, but there's no proof food is a factor. Likewise, no one's been able to prove stress causes ulcers.

Nor is there any ironclad evidence that bacteria causes ulcers, says gastroenterologist Chesley Hines, M.D. Although the bacteria are associated with ulcers, nobody knows if they're a cause or effect, Dr. Hines says.

"Ulcers have a tendency to heal on their own anyhow," Dr. Hines says. "They wax and wane—that's the nature of the beast." There's no known way to prevent ulcers other than continuous medication. Surgery is a last resort for stubborn ulcers, but here are some quick and easy ways to tame the beast.

Take your Tagamet or zap it with Zantac. Medications like Tagamet and Zantac are "for sure" quick cures for peptic ulcers, Dr. Hines says. These prescription drugs partially block the production of stomach acid, giving the stomach lining a chance to heal. Pain relief is almost instantaneous, he says, "and cure rates are very high. You can expect total healing of the wound in four to six weeks." Side effects are insignificant. Because ulcers can come back, you may need to take a maintenance dose. And because the drugs are so effective in relieving symptoms, you may think you can stop when the pain is gone. Don't: Give the ulcer time to heal.

DAYDREAM YOUR ULCER AWAY

Surgeon William Beaumont documented the impact of "fight-or-flight" stress on the stomach of one of his patients, a Civil War veteran. The former soldier had a wound that had never healed—a hole directly into his stomach. Dr. Beaumont could literally peek inside and see what was happening: When the soldier got angry, Dr. Beaumont could see an immediate bright-red flushing of the stomach lining. When the man was frightened, the lining would immediately blanch white.

The digestive system probably is the most susceptible to mental imagery of all the body's systems, says Martin Rossman, M.D., clinical associate at the University of California Medical School in San Francisco, codirector of the Academy for Guided Imagery in Mill Valley, California, and author of *Healing Yourself: A Step-by-Step Program for Better Health through Imagery.*

"Typically, our days are full of alarm signals, which increase acid secretion in the stomach, decrease blood flow to the digestive system, and increase its motility (muscle action)," Dr. Rossman says. "These reactions are all part of the fight-or-flight response. Certainly it's one of the most powerful stimulating responses the body has."

When you have an ulcer, you want to control your stomach's acid production. First relax using the method explained on page 376. When you've reached this relaxed state, begin to focus on your ulcer. Imagine what it looks like. "Then we play 'Fix the Picture,'" Dr. Rossman says. "What would this look like if it was all better?" So imagine your stomach lining perfectly pink and without holes.

Next, he says, "imagine a movie of the ulcer progressing to health." You may want to imagine it anatomically: first an ulcerous sore, then more blood flowing to it, bringing immune cells to scour and clean it. Then blood lays down a protective coating over the cleaned wound,

(continued)

DAYDREAM YOUR ULCER AWAY—*Continued*

and new pink healthy cells begin to grow over it. If you have problems figuring out what an ulcer looks like, look at pictures in an anatomy book or, better yet, medical journal ads.

Or if you're more abstractly inclined, Dr. Rossman suggests you might "imagine a fire in your stomach, and the healing process would be bringing cooling water down, through fire hoses or waterfalls or rivers, quenching the fire, then seeing regeneration or healing of the tissue." The more spiritually oriented person "might see a healing figure laying on hands, another might see white light coming in from their higher self or the universe."

"The key is to start with your own picture of what the problem is," he says. "Be receptive to the image your mind produces—an image of what your stomach lining would look like if it were perfectly healthy, and imagine a healing process to follow through from illness to health."

If you have trouble conjuring up your own image, you might want to try "The Mermaid," an all-purpose visualization for digestive problems described by Gerald Epstein, M.D., in his book *Healing Visualizations: Creating Health through Imagery*.

First close your eyes and breathe in and out three times. Imagine a mermaid with golden hair and a silvery blue body and tail. See her traveling through your digestive tract in a smooth, rhythmical manner. Have her touch the ulcer and see it heal completely. Then have her complete her journey to make sure everything else is in order. When she's finished, breathe out and open your eyes.

Do "The Mermaid" three times a day—early morning, twilight, and at bedtime—for up to 3 minutes. Repeat it in three cycles of 21 days on and 7 days off.

Trash the tobacco. Smoking not only doubles your chance of getting an ulcer, it slows healing and increases the likelihood your ulcer will return. Nicotine is a highly addictive drug and kicking it can take time, but the first step is as quick as stubbing out the one you've got going and tossing out the rest (see chapter 20).

Swallow an antacid. Over-the-counter antacids can heal an ulcer, because they can relieve symptoms and neutralize stomach acid. Long-term use has side effects, though, so antacids should be taken under your doctor's supervision.

Test out acid-churning foods. All food makes your stomach produce acid, some more than others. Coffee—with or without caffeine—is a known acid stimulant. So is milk—despite the fact it used to be *prescribed* for ulcers. It's an individual thing: You'll probably find that some foods make your ulcer symptoms flare up, while your friend with ulcers can eat those foods with impunity.

Bottle up the beer, cork the wine. Both stimulate stomach acid production. Interestingly, Dr. Hines says, spirits don't.

Take it easy with painkillers. Aspirin and other so-called nonsteroidal anti-inflammatory drugs like ibuprofen may increase your chances of getting a stomach ulcer. Heavy, long-term use of these drugs makes people with arthritis especially susceptible.

TURNING OFF LACTOSE INTOLERANCE

If you suffer from lactose intolerance, you'd rather not be a citizen of the Land of Milk and Honey. The honey part's okay, but hold the milk, please. It gives you gas, bloating, cramping, diarrhea, nausea, bad breath—things your fellow citizens in this idyllic land can be remarkably intolerant about.

Normally, the human body produces an enzyme, lact*ase,* to digest milk sugar, or lact*ose.* But because their lactase supplies are deficient, up to 30 million Americans are lactose intolerant.

It's not a serious condition, but it can be inconvenient and socially embarrassing. It's easy to treat with diet. Some people are more intolerant of lactose than others, so you can adjust these remedies to suit your own particular condition. The only way to do this is through trial and error—and a little time.

Today drink one glass of milk instead of your usual two. Day by day, drink and eat a decreasing amount of milk products. When your symptoms have disappeared or dropped to a tolerable level, that level of lactose is the amount you can comfortably handle.

Tonight eat dinner with your milk. You may find you can digest lactose more easily when you mix it with meals.

Drink your glass of milk a sip at a time. Your body may be able to handle lactose in timed sips instead of all-at-once chug-a-lugs. Rather than downing a whole glass of milk at once, try drinking small amounts with food throughout the day.

Spoon chocolate into your low-fat milk. Cocoa mysteriously makes milk more digestible for some people.

Have a dish of yogurt. The bacteria in yogurt help digest lactose.

Take a bite of good old cheese. Cheese aged six months or more has lost most of its lactose.

Drop in lactase. The enzyme is available in liquid to add to your milk, or in tablets to take. Some stores offer milk and other dairy products with the lactase already added.

Watch out for hidden lactose. Say you've done everything to cut back on lactose, and still you've got the symptoms. There's one more route to try before you head for the doctor: Read the labels on your vitamins and minerals and medications. Many of them contain lactose as a filler and binder.

VANQUISHING NAUSEA AND VOMITING

Nausea can be a natural predecessor of vomiting. Both may be the natural results of indigestion, overindulgence, pregnancy, overexercise, or illness. Nausea seems to last forever while you're experiencing it, while vomiting is over in seconds. Nausea and vomiting that last more than a couple of days should have a doctor's attention. Those two days can be long ones, though, so here are ways to help yourself make time pass faster and easier.

Let 'er rip. The fastest cure for nausea is vomiting. Depending on the cause of your nausea, vomiting once may take care of it, or you may need a few sessions. But still there's nothing like the relief from nausea one feels after vomiting. However, don't force yourself to vomit.

Spoon down some sugary syrup. No one knows why it works, but 1 or 2 tablespoons of cola syrup can settle a queasy stomach in a matter of minutes. So can an over-the-counter preparation called Emetrol, which doesn't contain the caffeine that irritates some people's stomachs.

Batten down the hatches with Bonine. Bonine is a chewable, over-the-counter antihistamine tablet used for motion sickness, but it also works against normal nausea.

Go with ginger. Capsules of powdered gingerroot are said to relieve nausea for some people. Or if it's a mild case, try flat ginger ale or gingersnap cookies.

Get on a bread-and-water diet. Light and easy does it. Clear, noncarbonated liquids are easiest on your nauseated stomach. Drink only small amounts at a time. Light, complex carbohydrate foods like unbuttered toast or crackers may also go down easily—and stay down. These are the kinds of foods that can also help prevent exercise-related nausea and vomiting.

Steer clear of antacids. They're not for common, non-disease-caused nausea, and they're certainly not clear liquids.

BANISHING THE BELCH

Little boys do it to gross out little girls. It can also be a quick and easy expression of appreciation for a good meal or a good beer. In some cultures, it's rude *not* to burp after dinner. Some people are master burpers, banging off a barrage of sound-barrier-breaking multi-octave belches on demand at parties. Others find themselves having belching accidents in polite society—during the boss's speech, the adagio, or communion.

The town of Wallace, Idaho, knows how to handle these disruptions: It's illegal to burp unless you first get a special permit from a doctor.

It can be embarrassing, it can be irritating to the belcher and belchees, but it's not dangerous. It has a complex medical name—eructation—but the cause is simple—air. A belch is itself a quick fix for excess stomach gas. The cures for too much belching are fast and easy.

Squelch your swallowing. Are you a compulsive swallower? Some people compensate for nervousness by unconsciously swallowing too often—saliva is full of tiny bubbles, and before you know it, your nervous swallows have led to big burps. Raise your swallowing consciousness; once you notice how much you swallow, burp relief is just a nonswallow away. If you have trouble controlling your swallowing, try holding a pencil in your teeth—it's hard to swallow with an open mouth.

Can the carbonation. There's a warranty on bubbly beverages: Belches guaranteed or your money back.

Chew with your mouth closed. And not just because your mother told you to, but because your open mouth acts like a vacuum, drawing in extra air. (Chewing gum, by the way, is a notorious air bubble producer.)

Eat slowly. When you gobble your food, you also gobble air. Slow down, and chew your food well.

Drink from glasses and cups. When you chug from cans and bottles you can see the air bubbles and hear them glug-glug their way down to the burp factory. Sipping from straws is another sure way to swallow your local atmosphere.

Eat middle-class. The richer the food, the more fat and oil it's likely to have—ingredients known to increase gastrointestinal gas.

Demand dentures that fit. Constantly using your tongue and jaws to fiddle around with poorly fitting dentures is a common cause of air swallowing.

HELPING HICCUPS DEPART IN HASTE

The act of hiccuping is a complex, spontaneous choreography involving the diaphragm, abdominal muscles, intercostal muscles (the ones between your ribs), major nerve pathways, and the brain, says hiccupologist (not his real title) Steven Shay, M.D., assistant chief of gastroenterology at Walter Reed Army Medical Center. The result is kind of like the Marx Brothers invading *Swan Lake*. The fastest remedies for hiccups aim at dropping the curtain on the bozos. Dr. Shay has provided his own remedies, but adds that "most people figure out their own ways that seem to work for them," and so we've included a few of them. And if nothing works, don't worry—most hiccups hiccup themselves out of existence in a few minutes.

Take a breath, bear down, and push. Pretend you're going to have a bowel movement. This stimulates the vagus nerve, which connects the diaphragm to the brain. (You may want to hover near a toilet when trying this method.)

Eat slowly. "I notice that hiccups come most often when people eat too fast, and especially when they're eating meat," Dr. Shay says.

Drink something. Do so as shortly after the hiccup as possible, Dr. Shay says. And nothing carbonated.

Rub your eyes really hard. Again, a vagus-nerve stimulator.

Swallow some sugar. Anywhere from a teaspoon to a tablespoon of sugar swallowed dry seems to help some people.

Drink upside down. Bend over and drink water from the opposite side of the glass.

Squeeze 'em. Try pulling your knees up to your chest and compressing it.

Suffocate 'em. That is, hold your breath as long as you can.

Stick your fingers in the back of your throat and wiggle them. This is another way to stimulate the vagus nerve. Dr. Shay has used this method in dangerous situations, as when a surgery patient coming out of anesthesia begins hiccuping, which can cause serious problems if not properly treated. A variation on this is to use a cotton swab instead of your fingers (but be careful not to swallow the swab) or lift the uvula with a spoon (the uvula is that little punching bag at the back of your throat).

Grab your tongue and pull firmly. This also stimulates the vagus nerve.

EAR PROBLEMS

N

o doubt about it. Ears aren't what they used to be. We pierce them. We poke at them. And we pound them daily with dangerously high decibels. We douse them with showers and dunk them relentlessly in oceans and swimming holes. No wonder they rebel! Or worse yet, tune out.

Well, here are some fast ear fixes that will make them perk up and listen. For example:

- In just 1 second, a tug on your earlobe can tell you what kind of ear infection you have.
- In just 1 minute, you can blow-dry potential swimmer's ear right out of your head.
- In just 1 hour, you can have surgery that ends the vertigo of Ménière's disease.

Hearing time is here.

PIERCING PROBLEMS AND OTHER EARACHES

By age six, 90 percent of all children have had at least one ear infection. And adults aren't immune, either. Colds, the flu, and allergies can often end up as a middle ear infection. And earlobes can end up pounding with pain as a result of too cheap or too heavy earrings.

You can walk around for weeks suffering from symptoms—redness, pain, fullness in the head, "hollow" hearing, even dizziness (depending on the type of infection). Left to heal on its own, an ear infection can last from seven to ten days or even longer. But you can knock the infection dead by taking fast action the moment it starts.

Pop a pill a day for seven days. A course of antibiotics is the fastest and surest way to halt an ear infection, says Peter Farrell, M.D., an otolaryngologist from eastern Pennsylvania. "While the antibiotics need to be taken for a week to insure that the infection doesn't return, you should be feeling better and be symptom-free within two or three days," he says.

Of course, it may take a day or two to even get to the doctor. Still, there's no need to go on suffering. Use the time to ease the pain as best you can.

Take a second to pull on your earlobe. You don't always need a doctor to tell whether you have an inner or outer ear infection, says John Harwick, M.D., an Allentown, Pennsylvania, otolaryngologist. You can do it yourself.

"A middle ear infection doesn't cause your ear to hurt when you pull on your earlobe, whereas an outer ear infection hurts more when you move your earlobe," Dr. Harwick says.

The pain accompanying an ear infection, particularly an outer ear infection, can sometimes be intense. How can you ease it quickly before you get to your doctor?

Reach into your medicine cabinet. Take an over-the-counter painkiller such as Tylenol until you get to the doctor, Dr. Harwick says. Take it according to package directions.

Warm the pain slowly. Laying a hot-water bottle or a heating pad against a painful outer ear also helps. "Heat increases the blood supply to the area, which provides pain relief," Dr. Harwick says. But remember: Just because you've eased the pain doesn't mean you're cured, he warns. You still need to see your doctor.

Remove earrings at once. If you have pierced ears, redness and swelling are a sign of infection that should not be ignored. Infection can result from piercing the cartilage. "If you get an infection in the cartilaginous part of your ear, you can end up in the hospital," warns Kathleen Yaremchuk, M.D., an otolaryngologist with the Henry Ford Hospital in Dearborn, Michigan. "The whole shape of your ear can be destroyed." It requires *immediate* medical attention.

Go for the gold. Painful and sore ears can also result from earrings made with inexpensive posts, such as chrome or nickel. They can cause contact dermatitis which can flare into an infection. Wearing earrings made with gold of at least 14 karats will avoid this problem, Dr. Yaremchuk says.

EVERYONE OUT OF THE POOL

It starts with itching. Next comes pain, then a hearing loss because the ear is stopped up with the swelling and debris. It's the classic sign of swimmer's ear, a flare-up in the ear canal caused by water retention, says Arnold Schuring, M.D., an otologist in Warren, Ohio. And you don't have to be a swimmer to get it.

Swimmer's ear can also result from showering or profuse sweating from running or a hard tennis game in intense humidity.

Put your finger to your ear. If you put your finger on the triangular piece of cartilage in front of the ear canal and it *really* hurts, you probably have swimmer's ear, Dr. Harwick says.

Drop in on your ear. For fast relief, drop three or four drops of a mixture of equal parts of white vinegar and water through an eyedropper or syringe. "Some people find that soothing," says Barry Hirsch, M.D., an otologist and neurotologist with the Eye and Ear Hospital of Pittsburgh. Or you can use plain rubbing alcohol.

Put a plug in it. "The first thing to do to prevent a recurrence is to keep water out of the ear, so wearing earplugs makes sense," Dr. Schuring says. If you don't have any or have nothing else available, you can use vaseline-coated cotton balls. Remember to wear these while showering if you are susceptible to water retention in your ears.

"For a dollar or two you can buy ear putty at a drugstore and use it to shape a plug that fits right into your ear." "Because you mold it to your ear, it fits better," Dr. Schuring says.

Plop in prevention. To dry ears after swimming or getting wet, use an over-the-counter antiseptic eardrop such as Ear Magic or Swim Ear. If used in the "itching" stage, it may also prevent infection. To get the drops into your ear, tilt your head so that the treated ear points upward. Pull the top of your ear upward and backward to coax the liquid into the ear canal. Now wiggle your ear, which helps get the drops down farther. Now return your head to upright to let the drops drain out.

Take a minute to blow-dry your ears. To dry your ears after a shower, use your hair blow dryer, suggests Dr. Yaremchuk. Make sure the blow dryer is set on low, and hold it about 18 inches away from the ear. Wave the dryer gently back and forth over the ear for a minute or less.

WHAT AN ITCH

Itchy ears can drive you crazy. It means you have dry skin in your ear, and that can also predispose you to swimmer's ear and other ear infections. The ear canal is easily aggravated by soap residue and too much cleaning. Itchy ears are more common as you get older because the natural oils in the ear canal dry out. Also, hearing aids can cause dryness and itching because of their contact with the sensitive ear skin and canal. Itchiness can even be triggered by allergy.

Spot check your diet. If you can't put a finger on the cause of your itchiness, it might be due to a food allergy, Dr. Harwick says. Wheat products, dairy products, red wine, and chocolate are common allergens. "Eliminate them from your diet and reintroduce them one at a time," he says. If the itching comes back after eating the food, you'll know what causes it and how to control it.

Lube once a week. Putting a drop of baby oil into your ear canal with a dropper once a week will put natural lubrication back into your ear canal.

WAXY BUILDUP?

For some people, earwax is the problem. It can be so vexing that it can lead to such unwise acts as poking a bobby pin, paperclip, or cotton swab in your ear to jar it loose. A bad move, doctors agree.

Don't touch! In most cases, leave earwax alone and it will do its job, Dr. Yaremchuk says. Sticky by design, earwax routinely dries up and falls out of the ear canal with the debris it's collected.

Soften the buildup. If your earwax collects and doesn't budge, put a few drops of mineral oil in your ears *twice* *daily for a few days*. This should soften the mass, which should then fall out on its own.

Use OTC drops with caution. "The problem with some of the over-the-counter eardrops for this purpose is that they are caustic. If you can't irrigate all the liquid out and wax is still trapped in there, you can get a bad case of contact dermatitis," Dr. Yaremchuk says.

If earwax stays lodged in your ear, see a physician.

EARS UNDER PRESSURE

You know the feeling. Your nose is all stuffed up; your head feels light; you feel your ears are going to explode. When you talk, your voice sounds like it's coming from another room. Ear congestion can be another miserable side effect of a cold, sore throat, or allergy.

When everything is working right, the eustachian tube, which connects the middle ear space to the back of your throat, equalizes the pressure on both sides of the eardrum. A cold, allergy, or throat infection causes it to swell. When it's swollen, air can't enter as readily. A similar thing happens when you're on an airplane that's descending: Your eustachian tube doesn't open. A vacuum results, producing pressure.

Chew, yawn, or swallow. All of these actions use the muscles that open the eustachian tube, so pressure can equalize.

Get 12 hours of relief with a 1-second action. You can take a 12-hour over-the-counter decongestant tablet or nasal spray the night before an early morning flight, or an hour before landing. Decongestants work by unplugging the sinuses that back up and block your ears.

Pinch your nostrils shut. While holding your nose, take mouthfuls of air. Use the muscles in your cheeks and throat (and not your chest or abdominal muscles) to force air into the back of your nose, as if you were swallowing with all your might. Do this until your ears "pop."

STOP THE WORLD, I WANT TO GET OFF!

You've just climbed *the* mountain—and that beautiful vista hits you as more dizzying than dazzling. The Big

Thunder Mountain roller coaster ride still has you rolling—and you got off it a half hour ago. The strobe lighting on the dance floor is making you reel—and you're sitting this one out.

Dizziness occurs when the sensory systems that control balance—such as your inner ear—deliver mixed messages to the brain. The brain just can't follow what the sinuses are telling it to do. If it happens on a boat, you call it motion sickness. But the truth is, it can happen almost anywhere your body must deal with a change in motion or decreased oxygen to the brain.

And dizziness has several faces. Maybe the world around you suddenly grays, your muscles go weak, and you just know you're going to pass out. Maybe keeping yourself upright or walking straight suddenly seems impossible. Or maybe you're standing stock still, but it feels like you're spinning, or like the world is atilt all around you. (This last example is what doctors call vertigo, a kind of dizziness that occurs when stimulation to a portion of your nervous system prompts a sensation of motion when there is no motion.)

An important question to ask yourself about dizziness is: Is this a single episode or a recurring problem? A single episode, perhaps accompanied by nausea and vomiting, may be part of or an after-effect of a viral infection. Frequent bouts of dizziness may result from:

- Ménière's disease, indicated by vertigo, with fluctuating hearing loss and ringing in the affected ear
- Benign recurrent vertigo, with symptoms similar to Ménière's disease, but without the hearing changes and ringing
- Benign positional vertigo, in which you experience brief, intense vertigo when you change positions (for example, sit up, lie down, or turn over in bed)
- Panic disorder, when vertigo is accompanied by hyperventilation and an overwhelming sense of panic or dread (see chapter 16).

Each of these conditions requires a doctor's diagnosis and treatment. What can you do to help yourself? Here's what our experts advise.

Duck into a darkened room. When you're having an

attack of dizziness, the best thing you can do is withdraw from unnecessary external stimuli. If you can't find a darkened room, close your eyes and lie down until you feel stable. That can take a few minutes to several hours, depending upon the nature of the problem.

Stare at your thumb. Or stare at some nonmoving object, such as a painting on the wall, or even a spot on the wall—anything that you can focus on and give your spinning world an anchor. Meanwhile, stay still. "This will make some types of dizziness go away," Dr. Harwick says.

Lie down. "The quickest thing to do is to lie down, but recline slowly," Dr. Schuring says.

Get busy. After the worst is over, and if you're not feeling too bad, increase your activity, Dr. Schuring says. Activity actually hastens the departure of dizziness.

Stop it before it starts. Take some over-the-counter anti-motion-sickness drug such as Dramamine. But it will be helpful only if taken *before* the symptoms begin, so it's most useful when you know you're going to be in a situation that typically makes you dizzy.

Check your diet. You may be eating yourself into a case of vertigo, according to ear specialist Joel F. Lehrer, M.D., of Teaneck, New Jersey.

In a study of 100 patients, all with dizziness and some also with hearing loss or ringing in the ears, Dr. Lehrer found certain metabolic abnormalities. Many of these patients were overweight and had high cholesterol and triglyceride levels in their blood. They were also insulin resistant, which means their cells had trouble using insulin, even when there were normal amounts in the blood. Only four, though, seemed to have a problem with low blood sugar, suggesting that it is overrated as a cause for vertigo.

When these patients were put on calorie-cutting, low-fat, low-sugar diets, their dizziness often disappeared. For many, this was the only treatment they needed. Ask your doctor if this might work for you.

Exercise for dizziness relief. Relief from dizziness caused by head injuries or problems with the inner ear can take months. So physical therapists are now speeding the process by weeks with special balance-restoring exercises that retrain the central nervous system. After assessing balance difficulties by asking patients to perform such tasks as climbing steps and sitting on large beach balls, therapists prescribe specific exercises designed to correct what is found.

For more information, check with your physician. He or she can put you in touch with a center or therapist practicing the techniques.

HIGH TECH • OUTPATIENT SURGERY ENDS MÉNIÈRE'S VERTIGO

In only an hour, a surgical procedure ends the vertigo that has caused a lifetime of dizziness for people with Ménière's disease.

Called Selective Chemical Vestibulectomy, the outpatient procedure chemically destroys the balance organ of the inner ear affected with Ménière's, without destroying the hearing of the affected ear, says Ronald Amedee, M.D., assistant professor of otolaryngology at Tulane University Medical Center.

A patient arrives at the hospital in the morning and is typically discharged later that day or early the next morning. The treatment consists of surgically placing a microscopic flake of dried streptomycin into the inner ear. Within the first 24 hours the flake dissolves and destroys the balance organ that has been sending the misinformation to the brain that results in dizziness.

Although considered by Dr. Amedee as "the first line of surgery," he stresses that only 15 to 20 percent of patients with Ménière's disease require surgical counseling. "The vast majority respond favorably to medical treatment, which consists of salt-restrictive diets, diuretics, and vestibular suppressants," Dr. Amedee says.

CLANG, CLANG WENT THE TROLLEY

About one in every five Americans hears sounds they would love to ignore but can't. You've probably experienced it yourself as a "ringing in your ears" or other strange noises in your head. Called tinnitus, this condition causes the sensation of sound, such as ringing, buzzing, or roaring, in the ears that doesn't exist in your surroundings.

"The overwhelming cause of tinnitus is exposure to

loud sound," says Jack Vernon, Ph.D., experimental psychologist with the Oregon Hearing Research Center in Portland.

Use a masking device for immediate relief. A masking device is anything that substitutes a genuine sound for the internal one being heard by a person with tinnitus. A portable cassette player with stereo headset is one example. "The most helpful is an ear-level hearing-aid masking device," says Gloria Reich, Ph.D., executive director of the American Tinnitus Association. It combines both a correction for the hearing loss that generally accompanies tinnitus, and a noise that is used to substitute or "mask" the internal noise. "The tinnitus masker and hearing aid are combined in the same case. It looks like a hearing aid."

Turn on your radio at bedtime. For some people, tinnitus makes sleep difficult. Listening to relaxing music can mask the tinnitus and help you fall asleep. If you have a clock radio, set it to turn off in an hour. By that time you should be asleep.

Just relax. Use relaxation therapy and biofeedback to reduce stress, which often exacerbates tinnitus, and to get you in better touch with your body, Dr. Reich suggests.

Seek pleasing surroundings. Be alert to environmental conditions that lessen the noise, Dr. Vernon says. He tells of one woman who entered a floral shop and felt her tinnitus stop. Looking around she noticed a recirculating water fountain. She put one in her bedroom and has slept well since.

Spend time with a professional. Although there may be some fast ways to mask tinnitus, there are no quick cures.

"People must realize nobody's going to pass a magic wand over your head and say, 'Presto! You're cured.' A lot of learning to cope with tinnitus is taking responsibility and doing something for yourself," Dr. Reich says.

Seek professional assistance in alleviating psychological results of tinnitus, such as depression or anxiety. Keep a positive attitude and assume control. "If people have the attitude that tinnitus is wrecking their lives, then it will. But if they think, 'This is something I can manage,' then they will," says Bill Reid, Ph.D., of

Beaverton, Oregon, a tinnitus counselor who happens to have tinnitus himself.

Tinnitus doesn't have one cause; many factors aggravate it, Dr. Reich says. Allergies to food and other things can make tinnitus worse in some people. They need to find someone who not only can diagnose this situation but also treat it. Temporomandibular disorder (TMD) can also aggravate tinnitus. Tinnitus is sometimes relieved when the TMD is corrected (see page 299).

"The bottom line is you need to be in the hands of someone knowledgeable and creative about solutions. If the first things you try don't work, keep seeking solutions," Dr. Reich says. For more information, you can write the American Tinnitus Association, P.O. Box 5, Portland, OR 97207.

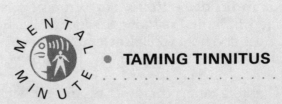

MENTAL MINUTE • TAMING TINNITUS

Fourteen years ago, Bill Reid developed tinnitus. He hears sounds that don't exist. "It's very disconcerting," Dr. Reid says. "Bells are ringing in your ears; whistles are going off. Plus, it makes you more sensitive to other noises."

For years none of the people he sought had a remedy that helped, so he began developing a technique of his own. Today, Dr. Reid, who is a tinnitus counselor, finds relief by taking himself back in time—a process he calls "an awareness bypass." The method, which Dr. Reid teaches to his clients in Beaverton, Oregon, is best done with the help of a professional counselor, but you can enlist a friend. Make an audio cassette of the session so you can practice over and over.

Dr. Reid starts by using a deep relaxation technique, such as the one that appears on page 376. It's important to get in a state of deep relaxation because of its effect on your mind. "When the brain wave activity is at the alpha state, a person is more in tune with his subconscious mind," Dr. Reid says.

(continued)

TAMING TINNITUS — *Continued*

When you've reached this deep state, you should be instructed to "go back in time, back to a time before you had tinnitus or a time when you weren't aware of it. What are you doing? Where are you? What natural sounds are you hearing?"

The idea is to get to a state where you can *feel* the natural sounds you are hearing, Dr. Reid explains. For example, *hear* the birds singing in the morning. *Feel* silence when you awake. Feel it! Breathe in. Let the feeling in. Hold onto it. This is the time you can mentally escape to where there is no tinnitus—where you will not be aware of tinnitus. Choose a word to remind yourself of this time when you didn't have tinnitus. Use the word to bring back this memory. "At some point each day, you'll experience a time, maybe a minute, maybe 2 or 3 minutes, maybe more, when you're not aware of the tinnitus," Dr. Reid says.

For positive results, Dr. Reid suggests you listen to your tape three times a day, but stresses that a positive, responsible attitude comes first. "Every person I've ever treated who was motivated got to the point where they could satisfactorily manage tinnitus."

BE SOUND SMART AND NOISE LEERY

Hearing's a lot like love: By the time you know it's slipping away, it's too late to get it back.

Hearing doesn't normally just suddenly disappear (although there are exceptions). More than 24 million Americans have some degree of hearing impairment. Another 20 million are exposed daily to noise levels capable of permanently damaging their hearing. And it's no longer just a problem for the elderly.

Audiologists report that today's American teenagers are experiencing premature hearing loss. Cited causes: loud rock concerts and prolonged listening to radios or cassettes through stereo headphones.

Noise becomes hazardous to your hearing when you're exposed to more than 85 decibels—the equivalent of routine traffic—for 8 or more hours per day, says John Steelnack, industrial hygienist with the Occupational Safety and

Health Administration (OSHA). That's not much more than the human voice, which measures 60 decibels. But, hearing at 115 decibels—the sound of a screaming infant, for instance—*for just 15 minutes* also puts you in the danger zone. Put two sources of noise together and their combined decibel level is augmented.

A refrigerator, for example, hums along at 50 decibels. A TV at normal volume, 65 decibels. A blender, 65 to 85 decibels. A vacuum cleaner, 70 to 80 decibels. An alarm clock ringing just 2 feet away is 80 decibels (no wonder you jump when it rings!). A hair dryer on high setting, 90 decibels. Combine just any two for a sustained time— watching TV and talking, for example—year in and year out and you're subjecting your ears to a lot of abuse! But there are quick and easy things you can do to be kind to your ears.

Cushion your appliances. Cushion blenders, food processors, mixers, and loud typewriters with a foam pad or even a towel, which helps absorb some sound. Also, when shopping for new appliances, buy the quietest model available. Ask the salesperson about the noise level. Manufacturers must state decibel level. Let the store know you're a noise-conscious shopper.

Buy the big picture. If you're shopping for a house, investigate the noise levels of the house at different times of the day. Certain noise-producing sources such as a nearby freeway can be obvious, but the range in noise may not be. If you view the house at 2:00 P.M. Sunday afternoon, you won't hear the 5:00 P.M. weekday traffic. Likewise, if the house is near an airport, it's possible you'll visit it between overhead flights. One hour's silence can be another hour's boom.

Wear ear protectors. By law, industries require employees who work around machinery and power tools to wear ear protectors. But how often do you see a home hobbiest doing the same? Woodworkers, for instance, use home shop tools that produce substantial noise, ranging from 65 to 115 decibels. "If you're using high pitched, whining power drills or saws, you should wear ear plugs," says Dr. Harwick. "If you use them once or twice without wearing ear protection, nothing permanent's going to happen. But if you keep doing that, eventually your hearing won't recover. It's prolonged repeated exposure to noise that causes permanent hearing loss."

Start a tranquillity garden. Do you find gardening relaxing? How about deafening? Power lawn mowers, electric pruning devices, weed whackers, and other motorized lawn care implements tear into vegetation with an ear-shattering vengeance.

"Homeowners should have an inexpensive pair of earplugs to use when sitting on their power lawn mower or using a power pruning device, " says Laurence Fechter, Ph.D., associate professor of toxicology with the Department of Environmental Health Sciences at Johns Hopkins University in Baltimore.

Make your office a pad. Obvious jobs such as factory work have federal hearing protection laws. So does office work, but the laws are often ignored. Yet a computer printer, for instance, might expose you to 85 decibels. You can protect your hearing at the office. Put an acoustic cover over printers or buy quieter models. Insist on drapes and carpeting to cushion the noise, and insulation around windows if your office overlooks a noisy freeway. And acoustically isolate soda and ice machines.

Beware the double whammy. Recent research has shown that exposure to loud noise in conjunction with certain chemicals increases hearing-loss risk over either factor alone. "People working in settings where they're simultaneously exposed to loud noise and to carbon monoxide or certain other chemicals that can interfere with oxygen delivery to the ear are the most vulnerable population," Dr. Fechter says.

Dance to a different drum. Pack your ear protectors along with your tights for aerobics class. Instructors have a tendency to over-amp the music, which can throw you a double whammy. The loud music alone is harmful enough. But, according to a Swedish study, the high decibels are even more harmful when you're exercising, because the oxygen in your blood normally available to sensory organs like the ears is now being diverted to the arm, leg, and heart muscles, says Rebecca Meredith, clinical audiologist.

Spread the word to your kids. A recent study discovered that high school musicians are at greatest risk among teenagers to suffer early hearing loss. "A considerable number of our young people are leaving high school at age 18 with a serious condition of hearing loss that could affect their ability to get employment," says Judy Montgomery, Ph.D., speech pathologist and director of special education for the Fountain Valley School District, who led the study.

The study showed that of the 1,500 California students tested, 6 percent of second graders, 8 percent of eighth graders, and 13 percent of high school seniors had some degree of hearing loss. Among those routinely exposed to noisier environments, such as band practice rooms, 26 percent had high-frequency hearing loss by age 18.

Does this mean we should discourage young musicians or ban rock 'n roll? No, no more than we should close noisy factories. The defense is the same—ear protectors. In fact, they're becoming quite the fashion.

Sport a pair of "ear shades." Many nationally known musicians have experienced hearing loss, and they're taking ear protection seriously. A California firm has responded by manufacturing Earshades, hip, trendy, fashion statements that protect the ear while sporting beads, feathers, and Day-Glo colors.

Take five. When attending concerts or sporting events, take a break for 5 minutes every hour. "Going out of the noisy environment to a quieter one lets your ears recuperate," Dr. Montgomery says.

Get up and go home. Leave any environment that's so loud it causes your ears to ring. Because noise-induced hearing loss originates in the higher frequencies, it's not detectable until it's too late, explains Dr. Montgomery. "Once the nerve cells are destroyed, they're gone."

HIGH TECH • **IMPLANTING AN ELECTRONIC INNER EAR**

Your inner ear is called the cochlea. Shaped like a snail shell and the size of a pea, it contains tiny hairs, waving back and forth in a sound-wave-conducting fluid. Each hair is connected to auditory nerve cells and transmits the electrical equivalent of a sound wave to the cells. But sometimes congenital defects, repeated infections, or serious accidents damage the cochlea, and the hairs can no longer relay the sound message. Hearing aids can often fill the gap, but for the profoundly deaf there was no remedy until the cochlear implant.

The implant is a marvel of microsurgery. After 2 to 3 hours of surgery and a four- to six-week wait for the implant to take hold, the profoundly deaf can experience permanent improvement in their hearing.

The device is made up of several parts that, when working together, are able to transmit sounds to the auditory nerve. A microphone rests behind the ear to pick up sound and send it to the speech processor, a cassette-size device you can wear on a strap or carry in your pocket. The processor codes the sound signal and sends it to the transmitter, which fits inside your outer ear like an earplug. The transmitter in turn relays the sound to a decoder implanted in the bone behind your ear. The decoder then sends electronic sound messages to the cochlear implant, which is a string of electrodes that coil inside your cochlea. These electrodes do the work that the tiny hairs can no longer do—send the electronic impulse to the auditory nerve cells and through them to the brain, which registers the sound.

With a successful implant, people regain some sensation of sound and are able to hear and monitor their own voice levels. "Most people

see some level of improvement, particularly in their ability to read lips," says Ralph Naunton, M.D., of the National Institute on Deafness and Other Communication Disorders, "And some are able to carry on a conversation with their eyes shut." They do not hear sounds in the same way as a hearing person—their hearing is now electronic, and they must learn to identify sounds in a new way.

There is continued improvement over time as people learn to listen to sounds. Some people learn to recognize environmental sounds such as doorbells, telephones, car horns, or fire alarms. And "the improvement is permanent, based on our 10 years of experience," Dr. Naunton says.

Use of the cochlear implant has been limited to the profoundly deaf who derive no benefit from conventional hearing aids, but who retain auditory nerve function.

In addition, according to Dr. Naunton, "There's growing evidence that direct electrical stimulation of the cochlea by the electrodes may protect nerve connections from further degeneration." In other words, the cochlear implant may not only help you hear better, but may prevent further hearing loss as well.

Because of the complexity of the cochlear implant, current costs total from $15,000 to $20,000, including postsurgery computerized programming.

● **HEARING BONES MADE OF GLASS**

A common cause of deafness is damage to the tiny sound-conducting bones of the middle ear—the malleus, incus, and stapes. The damage can come from recurrent ear infections, congenital defects, trauma (such as a car accident), or tumors.

For the last five years doctors have been fashioning glass replacements for the damaged bones. The implant can be shaped into a perfect fit for each individual. "This is essential to the level of hearing that can be attained," says Gerald Merwin, M.D., clinical professor of surgery/otolaryngology at the University of Florida in Gainesville.

The implant contains calcium and phosphorus in the same proportions as in bone, so it's compatible with the surrounding tissues.

This outpatient surgery takes about 1½ hours under general or local anesthesia and two to three weeks to heal before hearing is restored to normal or near-normal functioning. There is an 85 percent success rate for glass implants, although some persons may not tolerate it and at other times the operation must be repeated. The total cost is around $4,000.

"People are routinely exposed to noise and they ignore it," Dr. Yaremchuk says. "I saw children playing soccer by a railroad track. A train went by and every child covered his ears because the noise hurt. Every adult kept talking as if they didn't hear it. We train ourselves not to pay attention to noise. Although we ignore it, it's still doing its damage."

BOOSTING YOUR HEARING POWER

After 50 years of marriage, a couple decided to renew their marriage vows. At the altar the husband said, "I have loved you tried and true." To which the wife replied, "I'm tired of you, too!"

We can laugh at this joke because it is not at our expense. But hearing loss isn't funny. Sadder still, your hearing can fade away without your realizing it. That's a shame, because the sooner you detect hearing loss, the sooner you can do something about it. You don't have to resign yourself to living in a world without sound. Here are several fast, simple, and effective ways to help you compensate for the hearing abilities you may have lost:

Take the 10-second telephone test. Pick up the telephone receiver and listen carefully to the dial tone. Now switch ears. Does the dial tone sound louder? Softer?

Some cities offer telephone hearing screening tests using a series of tones. These tell how many you hear in each ear. Others are sponsored by a hospital or university. Such tests can sound the warning that your hearing is in jeopardy—remember, hearing loss can proceed so subtly that you may not notice the day-by-day deterioration.

The diagnosis of hearing loss, however, should be left to a physician.

Turn up the volume with a hearing aid. Hearing aids used to be synonymous with senility, but not anymore. Former President Ronald Reagan wears one and lent his name to an ad campaign fostering their use. Modern design has made them more unobtrusive and more reliable, says Samuel Varghese, M.D., otolaryngologist and director and founder of the Ear Institute of Cincinnati. For example, a miniature hearing aid, which can be laid close to the eardrum, is computerized so you can program it to adjust to different environments. "It virtually lasts forever because it can be pulled out from the ear canal and a fresh battery installed," Varghese says.

Buy a hearing ear dog. Hearing ear dogs help hearing impaired people. Dogs can be trained to distinguish between noises and can alert the owner to such sounds as a ringing telephone, a knock on the door, a baby crying. Dogs follow both voice and hand signals.

Electrify your hearing. Modern technology has come up with a wide range of electronic devices designed to alert people with hearing problems and help them communicate better. Besides the familiar closed-captioned TV shows and video cassettes with captions, a few of the more common ones are:

- Alerting devices: These help you know the phone's ringing, the baby's crying, there's someone at the door, it's time to get up. They may use a *flashing red light* with codes to tell you if it's the phone, the door, or the baby; a *loud sound;* or a *vibrator* that literally shakes you awake.

- Telephone aids: Some are handsets that *boost the sound;* other sound-amplifiers are portable. *Adapters* work with hearing aids that have T-switches by allowing them to pick up the magnetic field of the phone's sound signal. A *telecommunication device for deaf people (TDD)* has typewriter keyboards at each end; the talkers type instead of talk, and what they're saying is printed out. TDD systems can operate through *message relay service* for hearing people who don't have a TDD; many TDDs are portable.

- Systems for groups and large rooms: These literally bring the hearing impaired listener closer to the speaker. For these the hearing aid must have a T-switch. An *audio loop system* has a wire looping around the audience; the listener's hearing aid picks up the sound signal from the wire's magnetic field. *AM and FM* radio technology has been adapted to let listeners use personal headsets or portable radios (AM or FM); or tune in with their own hearing aids (FM). An *infrared system* emits light rays that transmit the sound to portable infrared-receiving headsets.

A visit to your community agency for the hearing impaired will be well worth your time. Other resources are audiology centers, universities, and manufacturers.

EMOTIONAL PROBLEMS

. . . .

f you're stressed out, depressed, angry, or phobic, you can spend 20 to 30 years lying on the psychoanalyst's couch remembering Mama and deciphering ink blots. Or you can turn things around in just a fraction of that time.

"There are alternatives to long-term therapy. A brief, focused approach can sometimes produce prompt relief," says Josef Weissberg, M.D., director of the Association for Short-Term Psychotherapy and president of the American Academy of Psychoanalysis. Many patients receiving short-term therapy see meaningful, lasting changes in a matter of weeks or months.

But small victories can begin happening even sooner.

- In just 5 minutes, you can control a panic attack.
- In just 30 minutes, you can give your self-esteem an effective boost.
- In just seven days, you can banish winter depression.

How?

By using self-help tips taken from short-term psychotherapy and using them as a frontal assault on emotional problems, you learn to take destructive habits, thoughts, or behaviors and replace them with new, constructive ones.

"In short-term psychotherapy you focus on a *specific* conflict, with an understanding between patient and doctor that treatment will be short," Dr. Weissberg says. "You attack that conflict which is underlying your present problem, rather than just talking about what's on your mind. You aren't interested in anything else," he says.

Using this approach, you can tackle those common emotional glitches that can keep your life from being as wonderful and carefree as you'd like it to be.

SNUFF ANGER BEFORE IT FLARES

You can learn to control outbursts of anger in a single day. Consider this universal anger-generator. It's rush hour and traffic stretches out to the horizon. You're tired. You're hungry. And now you're *furious*. Some line-jumping jerk has driven down the shoulder of the road to barrel past the waiting, overheating cars in order to squeeze in front of you!

You can let that anger stew until your blood pressure explodes through the roof, or you can defuse it instantly. Here's how.

Get physical. Go ahead and yell. It'll make you feel a lot better right away. Or punch the seat next to you. Expressing yourself physically may provide short-term relief for anger, says Roger Daldrup, Ph.D., a psychologist and professor of counseling at the University of Arizona who coauthored *Freedom from Anger*. Solving the underlying conflict that may be generating your anger could take longer, however.

Count and breathe. Take a deep breath and start counting. If 10 counts don't help, try taking two breaths and counting to 20. Feel the tension in your chest flow out as you exhale.

These are quick fixes for temporary frustration. But suppose it isn't some dope playing "rush-hour chicken" who has you steamed. Suppose it's your spouse or your boss that you want to call a total moron. Then what do you do? This anger is dangerous, and a blowup could have serious repercussions. Should you keep a lid on your anger while you wait for it to go away? The answer is no.

Express that anger immediately. "The myth is that we can forget anger, that it will go away," Dr. Daldrup says. "The hard evidence is that anger lasts and lasts. In fact, most people are walking around with a load of anger they've built up over the last 20, 30, or 40 years. This accumulation of anger is a heavy component in many diseases, including addictions. We pay for it one way or another," he says.

"Discharge your anger as it comes up. By doing that,

you won't be accumulating resentment and anger that someday will explode in a rage. Instead, there won't be any extra energy attached to it. When you feel angry

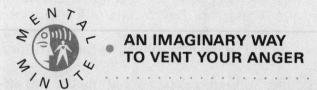

AN IMAGINARY WAY TO VENT YOUR ANGER

Most people walk around with 20 years' worth of anger churning in their guts. Here's one way to dump that load, says Dr. Roger J. Daldrup of the University of Arizona.

He suggests that his patients bash and swear at a "significant other" in their life who's causing the stress. These people can be parents, lovers, ex-spouses, current spouses, children, brothers, and sisters.

But not to their faces.

Here's how. First choose the person you'd like to have it out with.

Roll a piece of newspaper into a bat and take it with you into a quiet room. Place two chairs across from each other. Sit in one.

Now, imagine your opponent sitting in the chair across from you. Say out loud to that person, "I asked you here because I wanted to tell you how I feel."

Now, tell them exactly how angry you are, using the sentence form, "I resent you for . . ." or "I feel hurt that . . ." or "I feel angry when . . ."

Using the "you make me . . ." form expresses hurt, but it also keeps you in a pattern of blaming another person and withdrawing emotionally.

Saying "I feel . . ." or "I resent . . ." expresses your anger while giving you power by relating your feelings about an experience.

As you express your feelings, hit the chair where that imaginary person is sitting. Beat him until your system says you are finished—then do it for 15 minutes more.

When you are finished, tell your imagined person what you have accomplished—that you have vented your anger—and thank him for his cooperation.

you'll be able to say, 'I disagree with you' or 'I don't like what you are saying,' in a straightforward manner."

Express it appropriately. Even though it may feel good to snap at the object of your fury, don't. But don't play dead either. Speak up. Say, "Let's talk about our difference of opinion," or "Something is really bothering me." Your goal should be to bring down the heat so no one gets burned.

Don't accuse. You can explain what makes you angry without attacking the other person, Dr. Daldrup says. By using "I" language when expressing anger or hurt or disappointment you can tell the other person how you feel without directing any accusations. Say, "I feel angry when . . ." not "You make me angry. . . ." Using this approach makes you more powerful, Dr. Daldrup says.

If you can't say it, write it. If you are so upset that you might not be able to speak coherently, write a letter to the person who has angered you. You may decide not to mail the letter, but you will have emptied your anger.

ARRESTING YOUR ANXIETY

Another emotion, one usually generated by inner rather than outer demons, is anxiety. It comes in many forms, each one powerful. If just thinking about making a speech can make your palms sweat, your stomach knot, and your tongue tie, you may be experiencing performance anxiety. Others include social anxiety (shyness), information anxiety (the fear of looking dumb), and panic, which has some of anxiety's most intense symptoms. And then there are phobias, fears so strong that people will do anything to avoid the object that causes them. Bridges, elevators, open windows, dogs, simply leaving the house—all are fairly common causes of phobias. If you're afflicted with any of these anxieties, here's some fast relief.

Drugs work. Anxiety can be treated with drugs such as beta-blockers or benzodiazepines. You'll see the maximum improvement possible after about six weeks of taking them, with little additional improvement after that time span. But after withdrawal of benzodiazepines, symptoms may recur. In one study, 69 to 80 percent of people had a relapse of their anxiety within one year.

Treatment works better. Experts advise short-term, focused treatment to reduce anxiety, including meditation and relaxation, biofeedback, and exercise.

"Life is difficult enough without having to put up with fears," says Barbara Fleming, Ph.D., a clinical psychologist and director of the Phobia Clinic at University Hospitals of Cleveland. "Short-term focused treatment can be very helpful."

People who go to the clinic find that improvement can take from 12 to 20 sessions. And knowing that it won't take years and years of therapy to overcome anxiety, Dr. Fleming says, can be reassuring.

Reserve a specific time to think about your fear. Chronic worriers who spend an hour thinking about their problem will spend less time overall worrying, says psychologist Daniel Wegner, Ph.D., professor of psychology at the University of Virginia, Charlottesville.

Control your breathing. When you are relaxed, your breathing is slow and even. When you are anxious or upset, however, you tend to breathe irregularly. So as soon as you feel yourself getting uptight, say to yourself, "Stop." Then breathe, gently and not too deeply. Let your shoulders drop. Relax your hands. Repeat this technique once or twice more.

Take a brisk walk. Exercise, say the experts, will burn off the excess adrenaline that fuels your feelings of anxiety. Studies show a regular exercise program will help you bounce back faster in anxious situations. Exercise releases endorphins, a potent group of natural chemicals in the body that may block anxiety and depression.

Imagine yourself coping. Close your eyes and visualize yourself in the uncomfortable situation. In your mind, be as assertive or self-confident as you would like to be. Picturing yourself in control will help you become more assured when you face the real moment.

In a crisis, think challenge. Approach stressful, anxious situations thinking of opportunity, not obstacle. That positive outlook will give you a boost of energy.

Listen to the wind chime. There's nothing quite like the sound of wind on chimes when stress gets to a high pitch. The random melodic patterns can relax you, but choose chimes that are specially tuned so that each note harmonizes with the others, says Steven Halpern, Ph.D., a composer and the author of *Sound Health*. The best chimes are those made of copper or aluminum, 12 to 18 inches in length.

Toss out the caffeine. This stimulant has a definite effect on the central nervous system. It sharpens our thinking, dispels fatigue, heightens the senses, and gives us a lift. But it can be a mental-health nightmare. Caffeine overload can cause shaky hands, trembling muscles, jittery feelings, nervousness, restlessness, and headache —all of which can be diagnosed as an anxiety reaction.

GETTING UP FROM FEELING DOWN: DEPRESSION

Country and western songs will tell you, even cowgirls get the blues. And it's true. Almost no one is immune to the missing someone blues or the I-hate-my-job blues. This kind of depression is a universal emotion.

These down feelings are actually the lighter side of depression. Serious depression is a condition that alters your mental senses. Symptoms can include fatigue, insomnia or the opposite—excessive sleep, indecision, loss of sexual desire, changes in eating patterns, anxiety, phobias, guilt, hopelessness, helplessness, irritability, social withdrawal, and physical problems such as chest pains, nausea, coldness, sweating, and numbness of the hands or feet. While not as common as the blues, it's still fairly common. Between 20 and 50 percent of all adults experience depression sometime in their lives.

Traditional, insight-oriented psychotherapy, which takes years of work, hasn't been considered an efficient method of treatment, while antidepressant medications and short-term cognitive-behavior therapy have brought quicker results. Antidepressants offer relief to about 70 percent of depressed people who use them. But it may take trial and error to find the right medication and then maintenance therapy of from 6 to 18 months on drugs.

Cognitive-behavior therapy is the key to getting fast relief. It attacks the symptoms of depression quickly, at the first hint of a downward spiral. Though not every cognitive behavior technique will work for everyone, here are some strategies to try.

Unplug your negative thoughts and plug into something positive. One of the keys to overcoming depression is learning how to control your low moods and reverse them. Learn to switch off negative thinking just as you would a light switch. "I will never find anyone to marry me," is a very negative statement. A more positive and realistic thought is: "The way I feel and act now makes me unattractive, but I can change my behavior."

Put on your rose-colored glasses. People who see the world in the pink may be healthier, happier, and more successful than someone who is more realistic. Studies show people who are unfailingly positive in their views work harder and longer and are often rewarded for their perseverance. Realistic people are more likely to get depressed.

Treat yourself. Get a massage. Listen to music. Walk in the park. Call a friend. Establish a pattern of positive behavior for yourself. Try to do one extra pleasant thing for yourself every day.

Find a hobby. Learning to do something just for the sheer pleasure of doing it will provide enormous satisfaction. Take up astrophysics or the guitar—whatever pleases you. In the meantime, learning the hobby will take your mind off your problems.

Put on a happy face. Studies show that you can summon up new emotions by the expression on your face. So, when your heart is aching, smile and you may find your heart smiling with you.

Run, jog, or walk your way to happiness. Many depressed people stop exercising—and they feel guilty about it, adding to the already heavy emotional load. Exercise or aerobics classes or a personal daily walking program will improve your overall health as well as your mood.

Chuck that chocolate. Large amounts of sugar in your diet can cause your emotions to take a dive. Too much sugar causes an increased release of insulin, resulting in low blood sugar, which may lead to depression, nervousness, and weakness. Instead of eating candy, increase the amount of complex carbohydrates (like beans, whole grains, and vegetables) and protein (like poultry, fish, and dairy products) in your diet.

Eat breakfast. Studies show a deficiency of thiamine, vitamin B_6, and folate can make you irritable and depressed. So eat your whole-grain cereal (for thiamine) with a sliced banana on top (pyridoxine) and drink a big glass of orange juice (folate).

Ask your doctor about your medication. Sometimes it's a drug you are taking, not an illness, that's getting you down. Digitalis, for instance, was associated with depression in 11 of 18 heart patients studied at Mt. Sinai School of Medicine in New York. Other drugs that can cause depression include: steroids, centrally active antihypertensives, narcotics, anticonvulsants, prostaglandin inhibitors, hormonal agents, histamine blockers, and some sedatives. If you've noticed a change in your mood since beginning a new medication, talk to your doctor.

Give yourself a mental health day occasionally. If you wake up with the Monday morning blues and feel like staying in bed, go ahead and pull the covers over your head. Sometimes getting away from everything can be healthy. And while you're playing hooky, take in a happy movie, buy new clothing, straighten a messy drawer. Do something that makes you feel good and the feeling may carry you through to greet the next day with a smile.

Cry. Tears may be just what you need. Reserve a period for down time, when you can focus on your problem. Use your tears as the punctuation for your sadness. Impose a time limit on your crying, though, so you remain in control of your feelings. Then, get back to working on your positive self.

BECOMING YOUR OWN BEST SELF-BOOSTER

One by-product of depression is a "toxic" emotion called low self-esteem, says Harriet B. Braiker, Ph.D., a clinical psychologist in Los Angeles. The sort of self-talk she writes about are commonly voiced statements such as:

"I'm too old."

"I weigh too much."

"I'm intimidated by her."

"I'm not good enough to even apply for that job."

Yet everyone with blue moods shares these feelings

from time to time, she says in her book, *Getting Up When You're Feeling Down*. You can short-circuit this by-product of depression quickly by changing your thinking.

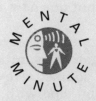

● TAKE STOCK OF YOUR CHOICES

When you feel stressed by one of life's unavoidable knocks, handle it with this very revealing Acceptance and Choice worksheet developed by Harriet B. Braiker, Ph.D. On one side of a sheet of paper state the unavoidable fact that's getting you down. Then, across from it, generate a list of your options—include as many choices as you can, even the pessimistic and the ridiculous.

Here's an example:
I accept that I can't change the fact that . . .

1. I will be 65 on my next birthday.

But I can choose to . . .

1. Be thankful I'm alive.
2. Remember the good times and plan new adventures such as a birthday party or a trip.
3. Forget my age. I feel like I'm still 39, and that was a great year.
4. Exercise to stay in good health and great shape.
5. Get involved with other people and stop thinking about myself.
6. Stay home and stay depressed.

When your worksheet is written, tape it to the bathroom mirror and circle the choices you like the best. When you start looking for the wrinkles and the gray hair, you can read over your choices.

The woman who generated the list above, a patient of Dr. Braiker's, also finds it helpful to repeat this sentence: "I can't change the fact that I'm getting older in years, but I can choose to keep a young attitude and make every precious year that I have to live count."

Dream up an imaginary best friend. Let them talk to you. Imaginary friends aren't just for kids, says psychologist Mary Gergen, Ph.D., an assistant professor at Pennsylvania State University. That imaginary friend can boost your self-esteem and provide emotional support. When Dr. Gergen polled her students, all but one admitted to using imaginary "social ghosts."

Plug yourself into an inspirational tape. For years, perhaps, you've been plugging into a negative, painful, and self-destructive mental description of yourself. Now you're going to replace that negative mental tape with a new one—a real tape, and a positive one. Record 30 minutes' worth of quotations from inspirational books or Bible passages that have meaning for you. Keep the tapes next to your bed and make those good words the first thing you hear in the morning and the last thing you hear at night. Saturate your mind with these positive thoughts.

Make a list. Right next to your "to do" list, make a list of your daily accomplishments. Compiling your achievements will give you a list that's bound to boost your self-esteem. The result? You'll become less critical of yourself.

LIGHTENING UP SEASONAL AFFECTIVE DISORDER

Sometimes, our moods and emotions are quite predictable. For some people, the season of the year best predicts their emotions. In the summer, they're sunny, outgoing, warm. In wintertime, though, watch out. As the days get darker, so do their personalities. They feel—and react—a lot like bears. They want to eat a lot, then hibernate until springtime. Their mood is melancholy from late September or early October until late March or early April.

Experts call this phenomenon seasonal affective disorder or SAD. SAD is another form of depression which affects about 20 percent of the U.S. population. The major difference between depression caused by the coldest season of the year and classical depression is this: People with SAD feel good in the summer and awful in the winter. Also, most SAD sufferers eat everything in sight and want to sleep all the time.

Shedding some light on the problem is the fastest

and easiest cure for winter depression. You can wait the problem out—and spend six months of misery. You can pop an antidepressant drug and wait three weeks for relief from depression. But it takes only a week of phototherapy—light therapy—to cure most winter-depressed people, says Karen Stewart, Ph.D., a psychologist at Thomas Jefferson University's Jefferson Medical College in Philadelphia, who treats people with SAD and researches winter depression.

Bask in manmade sunlight. An hour or two a day can alter a person's light-sensitive body rhythms so that they no longer feel perpetually tired. These special lights register a minimum of 2,500 lux (a lux is a unit of light intensity) compared with 100,000 lux from summer sunshine and 300 to 500 lux from ordinary lamps in the living room. Phototherapy clinics often loan special lamps to patients, so they don't have to visit the therapist for each treatment. Note: Do not use tanning lights to simulate summer sunlight. In addition to the risk of sunburn and skin cancer, tanning lights can cause eye burns.

Trip to the light fantastic. Fly to a tropical island or spend a week in the fantastic Florida sunshine to get a bit of fast relief for the wintertime blues. The bright sun works as well as special lights, although most people have to return to phototherapy lights when they get home.

Migrate to the Sun Belt. Packing up house and home may seem like a radical option, but compared with dealing with half-years of gloomy winter moods, it's fast and permanent.

Pour yourself a drink. A drink of vitamin D-enriched milk, that is. Or take a vitamin D supplement. One study shows that vitamin D may keep us in sync with the sun, perhaps triggering the release of thyroid-stimulating hormone, insulin, and digestive acids at optimal times. It may, in other words, be a key to how our internal body clocks work, helping to regulate our mental health and temper our tendency toward winter depression.

TAKING CONTROL OF A PANIC ATTACK

One of the most frightening emotional problems of all is the panic attack. You feel an unexplainable sense of impending doom. Your pulse rate shoots up and you feel your heart pound. Your chest feels tight—as if you are about to suffocate. You feel hot and cold. Your body shakes. You may imagine you are dying.

For the estimated 5 percent of all Americans who have panic attacks, the cause is uncertain, although susceptibility to panic attacks seems to run in families. They are more common in women than men.

A full course of treatment in a clinic can take from 12 to 20 sessions, Dr. Fleming says. Very significant improvements can occur in that span, but you can start to find relief in just a few minutes with a few quick tips and ways to reduce or prevent future attacks.

First, go ahead and panic. That's not a joke. Let the symptoms float through your body. The physiological portion of the attack—the symptoms—will last from 20 seconds to a couple of minutes if you don't fight them. Fighting back—trying to stop the symptoms or becoming self-conscious about what is happening—may prolong the symptoms. So, go ahead and recognize the attack. Tell yourself, "it feels awful, but it won't hurt me." Research shows if you can learn this step, a panic attack is likely to be milder and go away faster.

Control your breathing. You may have been breathing since you left Mom's womb, but it doesn't mean you've been doing it right all these years. A lot of the symptoms of panic may be related to hyperventilation, Dr. Fleming says. Because many people breathe lightly— they're shallow breathers—it doesn't take much to tip them into hyperventilation. When panic strikes, suddenly they start taking faster breaths and bang!—their panic takes control.

"We teach our patients to slow down their breathing and to breathe from their diaphragm," says Tim Brown, Psy.D., associate director of the State University of New York's Phobia and Anxiety Disorders Clinic in Albany. "They pace their breathing to a count to make them conscious of how fast they are breathing. Ideally, we try to get them to 8 to 14 breaths a minute."

To learn how to breathe diaphragmatically, place your hand between your chest and your navel. "The movement should be coming from the lower part of your hand—

from your stomach," he says. "Breathing through the nose rather than the mouth helps. So does using imagery: Imagine that a balloon is in your stomach and you are slowly inflating and deflating it."

His patients practice slow, diaphragmatic breathing twice a day for 10 to 15 minutes at a time. "Initially, we have them practice in a quiet room," Dr. Brown says. "But as they get more proficient, we encourage them to practice in other situations, like in their cars while driving so they can focus their thoughts on their breathing. And by doing that, they can control their hyperventilation." If you practice this method regularly, you could be on your way to more effective breathing—and fewer bouts of hyperventilation.

Burn off the adrenaline. Excess adrenaline produced by your body's fight-or-flight response may be causing the hyperventilation and palpitations. A brisk walk will help dissipate that adrenaline.

Anxiety is often the culprit in panic or hyperventilation attacks. And exercise is a great way to decrease anxiety. Many experts suggest that a daily workout of at least 20 minutes not only improves the body but also does wonders for the mind.

Lower your expectations of disaster. In just 12 weeks, Dr. Brown and his colleagues teach panickers to control their attacks (panic and hyperventilation) by teaching them how to slow their breathing as well as reduce their negative expectations. "A major component of our 12-week treatment program is teaching them to change their fearful thoughts regarding the sensations of anxiety," Dr. Brown says. In other words, patients learn that the symptoms of anxiety, while unpleasant, don't lead to harmful consequences such as heart attack, stroke, or loss of control.

"Most panic disorder patients catastrophically interpret the symptoms to be more harmful than they actually are," he says. Often, the hyperventilation itself leads to its own brand of mountain-out-of-molehill anxiety. "One concern often reported by panic disorder patients is that their panic attacks will result in heart failure," Dr. Brown adds. "Breathing and other bodily functions and sensations become their focus; they become very anxious and stressed in response to changes in their internal bodily state."

Make your vices vanish. Caffeine and alcohol add fuel to the fires of hyperventilation. "Both can produce sensations that, when interpreted catastrophically, can result in panic or anxiety," Dr. Brown says.

Splash your face with cold water. The sudden shock of cold will help distract your mind from your physical symptoms.

Bag your breathing. Of course, "one can't mention hyperventilation without mentioning that familiar brown paper bag," Dr. Brown adds. "If only a short-term solution, it helps restore the proper balance between carbon dioxide and oxygen."

When some people get frightened, they breathe rapidly and deeply, causing them to breathe out a large amount of carbon dioxide. Excessive loss of CO_2 causes the blood to become alkaline, resulting in the symptoms of a panic attack. Breathing into a paper bag results in your breathing a higher carbon dioxide content. But it doesn't change the underlying problem. That's in your head, not your lungs.

Sniff a peach. Certain fragrances can lift spirits and lower blood pressure, according to research at Yale University. Peach odor, researchers report, can sometimes calm a panic attack.

PHOBIA-FIGHTING STRATEGIES

Maybe it's elevators you don't like. Or maybe it's bridges that give you the shivers. Or airplanes. Or black cats. Or highways.

When you start avoiding something because you can't handle the fear, you may have a phobia, Dr. Fleming says. Your elevator phobia may not trouble you if you work in a three-story building, but what happens when your company moves to a 32-story building? And your office is on the top floor? Suddenly you're faced with the choice of looking for another job or overcoming your phobia.

Even if you're not facing such extreme circumstances, it's still a good idea to work on conquering your fear—simply because phobias tend to spread. A fear of elevators today can become a fear of enclosed spaces tomorrow.

Some phobias need professional help. Some may respond best to medications such as antidepressants, anti-motion-sickness drugs, antihistamines, or anti-anxiety medications. This kind of therapy can take from one to four years to work.

Face your fear. Some phobias can be nipped in the bud by following the maxim: "When you fall off the horse, get right back on."

"Clichés become clichés because they have an element of truth to them," says Dr. Fleming. "If you have a bad experience and you begin to avoid the situation, it makes it all the more frightening. The best thing you can do is try the thing you are afraid of."

Begin by sneaking up on it. In the case of elevator fright, work on getting comfortable with the elevator one step at a time. Practice each step until you're comfortable with it before moving on. Step one: Look at the elevator doors. Step two: Walk on and off. Step three: Take a short ride. Before long you'll be getting off on the 32nd floor.

UNDOING PROCRASTINATION

If your style is to delay tasks—even though you ultimately meet your deadlines—procrastination could be your problem. The stress of procrastination may be costly, increasing your risk of ulcers and headaches.

As a procrastinator, you'll probably want to put off solving this problem. But taking these few short steps could immediately start reducing your stress.

Prioritize your deadlines. This is the advice from Jane Burka, Ph.D., a Berkeley, California, psychologist and coauthor of *Procrastination: Why You Do It, What to Do about It*. Decide which deadlines are important and which are flexible. Self-imposed deadlines, such as painting the living room before Christmas, are flexible. Filling out your income tax form before April 15 is not. Put this kind of "must do" task at the top of your list of priorities.

Set short-term deadlines. Assess the time you need to complete an entire project. Next, break the job into steps you can accomplish in 15 minutes. People can stand to do most anything for 15 minutes, according to Dr.

Burka. Finish that small piece and make a note of what needs to be done next.

Bore yourself silly. When you really feel as if you can't do anything, don't. Just sit in a chair and do nothing. After a while you'll be so bored that you'll be more willing to start the work you've been putting off, says psychologist Michael LeBoeuf, author of *Imagineering*.

LEARNING TO BE LESS THAN PERFECT

Maybe you don't put work off for tomorrow. Maybe you start your work immediately, so that you can have every minute possible to be sure the job is done perfectly.

Well, nobody's perfect. Some people just *think* they have to be. They think they have to be at the top of everything they try, just to be worthwhile. They concentrate so much on not failing that they forget to see their accomplishments. They don't take the time to enjoy their success because they're too busy moving on to their next project.

One study of more than 700 men and women showed that perfectionists have far from perfect lives. They tend to be distressed and dissatisfied with their careers and personal lives. And despite their perfectionism, they weren't any more successful than their nonperfectionist peers.

You can concentrate on figuring out why you aren't so perfect (the perfectionist's logical choice) or you can concentrate on changing your behavior—and make a quick change with a few steps.

Stop and note when you aren't satisfied with what you do. Quit judging yourself so harshly when you don't meet your goals. Give yourself permission to be imperfect. Learn to settle for 90 percent.

Concentrate on the task at hand, not on the outcome. Tell yourself, "Here I go again. I'm worrying about the future. Let me do my best." Then, do it.

STEPPING UP WHEN YOU ARE FEELING SHY

Getting things perfect and making the impression of being perfect have a lot in common with shyness. Picture yourself standing at a door knowing that a group of strangers is just on the other side. Even though you hear muffled laughter and other happy party sounds, you still have a hard time stepping over the threshold. What if you don't make a perfect impression?

This is an attack of shyness. It's a common emotion. But most shyness can be managed with a few quick tricks.

Rehearse your opening line. Hurdle the biggest shyness barrier to joining the group by practicing your opening line before you get into the situation, says Jonathan Cheek, Ph.D. A psychology professor at Wellesley College who has researched shyness for 10 years, he's also the author of *Conquering Shyness*.

Any line will do, he says, but try an easy one: "How long have you been here?" "Great shoes. Where did you find them?" "What do you do for a living?"

"Shy people tend to be so judgmental of themselves," Dr. Cheek says. They are very worried about using clichés or about saying something superficial. They start thinking to themselves, 'If I break the silence and do talk, it had better be perfect.'

"The art of small talk is the art of talking in clichés. Small talk is how people warm up to each other."

Step right up. Approach the group a little closer than you ordinarily feel comfortable with, Dr. Cheek says. Studies show that shy people tend to stand too far away from strangers to be included in group discussion, so they end up feeling left out.

And speak right up. Ask questions that demand something longer than a yes or no answer. Ask a follow-up question. If you focus your attention on your social interaction and away from self-criticism, shyness will melt away without your even being aware of what has happened.

Use body language, too. Make eye contact. Uncross your arms and open your body to the group.

Using these fast, simple steps, you can begin to avoid—or lessen the impact of—some of life's emotional potholes. You can't avoid some of them. There are always going to be times when your day-to-day experiences splash back into your face, making you cry. Or rant and rage. Or feel shy. But practicing these techniques can mean less stress and more happiness in the long run.

QUICK CONFIDENCE BUILDERS
FOR PUBLIC SPEAKING

Unaccustomed as you are to public speaking, you can still look and sound like a pro. Here are some quick fixes from John F. Noonan, president of Toastmasters International.

Visualize yourself doing a good job. Think positively— know that you will succeed. Picture the audience responding with warm applause.

Make friends with the audience. Introduce yourself to as many people in the audience as possible before you give your speech. Just introduce yourself and ask each where they are from or what brought them to the auditorium. Once you've met some of your audience, "You'll look out at a group of friends instead of a group of strangers," Noonan says.

Take a fast walk around the room. Do this before you start your talk. If you're backstage where the audience can't see you, do some jumping jacks or run in place for 60 seconds. Noonan has seen brief, vigorous exercise used to chase away those tummy butterflies. It works. Fast. Here's an example that Noonan likes to give.

"We had the world championships of public speaking in Philadelphia in 1982," says Noonan. "There were nine contestants, and just as the moderator was introducing contestant number five, he glanced at the speaker's table and number five wasn't there. The script said to introduce him, so the speaker did. And just as he said number five's name, number five came crawling out from under the table. He was under there doing pushups. And he was the guy who won the championships."

EYE PROBLEMS

The expression "in the blink of an eye" says things are happening fast.

And how often do you blink? Once every 5 seconds or less. Between blinks, when your eyes are open, light zips through the lens to your retina at 132,856 miles per second. Your retina can see up to 60 "pictures" per second.

That's how fast your eyes work. You can work almost that quickly to head off eye problems.

- In 5 seconds of looking out the window, you can solve a bad case of eyestrain.
- In 10 seconds, you can take a test that predicts a sight-threatening disease called macular degeneration.
- In 5 minutes, you can do an eye exercise to improve your eye/hand coordination.

Doctors are using high-tech approaches to fix eye problems faster, too. If a cataract should regrow over your artificial lens implant, for example, your doctor can zap it with a laser, restoring your eyesight instantaneously. To prevent scar tissue from forming after retina surgery, doctors have developed a spongelike contact lens impregnated with timed-release medication that begins working at once. Developed by an ophthalmology professor at the University of California, the lens is designed to dissolve after its job is done—in anywhere from 8 hours to three days.

CLEARING UP CATARACTS

A cataract is a painless, cloudy formation over the lens of the eye that can lead to blindness if left untreated. Some

41 million Americans over the age of 40 have cataracts. Aging, diabetes, exposure to X-rays and ultraviolet radiation, and use of steroid drugs may contribute to cataract formation.

In the bad old days, surgeons waited until a cataract was "ripe," or completely opaque, to remove it. Today, surgeons can remove cataracts as soon as they interfere with daily life. The operation takes about an hour and causes little or no pain. At the same time, the surgeon can implant an artificial lens, called an intraocular lens, that restores vision. Some people who have had cataracts removed still have to wear glasses, however.

Your doctor's high-speed techniques can fix cataracts, but you can decrease your chances of getting them or at least slow their development with a few quick preventive steps.

Wear sunglasses to cut your risk immediately. Studies show that regular use of glasses made with lenses that screen ultraviolet rays from the eyes reduces the risk of cataracts and slows their growth. Look for sunglasses designated Z80.3. These will filter out 95 percent of the harmful rays.

Eat a snack rich in vitamin E or vitamin C. Preliminary studies suggest that both vitamin E (found in such foods as wheat germ, sunflower seeds, almonds, cod-liver oil, and salmon) and vitamin C (found in fresh orange juice, broccoli, spinach, grapefruit, and strawberries, for example) may slow the growth of cataracts.

Snuff out your cigarette. Researchers at Johns Hopkins University report that cigarette smoking increases your risk of developing a common form of cataracts.

HIGH TECH • **LASER SCAN MAY DELAY CATARACTS**

Researchers at Joslin Diabetes Center in Boston are testing a low-level laser device that can spot the first cataract-producing proteins and measure how fast they are growing. After the 5-second test, the results are analyzed and reported to your doctor. With an experimental drug that may stop or reverse protein production, scientists hope to delay cataracts and the surgery necessary to remove them by 15 to 20 years.

SHOCK WAVES FOLLOWING LENS REPLACEMENT RESTORE VISION INSTANTLY

*Z*ap! If, after cataract surgery, your replacement lens becomes clouded, a new, quick procedure with a laser beam can instantly restore your vision.

Commonly, an artificial lens is implanted in the eye following cataract surgery, restoring vision to good or near perfect. But, in about half of all cases, the capsule that encloses the lens clouds over. Traditionally, follow-up surgery had to be done to clear vision.

Now, a quick-pulse laser creates a shock wave in the eye. That makes a tiny hole in the center of the clouded capsule, restoring sight instantly. You need no further treatment or recovery time.

GETTING A GRIP ON GLAUCOMA

Glaucoma is a painless—but dangerous—eye disease that your eye doctor will look for at every checkup. Glaucoma occurs when the fluid normally produced by the eye cannot drain away as it should. Instead, it is trapped within the eye. Pressure builds, eventually reducing blood flow to the retina and strangling the optic nerve. Untreated, glaucoma causes blindness. Symptoms include headaches, frequent eyeglass prescription changes, a decrease in peripheral vision, difficulty adjusting to darkness, swelling, redness, and the appearance of colored haloes around lights. Glaucoma occurs usually in people over age 40, but it can appear at any age.

Your doctor has some fast ways to detect glaucoma. One is a video-game-like test that measures the sensitivity of your retina to light. Another 2- to 3-minute test uses a special video camera to "map" the sensitivity of your retina so that your doctor will have a comparison for each of your eye checkups.

Slip in a prescription-drug dispenser. If your doctor prescribes pilocarpine, one of several glaucoma drugs, you can get a tiny contact-lens-like wafer that sits on the sclera under the lower eyelid and dispenses a prescribed amount of medicine, making eye pressure control easier and exact. This new medication delivery system is especially time-saving for people who are supposed to use eyedrops up to four times a day.

Ask your doctor about laser surgery. Traditional glaucoma surgery, called iridotomy, cut the iris, allowing excess fluid to drain. Now the same procedure can be done much faster, as well as more safely and effectively, with a laser. This kind of surgery has become standard office procedure.

Your doctor is the only one who can treat glaucoma with prescriptions or surgery, but there is a quick self-help measure you can try.

Take a brisk walk to reduce eye pressure. A study at Oregon Health Sciences University in Portland showed that after treadmill walking, eye pressure dropped by 30 percent. Researchers speculate that the burst of adrenaline that comes with exercise, such as walking, may lower pressure.

HIGH TECH • CURING GLAUCOMA WITH A TINY PLASTIC FAUCET

Glaucoma victims whose eye pressure resists control by drugs or surgery can now have a tiny device called a Molteno implant inserted in their eyes. Fluid automatically flows out of the eye whenever pressure starts to build up inside.

The implant is a ½-inch circular acrylic anchoring plate that is attached to a ¾-inch silicone drainage tub. The procedure takes about 40 minutes and the hospital stay is only one day.

The implant doesn't show unless you lift your upper lid. Redness from the surgery lasts about ten days to two weeks and vision returns to normal about that quickly.

SLOWING MACULAR DEGENERATION

One of the most common causes of impaired vision and blindness in people over 50 is a disorder called macular degeneration. The macula lies near the center of the retina at the back of the eye. Because it is the area with the densest concentration of rods and cones (nerve cells that detect color and light), the macula detects sharp detail at the center of the field of vision.

As we age, the small blood vessels of the eye can become constricted, diminishing the blood supply to the retina. Also, in some cases these vessels can start to leak fluid and generate scar tissue. The result is blurred or obstructed central vision. Peripheral vision remains unaffected.

Take a 10-second test. If you have macular degeneration, you gradually lose your reading vision. Eye doctors suggest people over 50 try this 10-second test daily: Cover one eye at a time and look at a straight vertical line. If the line looks wavy or broken, or if you see a black spot, see your eye doctor.

Try a 60-second test. Doctors at Johns Hopkins University Medical School are experimenting with a powerful predictor of who will develop macular degeneration. Special eyedrops make your eyes supersensitive to light. Then you sit in a darkened room and your doctor gives you a target of four dots in a diamond shape to stare at. A red light in the center of the diamond flashes off and on. Each flash is dimmer than the last. You press a buzzer each time you see a flash. The last—and faintest—flash measures your macula's sensitivity.

Follow Bugs Bunny. Eat all the carrots you want. A study at the University of Illinois suggests that daily consumption of fruits and vegetables rich in vitamin A (carrots, squash, pumpkin, brussels sprouts) may be linked to a lower risk of macular degeneration. In a survey of more than 3,000 people, those who rarely ate fruits and vegetables rich in vitamin A were significantly more likely to develop the condition than those who ate such foods daily. The risk seemed to decrease with each additional day that fruits or vegetables were consumed.

HOW DRY EYE AM

Some eye problems can be caused by the environment as well as by illness. Dry eyes is one of them. When you blink, a film of tears is supposed to spread over your eyes. Sometimes, though, your tears don't moisten your eyes enough.

Aging, dermatitis, rheumatoid arthritis, allergies to

eyedrops, or a hot, arid climate could be to blame. Dry eyes can also be caused by an eye infection, a vitamin A deficiency, or some common medications such as decongestants, antihistamines, tranquilizers, antidepressants, and heart and blood pressure medicines. Be aware, too, that dry eyes can signal a serious eye problem, so you'll need to see an ophthalmologist for a diagnosis if your dryness persists.

Some nine million people in the United States have a chronic dry eye problem, with women outnumbering men by about ten to one. If untreated, in extreme cases the condition can cause damage to the cornea or loss of sight.

Mild, temporary dryness can be eliminated as quickly as you might wipe away a tear. Here's how.

Think blink. Making sure you blink often enough may sound easy, but it's not. When your eyes are riveted to the TV or computer screen or focusing on a project, you may forget to blink. After a while, the surface of your eyes dries out and becomes irritated. Make a point to blink regularly.

Drop in artificial tears. Over-the-counter eyedrops, which come in about 30 different brands, may help lubricate your eyes and prevent infections.

Sleep on your dry eye problem. Dab on one of the several over-the-counter combination tear-replacement/moisture-sealing ointments at bedtime and your eyes will be moister by morning. Most of these ointments contain petrolatum and mineral oil.

Flip on the humidifier. Add a little moisture to your environment and the work of moisturizing your eyes becomes a little easier.

Squeeze on some vitamin A ointment. One study at the Massachusetts Eye and Ear Infirmary in Boston showed that applying vitamin A directly to the eye may stimulate mucus-producing cells. Check with your doctor to see if a prescription ointment is available.

Snap on an airtight chamber. Try something new—a pair of special glasses that have plastic sides around each lens, forming an airtight chamber. As your tears evaporate, the air inside becomes humid, thus slowing down further evaporation. Moisture chamber glasses are available with and without prescription lenses at your optometrist's office.

Soak your dry eyes. Dip a washcloth in warm water. Wring it out and hold it over your eyes for a few minutes. The moist heat can unclog sluggish glands and induce your eyes to lubricate naturally.

Put in a pellet. If your dry eyes are a symptom of Sjögren's syndrome, one of the diseases that causes dry eyes, your doctor can prescribe lubricating pellets called Lacrisert. Each day, you insert a pellet under your lower lid; as it dissolves, it lubricates your eyes.

Pop in dry-eye contact lenses. People who complain of dry eyes often can't wear contact lenses because there isn't enough moisture in their eyes to make wearing the lenses comfortable. Now, for some, so-called bandage lenses can lessen dry-eye discomfort.

TAKING THE ITCH OUT

Allergies or infection can make your eyes itchy. Sometimes a sty will give you the urge to rub and massage the itch away.

When the itch isn't caused by an infection or a sty, think fast and try the following remedies.

Soothe with eyedrops. For fast relief from allergy-caused itching, use over-the-counter eyedrops containing naphazoline.

Press on a compress. A warm or cold compress against the closed eye may help relieve the itch.

Slice a cucumber. Then close your eyes and cover them for a moment with the cucumber slices. This will cool the itch a while.

IMPROVING YOUR NIGHT VISION

For most people, it takes about 20 minutes to see in the dark. Others, however, cannot adjust to darkness. They have an eye problem called night blindness.

In the United States, most night vision problems are caused by aging, says Arol Augsburger, O.D., an optometrist and researcher at Ohio State University. "The natural lens of the eye becomes less clear and grows more cloudy, eventually developing cataracts. It's in that intermediate stage, between clear and cataracts, that we have a dirty optical system that makes it difficult to see under dim lighting. In a true sense, it's not night blindness but a hazing of the vision. The cloudiness scatters the light, making it hard to see."

True night blindness needs a doctor's attention because it could be caused by disease such as retinitis pigmentosa, a deficiency of the pigment in the eyes, Dr. Augsburger says. But some problems seeing in the dark can be reduced by following a few quick tips.

Eat like Peter Rabbit. Eating foods rich in vitamin A or beta-carotene, such as chicken and calf's liver, mixed vegetables, kale, cantaloupe, sweet potatoes, collard greens, spinach, and of course, carrots, helps you see in dim light and also prevents xerophthalmia, a serious dry-eye condition that can lead to blindness.

"You need an array of vitamins and minerals to make the photochemical processes in the retina work properly," Dr. Augsburger says. "If you have a reasonable diet that contains vitamin A, as well as other nutrients, then you have what you need. Adding extra vitamin A doesn't make you see super well."

Glance sideways. When the glare of oncoming headlights dims your own vision, look to the side of the lights, where the glare isn't as intense, Dr. Augsburger says.

Wash your glasses. Gunk on the inside or outside or your lenses can scatter light, making your vision problem worse.

Wash your windshield. And don't forget to wash the inside, too, Dr. Augsburger says. Debris on the glass makes it harder to see, especially at night.

CONQUERING CONJUNCTIVITIS

One eye problem you can control easily is conjunctivitis, commonly called pinkeye. It's an inflammation of the conjunctiva, the membrane covering the eye and eyelid, that makes the eyes watery and red-rimmed, Dr. Augsburger says. If it's caused by a virus or bacteria, it usually will clear up by itself in ten days to two weeks. Allergic conjunctivitis lasts longer and itches intensely—it's often seasonal and is treated like an allergy; that is, by avoiding the allergen and using antihistamines.

"The problem is, your eyes don't look very good," Dr. Augsburger says. "Your lids stick together and there's all this gooey stuff that can spread the disease."

So you can trot off to the doctor and get an antibiotic, which should eliminate the problem in about five days (if the cause is bacteria). Especially see a doctor if it's getting worse instead of better after five days, or if you have considerable pain or yellowish or greenish discharge. But there are fast, easy steps you can take to relieve the irritation and to prevent spreading the infection to others in your household.

Compress your conjunctiva. Apply a warm, wet washcloth for a few minutes three or four times a day. This immediately soothes the irritation. If you have allergic conjunctivitis, use a cold compress to relieve the itch.

Clean out the crust. In conjunctivitis, a crust forms along your eyelids. A soft, moistened cotton ball will wash away the crust and keep the area clean.

I-Scrub your eyes. If the cotton ball doesn't work, try I-Scrub, a nonprescription solution that includes a mild detergent.

Wash your hands. And make sure everyone else washes theirs, to avoid spreading the conjunctivitis germs. If they've touched some of the germs, they may rub their eyes and infect themselves.

Keep your washcloth, clothing, and towels separate. To avoid spreading the infection, don't share your personal items with anyone else.

TAKING THE STING OUT OF STIES

A sty is a bacterial infection at the root of an eyelash. They're more common during childhood, but they can happen to anyone at any time. Their beginnings are marked by slight discomfort when blinking; soon the lid becomes red and swollen. A small boil pops up. A doctor can give you antibiotic eyedrops to get rid of the infection.

If you do nothing, Dr. Augsburger says, 90 percent of all sties will go away in one to three weeks. The sty will rupture by itself, drain, and heal. But if you don't want to wait while nature takes its time, there is one thing you can do to speed the process.

Apply a soft, warm, moist cloth. The warm, moist

heat will raise the temperature of your eyelid, soften the skin, and speed draining. Do this for 10 minutes, four times a day. The sty will probably disappear in a couple of days, Dr. Augsburger says. If it doesn't, see a doctor. Don't squeeze the sty in hopes of rupturing it, he warns. That could force pus into your eyelid, causing blood poisoning.

ERASING DARK CIRCLES AND REJUVENATING RED EYES

After a late night out, your head aches, your mouth feels as if you've been chewing on a shag rug, and your eyes are red-rimmed orbs underscored by dark circles.

Dark circles under your eyes are really small veins returning blue blood to your heart. Usually visible when you're tired, they also appear when you are ill or pale or have lost a lot of weight. Some people, however, simply inherit the tendency toward dark circles. And when children develop these dark shadows, it often indicates an allergy. Redness can be caused by fatigue, a bacterial invasion (see "Conquering Conjunctivitis" earlier in this chapter), or an injury.

Help is as near as your bathroom.

Whiten up with drops. If fatigue is the culprit, use commercial eyedrops to constrict the blood vessels and whiten your eyes.

Wipe out redness with witch hazel. Saturate two cotton balls with witch hazel, squeezing the excess out so it won't drip. Put your feet up and place the cool, moist cotton balls over your closed eyelids, taking care not to get the liquid in your eyes. Rest for half an hour. If you don't have witch hazel, try two tea bags that have been steeped in cold water.

Paint your eyes pale. If you inherited your dark circles, try a specially modified makeup base or glasses with tinted lenses to help disguise the darkness.

Shoo the allergens out of the house. If your child has dark circles caused by allergy, find the source and get rid of it. An allergy can be caused by house dust, cat or dog dander, or foods such as wheat, milk, or chocolate.

Sleep tight. If late nights painting the town red are painting your eyes technicolor, reexamine your lifestyle to include adequate sleep and healthy diet.

TAKING THE PUFF OUT OF YOUR EYES

Puffy circles around the eyes are caused by too much fluid in the skin. Anytime your blood has to move uphill to get back to your heart—you scrub the floor on your hands and knees, you get on all fours to play a game of marbles—there's a tendency toward swelling. Sleeping can make fluid collect in your face and around your eyes. Allergies can also cause puffiness.

Sit up. No matter what else you do, sitting up is the simplest, easiest way to make gravity work for you.

Use ice or a cold washcloth. For an even faster solution to the puffy problem, don't wait for gravity to work its magic. A cold compress—ice wrapped in a towel or a cold washcloth—over your eyes will speed recovery.

WHAT TO DO WHEN YOUR ARMS GET TOO SHORT

"The most universal eye problem is presbyopia," Dr. Augsburger says. Presbyopia, the loss of close focus vision, strikes most people at about age 40 and is marked by the need to hold a book or newspaper farther and farther away from the eyes.

"Our population is graying. From the day we are born, the focusing lenses in our eyes become less flexible, less and less elastic. It becomes more difficult to see close up. We begin to need reading glasses or bifocals to make up for the inelasticity," he says.

Take this test. Open a telephone book and choose some numbers. Keep your glasses on if you normally wear them. Move the book away from your body until you can focus on the numbers. If you must fully extend your arm or bend it only slightly, you may have presbyopia. Your optometrist can give you a more precise test. Normally, people can read things clearly 14 to 16 inches away.

Pick up a pair of dime store glasses. If your doctor says your problem is simply vision loss caused by presbyopia, you can get over-the-counter glasses at your local five-and-dime or drugstore. Ready-to-wear specs are perfect and fast for part-time use. These off-the-rack reading glasses have glass or plastic, tinted or untinted lenses. They are available in bifocal and trifocal and come in a variety of frame styles.

Order bifocal contact lenses. This new type of bifocal contacts has areas for different vision capabilities arranged in a circle, like a bull's-eye, on the lenses. By looking through the center of the lens, you can see distance. The surrounding area gives a close-up view. It takes one to four weeks to learn how to get the focus you need, but once the technique has been mastered, you have nearly perfect vision. The overall success rate is about 60 percent, Dr. Augsburger says.

FAST AID FOR INJURIES

It can happen in a second—an eye injury caused by a rock thrown from a lawn mower or by a tennis racquet or baseball bat swung thoughtlessly. Swimmers can have eye problems from the chemicals used to disinfect swimming pools.

Quick action means quick relief. Here are some fast-action strategies to use.

Slap on a cold compress. The proverbial steak over the black eye is a great make-do, fast remedy for a bruise on the cheek, eyelid, or eyebrow. An icebag works just as well, though, to prevent the spread of the bruise. Any blow hard enough to blacken the eye could damage the eyeball, so see your ophthalmologist, too.

Rinse out the burn. If a household chemical splashes into your eyes, grab the spray nozzle from the kitchen sink to rinse the chemical out of your eyes. Position your head so the injured eye is on the lower side, then, using a gentle spray, flush the eyes for 5 to 10 minutes. Then, seek professional help immediately.

Snap on high-impact glasses. The best quick cure is a preventive. Impact-resistant glasses, which cost from $15 to $40, should be worn by anyone running power equipment, such as a lawn mower or carpentry tools. They're protection for people spraying chemicals or paint. And there's a variety specifically designed to provide eye protection during sports.

Wear goggles. The chlorine that disinfects the pool you swim in can make your eyes feel dry and scratchy. Microbes in fresh water can cause infections. Pull on a pair of watertight swimming goggles to protect your eyes when you take a dip.

REMOVING SPECKS FROM YOUR EYE

An eyelash, a speck of dust, or a grain of sand can feel the size of a log when it's in your eye. Fortunately, most foreign objects will be flushed out naturally by tears. Some, however, are not. See if one of these simple tricks will wash the speck out.

Flush your eye. Wash your hands thoroughly. Pull the upper eyelid down over the lower lid and then let it slide back. This will produce tears and may flush out the particle. Or, aid those tears. Grab a bottle of sterile saline solution, the kind you wet your contact lenses with, and squeeze it over your eyeball. If you don't have this solution, fill an eyedropper with warm water. Or you can make a simple irrigation solution by dissolving ½ teaspoon of salt in an 8-ounce glass of water.

Pick the foreign object out of your eye. If you can see an object and it's not embedded, but it won't flush out of your eye, have someone pick it off with the corner of a clean, moistened cloth, handkerchief, or paper tissue. Don't use a cotton swab, because loose fibers will come off and stick to the eye.

If the object seems embedded in your eye, do not rub your eye. See a doctor immediately.

STOPPING EYESTRAIN

One of the most common causes of eye problems today stares us in the eyes when we sit down to work. It's a computer screen. The disease it causes is called "repetitive stress injury," says Lowell Glatt, O.D., a New York City optometrist and member of the committee on environmental vision of the American Optometric Association.

"What happens is this: You sit down and lock your eyes on the computer screen," Dr. Glatt says. "You sit there for hours, processing information into the computer, concentrating on the screen 26 inches from your face."

After a while, your eyes get tired, you get a headache, and you have a hard time focusing your eyes when you shift them from the computer. Your eyes may feel dry and they may burn.

And it's not just computers that cause the problem.

Any kind of work that demands close, continuous concentration can cause the same symptoms. Computers have been targeted as the culprits, however, because they've become a staple in many offices.

Relief from repetitive stress injury to the eyes is as easy and as fast as a blink. In fact, that's the first thing Dr. Glatt recommends.

Blink . . . then blink again. Staring at a screen can almost shut down the blinking mechanism, allowing the surface of your eyes to dry out and become irritated. Concentrate on blinking more often when you have to do close work.

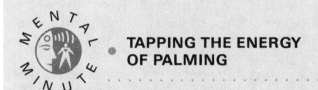

TAPPING THE ENERGY OF PALMING

When you are "palming" your eyes, according to Janet Goodrich, Ph.D., a Reichian therapist, there is no outside light to stimulate your visual system. Instead, your imagination creates light and colored images that relax and reenergize your eyes.

Here's how.

Hold your hands, palms up, in front of you. If you like, you can rest your elbows on a pillow on your lap or on a tabletop for extra support. Breathe deeply, letting your breath expand your abdomen. Yawn. Rub your hands briskly together, then place them, slightly cupped, over your eyes. The cupped part of your palms should be over your eyes and the bony part of your hands, just above the wrist, should rest on top of your cheekbones. Cross your fingers over the top of your nose and rest your fingertips against your forehead. Keep your eyes closed.

Dr. Goodrich suggests you begin by imagining a blue sun in the center of the Earth. Breathe deeply as you visualize this image. See the different blue hues—cobalt, aquamarine, and indigo—that radiate from the sun. The color covers your feet and flows into your legs, moving up through your chest and into your shoulders. The blue light

(continued)

covers your hands, swirling into your palms. Light floods your eyes and brain, then flows to the visual center at the back of your head.

Keeping your eyes closed, take your palms away from your eyes. Stretch. Yawn. When you are ready, open your eyes.

You can use other images while palming. For instance, you can picture yourself walking in an open field, smelling the grass and leaves. See yourself picking an apple from a tree and shining it on your sleeve. Take a bite and taste the juice as it fills your mouth. Toss the apple toward the blue sky, then watch it change into a red rubber ball as you catch it. Toss the ball into the distance and follow it with your nose as it gets smaller and smaller and finally disappears on the horizon. Bring the ball back. This mental exercise, according to Dr. Goodrich, will flex your imagination and improve the saccadic movement, the ability of the eye to move from picture to picture or word to word when reading.

Stare off into space. Every once in a while—from every 20 minutes to every hour, depending on your own needs—look across the room. It may take only a glance, a couple of seconds away from your computer screen, to allow your eyes a chance to refocus and rest. You'll go back to work with refreshed, more productive eyes.

Switch glasses. If you wear bifocals, you've probably already noticed you have to turn your head to the side each time you want to read the information you're typing into the computer. Then you have to swing your head back to see the screen. Your optician can grind a pair of occupational lenses that puts your close-up lens on the side instead of at the bottom of your glasses. That way, you can just glance to the side when work demands. Or you can get a pair of close-up lenses that attaches to your regular glasses like flip-up sunglasses. Flip them down to work, flip them up after hours.

Make yourself an air screen. If you're blinking and your eyes still feel as hot as Cherries Jubilee, your computer could be fanning the flames. As the fan inside the computer blows to cool the computer's inner workings, it also blows a steady stream of air—drying air—toward your eyes. Tape a piece of cardboard to the top of your monitor so it baffles the air away from your eyes, toward the ceiling.

Flip off the light. If your vision problems and eyestrain are at their worst after watching the bright screen, rethink the lighting around your work area. The background light level should be low and offer contrast. You shouldn't see any bright sources of direct or reflected light in the screen.

Install a glare screen. Add a screen to minimize the amount of glare reflected back into your eyes.

Wipe the dust off your screen. Your eyes must work harder when they're trying to see past dirt, smears, and fingerprints. Give your computer screen a 2-second wiping with a damp cloth.

Request polarizing lenses. To cut screen glare, ask for this type of lens when you get new glasses.

FAST EXERCISES FOR YOUR EYES

Exercising your eyes can rehabilitate your eyesight, according to some behavioral optometrists. It can offset fatigue and eyestrain for those who toil on word processors. It can be used to improve learning skills and on-the-job performance. Athletes can train their eyes to improve their focus and visual concentration. Here are some quick exercises you can try to improve your brain-to-nerve-to-muscle connection.

Zoom in on the fine print. If you work at a video display terminal, try this. Tack a page of newsprint to a wall about 8 feet from your chair. Every 10 minutes or so, interrupt your work to look at the newspaper. Bring the print into focus, then look back at the words on your screen. Shift your focus back and forth for 30 seconds. Do this six times an hour. This exercise may eliminate the blurred vision you experience at the end of your workday.

Read your thumb. Hold your thumb at arm's length. Move it in circles, X's, and crosses. Pull your thumb closer, then push it away. Follow it with your eyes. As you do this, keep as much of the room as possible in your field of vision. Continue the exercise with one eye closed. Repeat with the other eye. This can improve your peripheral vision.

Watch the bouncing ball. If you play tennis, squash, racquetball, or handball, ask your partner to give you some help. Stand 3 to 5 feet from a blank wall. Get your partner to stand behind you and toss the ball against the wall. When the ball bounces off the wall, catch it. This will improve eye/hand coordination.

Train your brain. Put three colored beads on a string 6 feet long. Fasten one end of the string to a wall at eye level and hold the other end of the string to your nose. Slide one bead close to the wall, place the second 4 feet from your nose, and place the third 16 inches from your nose.

Look at the far bead. Two strings forming a "V" will come together at the bead. Shift your eyes to the middle bead. There will be an "X" where the beads come together. Shift from the "V" to the"X" and back again. If your eyes are working together, you should see the strings crossing when your eyes focus on a bead. If your eyes aren't working together, you'll see different patterns or one string. This exercise teaches your eyes to work together and your brain to not shut off one eye's vision.

. . . .

PICKING UP DROOPY LIDS

Aging is the cause of many eye problems, including droopy lids. In adults, droopy lids, a condition called ptosis, are a sign of muscle weakness in the lid. It also can be caused by nerve or muscle damage from an injury, by a disease such as diabetes, or by a stroke.

Lift your lids with a piece of tape. Nonsurgical eye-lift tape, invented by a Santa Monica, California, plastic surgeon, invisibly takes up the slack in sagging eyelids. Anyone can benefit from this quick fix, which takes only moments to apply. The product is great for people who are undecided about surgery, who can't undergo surgery for medical reasons, or who can't afford surgery. And it's faster than surgery. For a price list and information on where to find the tape, write Harold D. Clavin, M.D., Clavin Laboratories, 2001 Santa Monica Boulevard, Suite 890 West, Santa Monica, CA 90404.

FATIGUE

Yes ma'am, this is the Fatigue Squad. Sergeant Toopooped Topop speaking. What's that? You can't get out of bed in the morning? You're falling asleep in your corn flakes? You yawned in your boss's face? And yesterday evening you dozed off while your husband was telling you about the pay raise and promotion he got? Hmmm . . . this sounds serious, ma'am. We'll send somebody right over. What's your address? Ma'am? Hello? Wake up, ma'am . . ."

If you're tired all the time, it could be just that you're not getting enough sleep. Fatigue can also be a signal of a physical illness or poor eating habits or a drug reaction. There are many possible causes for fatigue, and so you might have to do a little detective work to figure out why you're so darn tired.

But once you've pinpointed the cause, there's plenty you can do to help yourself. For example:

- With a few simple lifestyle changes that take no time at all, you can cure energy-robbing insomnia.
- With a 1-minute phone call, you can eliminate a potent but often unsuspected cause of fatigue.
- By taking a 15-minute vacation, you can leave that tired feeling behind.

Are you still with us? Good. It's time for a quick fix for your fatigue.

SLEEPING IT OFF

It seems so obvious, but if you haven't slept well the night before, you're very likely to feel tired the day after.

Half of all Americans have trouble dozing off at some time in their lives, and an astonishing 35 million of us have chronic insomnia. Scientists believe sleep disturbance is a common response to changes in our lives, from trouble at the office to serious illness. For most of us, normal sleep patterns return after the daytime problem that is the source of worry goes away or gets better.

If occasional sleeplessness troubles you, follow these simple suggestions from Patricia Prinz, Ph.D., associate professor of psychiatry and behavioral sciences at the University of Washington School of Medicine.

- Try not to drink coffee, cola, or other caffeine drinks after 6:00 or 7:00 P.M.
- Go to bed at the same time every night.
- Get regular, moderate exercise.
- Better skip alcohol after dinner. Booze interferes with sound sleep.

DIETING WITHOUT LOSING YOUR EDGE

They don't call them crash diets for nothing. Diet or not, you *have* to eat if you don't want to wind up nose down on the pavement. Simply put, crash or fad diets can leave you feeling fatigued.

Because they offer so little in the way of balanced nutrition, crash diets can turn your muscle mass into mush. The destruction becomes so pronounced after a short time that the muscle tissue can no longer efficiently process calcium, according to studies done at the University of Toronto. If you're on that kind of diet, your body will not be able to function properly. It will slow down and conserve energy by making *you* slow down.

To get a good start on a diet that will leave you feeling fresh and exhilarated, bear in mind the following basic rules.

- Eat a variety of foods. Avoid diet plans that force you to live on one specific kind of food, like grapefruit. We need a wide variety of nutrients from all kinds of food. No one food supplies you with all the nutrients your body needs to maintain health.
- Women in general shouldn't eat fewer than 1,200 calories a day; men, not fewer than 1,500 calories.

According to diet and nutrition experts at Stanford University, you can't get all the nutrients you need if you eat fewer than those amounts.

If you cut 250 calories a day from your diet, you should lose about a half pound a week.

- Don't eat big meals late at night. You probably won't be able to burn off the calories as quickly by bedtime as you would earlier in the day.
- Don't skip meals. If you do, you'll only be hungrier later. When you do sit down to eat, you probably will eat more than you should.

EXERCISING YOUR RIGHT TO MORE ENERGY

If your body isn't exercised regularly, it probably doesn't use oxygen very efficiently. Your muscles need that oxygen, or they don't work as long or as hard as they can. The result of all this sitting around: When you need muscle power, you don't get it, and you tire quickly.

What's more, even as your muscle sags, so, too, does your self-image. Your emotional state can become a mirror image of your physical condition, adding to your fatigue.

That's why exercise benefits you in two ways. First, it improves your physical condition, enabling your body to more efficiently deliver oxygen to your muscles, increasing your endurance. Second, exercise stimulates an overall feeling of well-being.

Studies show that as you exercise, your body becomes better able to handle the everyday emotional and physical stresses of life, says Ralph Wharton, M.D., clinical professor of psychiatry at Columbia University. "The question is, what does exercise do in a neurochemical sense? We don't know exactly," he says. "But we do know that, whatever exercise does for the brain, it also seems to do for the ego. When people exercise, they see themselves running or swimming well. They feel a certain mastery over their personal environment."

SQUELCHING FATIGUING SIDE EFFECTS

You get plenty of sleep, you jog around the park, but you still feel exhausted, like you just can't get started. Maybe your fatigue is coming from outside your body.

A number of drugs—including antihistamines, pain relievers, diuretics, antihypertensives, antibiotics, oral contraceptives, and anticonvulsants—can sometimes cause fatigue as a side effect.

If you are taking a drug and you think it makes you feel drowsy, the first thing to do is to call the pharmacist who sold you the product, says William N. Tindall, Ph.D., vice president of professional affairs for the National Association of Retail Druggists.

"The pharmacist will have your complete drug history and will be able to tell whether the drug you are taking is causing your drowsiness, or whether two drugs in combination are having that effect. Remember, the other drug could be a nonprescription drug, so be sure to tell the pharmacist which drugs you're taking. Then, the pharmacist will call the doctor and together they'll decide the best thing to do."

What they might do, Dr. Tindall says, is substitute another drug. "With all the drugs on the market, they can usually find something that isn't as hard on the patient."

Whatever you do, *don't* stop taking a prescription drug without consulting your physician first.

TURNING OFF TENSION

It takes a lot of energy to deal with the pressures of everyday life. After expending all that energy, you may be left with a gnawing, overwhelming sense of fatigue.

Not all the stresses of life leave us feeling emotionally drained. "It takes a certain kind of stress, in which you have no choices, no options, no alternatives," says Harvey L. Alpern, M.D., a board-certified cardiologist in Los Angeles. "The classic example is the woman who finds herself in a dead-end job. She has a tough boss that she can't talk back to. She has to do the same, repetitive things day after day. She has no sense of control. She may have a family who needs her, so she has even more work to do when she gets home. She is trapped. This woman may suffer fatigue."

If you're stuck in that kind of situation, maybe it seems like there's nothing you can do. But according to

Dr. Alpern, the symptoms of fatigue associated with stress can often be alleviated by asking your doctor, or consult a stress therapist, about relaxation techniques. They may take only 10 or 15 minutes to learn.

Once you know the techniques, use them to take a couple of 10- or 15-minute "vacations" from your work around the home or office every day. "Doing these exercises and paying attention to your feelings can break that all-day feeling of tension," Dr. Alpern says.

IRONING UP WHEN YOU'RE RUN DOWN

Take the iron out of a bridge, and it'll collapse. Run low on iron in your blood, and maybe *you'll* collapse. Iron deficiency can lead to anemia, which in turn can lead to fatigue.

Even if our diet is iron-rich, we might have trouble holding on to it. In women, heavy menstrual flow may deplete the body's stores of iron, resulting in frequent fatigue, says James D. Cook, M.D., head of the Division of Hematology at the University of Kansas Medical Center. Men, on the other hand, may suffer iron deficiency due to gastrointestinal bleeding. Such bleeding might be virtually unnoticeable yet sufficient to cause anemia.

Pregnant women and children going through rapid growth periods often need more iron than the rest of us. If this need is not met, they, too, may have iron-deficiency anemia and that washed-out feeling.

The Recommended Dietary Allowance (RDA) for males and for females over age 51 is 10 milligrams. For females ages 11 to 50, the RDA is 15 milligrams. Among the best food sources of iron are beef liver, dark meat turkey, lean ground beef, lima beans, sunflower seeds, prunes, broccoli, and spinach. If you're supplementing, stick to the RDA unless your doctor tells you otherwise. Iron in large amounts can be harmful.

CLIMBING OUT OF A DEPRESSING HOLE

Your only son is about to marry an intelligent, beautiful young woman. She's the kind of person you would have picked yourself for someone as special as your boy. There's every reason for joy in your life, but that's not how you feel. You're very sad and very tired. And, suddenly, this wedding is becoming a problem.

"Fatigue often is a warning signal of a failure to master a problem," Dr. Wharton says. "Sometimes there is anticipation of a conflict, and other times the conflict is ongoing."

Another reason why a depressed person might feel exhausted is lack of sleep.

"Many depressed people may have serious trouble sleeping," Dr. Wharton says, "or they'll have recurring nightmares. The sleep disturbance is part of the depressive cycle. They'll wake up feeling tired. In fact, they've been sleeping, but they've been having very troublesome dreams, which can be as exhausting as if they were struggling during the day, digging a ditch. They're digging a deeper and deeper emotional hole, and never getting out of it."

But you can start getting out of this hole if you begin to understand why you feel depressed. "It's often possible to see what you can do to prevent trouble in the future, to prevent this emotional fatigue reaction that makes everything an effort," Dr. Wharton says.

But there's more to getting better than recognizing what makes you depressed. Once you know the underlying cause of your emotional downturn, you then have to change the way you react to the situation or, failing that, change the situation. For either option, you might need the emotional help of a trained mental-health practitioner.

"Sometimes getting better means taking a look at how you have dealt with crises in the past and learning ways to cope with the new crisis," Dr. Wharton says. "Other times it requires an exploration of one's whole past. But the good news is that fatigue of this sort is usually treatable." (See chapter 16 for more on depression and fatigue.)

CHECKING UP ON FATIGUE

Chronic weariness, along with thirst and general weakness, can signify the onset of diabetes. Nonstop fatigue might also be the first sign of hepatitis, a thyroid disorder, mononucleosis, tuberculosis, or infection. And one of the first warning signs—occasionally, it's the only signal—of heart disease may be fatigue. For all these reasons and more, unexplained fatigue should always be checked out by a doctor.

WHEN TIREDNESS IS A DISEASE: A SPECIAL MEDICAL CARE UPDATE ON CHRONIC FATIGUE SYNDROME

Chronic fatigue syndrome (CFS) is an illness of continual dog-tiredness, achy muscles, fever, drowsiness, and the blahs that lasts months, even years. And tens of thousands of Americans may have it.

But although scientists don't yet know exactly what causes CFS, there's new hope for dealing with it. Finally, after a lot of confusion about what CFS really is and even whether it actually exists, medical experts are pinning it down and learning more about how to curb it. And they've put out the good word: CFS is not a fatal disease, and most people who suffer from it get better when they learn how to fight it.

WHO HAS IT, WHO DOESN'T

About one in five people who walk into a doctor's office complains that fatigue is disrupting his life. Yet only 3 to 5 percent fit the criteria of CFS that were devised by more than a dozen experts, along with the Centers for Disease Control (CDC) in Atlanta.

According to these criteria, people who truly have CFS are those who:

- Have suffered a debilitating fatigue (or easy fatigability) that's lasted at least six months
- Have ruled out (with their doctor's help) any other physical or psychiatric diseases that may mimic CFS symptoms, like acute nonviral infections, depression, hormonal disorders, drug abuse, or exposure to toxic agents
- Have at least 8 of the following 11 symptoms recurring or persisting for six months or more

Chills or mild fever

A sore throat

Painful or swollen lymph glands

Unexplained general muscle weakness

Muscle discomfort

Fatigue for at least 24 hours after previously tolerated exercise

A headache unlike any previous pain

Joint pain without joint swelling or redness

Complaints of forgetfulness, excessive irritability, confusion, inability to concentrate, or depression

Disturbed sleep

Quick onset of symptoms within a few hours or days

Such symptoms are common to a variety of diseases, and chronic fatigue alone does not a CFS diagnosis make. So it's important to meet fully the CDC's criteria before your doctor can declare you a bona fide CFS victim. After all, some of us, because of our lifestyles, *should* be tired. A mother of three who gets only 4 hours of sleep each night is bound to be physically exhausted. Psychological stresses can also make you tired.

Besides having specific criteria for diagnosing CFS, scientists also know that many CFS sufferers have common traits. Some people with CFS often have several abnormal immune system responses. Some, for example, have high levels of antibodies in their blood, normally a sign of the presence of bacterial or viral agents. Some CFS sufferers say that their fatigue started abruptly when they had a specific infection, such as the flu. They may even be able to name the exact day they took sick.

The syndrome often begins during a stressful time, such as during a divorce, a career change, or a death in the family. Also, many CFS people say they're depressed, but it isn't clear whether the depression caused CFS or developed later when "patients are sick and tired of being tired," says Stephen Strauss, M.D., chief of medical virology at the National Institute of Allergy and Infectious Diseases.

CFS sufferers also are more likely to suffer from

various allergies, and their immune systems may not produce the normal amount of chemicals that regulate the body's defensive responses to disease.

IN SEARCH OF A CAUSE

Over the years, doctors have come up with unproven and dubious explanations for the malaise: iron-poor blood (anemia), low blood sugar (hypoglycemia), environmental allergy (twentieth-century disease), or systemic yeast infection (candidiasis).

At one time, scientists considered Epstein-Barr virus (EBV) as a possible cause of CFS, since many—but not all—CFS sufferers have EBV in their blood. Some researchers believe that EBV may cause the syndrome in people who never recovered from mononucleosis. Others hypothesize that EBV or other viruses slumbering in the body somehow are reawakened to cause the symptoms. New evidence, however, indicates that EBV alone doesn't appear to be the culprit. One of the latest studies found that 23 of 30 people with CFS had evidence of a retrovirus infection—and so did many of their healthy friends and relatives, which means CFS *could* be contagious. (Retroviruses commonly disrupt the immune system.) But these study results are "extremely preliminary and do *not* by themselves prove that CFS is caused by the retrovirus or that CFS is contagious," says Walter J. Gunn, Ph.D., principal investigator of the CFS surveillance system at the CDC.

Most patients with CFS have features that overlap with the disorder call fibromyalgia, which is also associated with fatigue and muscle and joint pain. Some experts believe that CFS and fibromyalgia may actually be the same condition in many cases. If the two syndromes are the same, then the number of chronic fatigue syndrome patients may be enormous, since three million to six million Americans have been diagnosed as having fibromyalgia.

To study CFS and to try to zero in on possible causes, the CDC has asked doctors in Atlanta, Grand Rapids, Reno, and Wichita to gather detailed information about the onset of CFS, what symptoms they see, and the course of the illness. "Some things point to a virus, but we are looking at everything—pesticides, fertilizers, varnishes, paints, household construction, and insect bites," Dr. Gunn says. "We now have a solid group of patients who meet the case definition, and we hope to find some common cause."

GETTING A DIAGNOSIS

So if you believe you meet the CDC's criteria for chronic fatigue syndrome, you should be tested and have an adequate workup. Your family physician's office is probably the best place to start the investigation. With some simple tests, your doctor should be able to rule out other illnesses that may look like CFS.

Most people with CFS end up seeing several specialists, such as a rheumatologist, an orthopedist, a neurologist, and a psychiatrist, to exclude other causes of the flulike symptoms. University medical centers usually can provide all the consultants necessary to diagnose the syndrome.

Because it's not a simple disease to identify, some doctors are overdiagnosing the illness, leading patients who have not had appropriate workups to believe they have the syndrome. And some doctors who don't know exactly what CFS is are underdiagnosing it.

"Only about 50 percent of the people who are told that they have chronic fatigue syndrome actually have it according to the CDC criteria," says John Renner, M.D., a clinical professor of family medicine at the University of Missouri at Kansas City. He's seen the medical records of hundreds of patients diagnosed with the syndrome.

"This is a complicated illness," he says. "First and foremost, it is something that takes a sophisticated medical workup, which includes immune studies (like blood work that looks at antibodies) and all the tests necessary to rule out other diseases. You want someone who understands the sciences of infectious diseases and immunology. If there's any doubt in your primary physician's mind, don't hesitate to consult an immunologist. You probably will want to get a second opinion."

IT'S NOT ALL IN YOUR HEAD

One myth that CFS experts are trying to dispel is that the illness is all psychological. It's true that most people with

CFS become depressed during their illness. But then so do most people with chronic illnesses. The question is whether they have a history of depression before the flulike symptoms appear.

When doctors treat fatigue as just a trivial psychological problem, they do CFS sufferers a disservice. The kind of fatigue they feel is serious and unrelenting. "I can drive to the grocery store and fill a lightweight plastic bag with food, and that's it for the day," says Nanette, a CFS patient. "The quality of my life has been reduced tremendously. I can get people to buy groceries for me and to do my housework. But I can't get someone to help me concentrate or think clearly."

Many illnesses have gone through stages of skepticism only to become fully recognized later, including multiple sclerosis, Legionnaires' disease, lupus, and AIDS.

"Rather than saying that chronic fatigue syndrome is all in the patient's head, the skeptics need to listen to their patients more intently. The patients know their bodies and their emotions," says Orvalene Prewitt, a cofounder of the National Chronic Fatigue Syndrome Association in Kansas City, Missouri. "We need to pursue all avenues to find an answer for this baffling flulike illness. Both the public and doctors need to know that there are people out there who really are sick."

FIGHTING BACK

There's no proven cure yet for CFS, but there are treatments that often can help reduce the symptoms. And there's plenty of ongoing research to test new therapies. In part because of the symptomatic treatments, those who meet the CDC criteria usually do not get progressively worse, and many have gradually improved over time.

Most experts say that the following are your best bets for treating symptoms:

Get adequate amounts of rest. Measured doses of taking-it-easy do alleviate some symptoms.

Eat right. CFS is not associated with vitamin or mineral deficiencies, but eating meals with adequate amounts of nutrients (including calories) does make a difference in how some CFS sufferers feel. Some report feeling better when the diet is low in sugar and fat.

Do a small amount of exercise every day. Even if it's just stretching. Chronic overexertion tends to worsen symptoms and may prolong the course of the disease. But most experts do not believe people will get better faster if they stay in bed. That can be psychologically and physically devastating.

Ration your limited energy. "Every day, I think of energy credits," Nanette says. "The first credits I use are always for myself—I wash my hair, paint my nails. Then I balance out the rest over the day."

Ease your pain. If you are in a lot of pain, ask your doctor about pain medication.

Get emotional help. Chronic illness really takes a toll on your emotions. You need to know how to deal emotionally with the disease. You can seek counseling or get support from CFS patient groups. "I went to a support group and found others like myself," Nanette says. "I also saw I needed some help on how to adjust to being chronically ill. After I had stopped working, I didn't call my friends to chat or get involved in any activities. Now I've become the leader of the support group. Helping others helps me feel good."

Those patients who can maintain a positive attitude seem to cope the best. "I focus on living a balanced life and increasing my stamina," Nanette says. "Now I really appreciate the company of others. I'm not waiting to catch up with life. I do things in moderation, but I don't miss out on too much."

Ask about tricyclic antidepressants. To help CFS sufferers, doctors have tried various drugs to help boost the immune system or to attack specific viruses. It's unclear, though, whether these medications can really help, because they haven't been tested. One drug that was tested, the antiviral called acyclovir, was found ineffective.

But one type of drug—tricyclic antidepressants—appears, theoretically, to be designed specifically for this syndrome. "Depressive symptoms are part of the illness, but alleviating depression is not the only reason to use antidepressants," says James F. Jones, M.D., of the National

Jewish Center for Immunology and Respiratory Medicine in Denver.

"Tricyclic antidepressants have a number of pharmacological activities," he says. "They are potent antihistamines, which may help ameliorate allergies. They also are sedating, which can help patients get a good night's sleep. And they have anti-inflammatory effects." Dr. Jones has been able to relieve the symptoms of 70 percent of his CFS patients using one-tenth the dose of antidepressant generally prescribed to treat depression. He points out that antidepressants have not been evaluated in controlled trials of CFS patients.

Shun the snake-oil peddlers. There are plenty of them in the CFS wilderness—the mystery of the disease and lack of a cure brings them out from under the rocks with unproven therapies promoted as sure cures. "Be wary of so-called chronic fatigue syndrome specialists who suggest you fly across the country to see them," Dr. Renner says. "They are likely to put you on a bizarre treatment." The list of unsubstantiated therapies promoted as effective includes injections of hydrogen peroxide, homeopathic remedies, high colonics, and large doses of vitamin C or other food supplements.

"Until a cure is found, focus on safe, best-bet treatments," Dr. Renner says. "And remember that most people with CFS do learn to cope with it and they usually get better."

C H A P T E R

19

FOOT PROBLEMS

t would be nice if you could just walk away from foot problems. And actually, walking, in general, *is* a good way to help keep feet healthy.

"Any time you stimulate your cardiovascular system, you help your feet by keeping the blood circulating," says Joseph Ellis, D.P.M., a podiatrist and consultant to the University of California at San Diego.

If you choose to ignore foot problems, they usually stay put. Yet, with the right moves, everything from athlete's foot to plantar warts can be cured faster than Carl Lewis running a 100-meter race. Okay, maybe not that fast. But still fast. Consider that:

- In just 10 minutes, you can relieve bunion pain with a warm soak.
- In just 15 minutes, a special paste can dissolve calluses.
- In just four days, you can banish corns with wine.

Quick-acting remedies are pretty amazing when you consider the structure of the human foot. Each one comes equipped with 26 bones. And then there are all those joints, ligaments, tendons, and muscles.

You will ask a lot of your feet, walking approximately 115,000 miles during your lifetime — the equivalent of four strolls around the Earth's circumference. No wonder your feet occasionally demand some fast action!

EASE THE PAIN OF BUNIONS

A bunion is a troublesome growth of bone on the outside of the big toe. Pain comes from walking improperly or because your shoe is pressing against that out-of-place bone.

If you're younger than 30, chances are your bunions are inherited, and like relatives you don't like, they're difficult to get rid of. If you're 40-something plus, they're like unwanted friends you wish you hadn't met.

Wear kinder, gentler shoes. Soft shoes can immediately ease the pain, especially if they're extra wide around the toes.

Line your shoes with a soft orthotic device. These products can help absorb shock and take pressure off sore spots.

Soak your feet in warm water. A 10-minute warm soak will give quick, temporary relief from all kinds of foot ailments, bunions included. Also, you can speed up healing of mild bunions with whirlpool baths and ultrasound.

Take aspirin. But don't overdo it. It's a temporary solution at best. Follow the instructions on the bottle. If pain-relieving methods don't work, see your doctor.

Opt for bunion surgery. This long-term solution takes only 30 to 40 minutes. "Generally you're walking within a day or two," Dr. Ellis says.

HIGH TECH

QUICK RECOVERY WITH NEW BUNION SURGERY

Walk away after bunion surgery?

Yes, it's now possible.

By combining bioengineering and a single screw, it's not only possible to get back on your feet quickly after bunion surgery, it's also possible to do so almost free of pain.

With traditional surgery to correct that out-of-place bone on the side of your big toe, you could just about count on four to five days in the hospital. And you would have to wear a cast and limit your walking for several months.

The new surgery is done on an outpatient basis—no hospital stay. And you're back in normal shoes in about three weeks.

You can thank the surgical screw for much of this—it keeps the realigned bones in place after surgery. You'll have to have follow-up visits, and the screw must be removed four to seven months later. But in the meantime you can walk with relatively little pain.

COOL ADVICE FOR BURNING FEET

"There are probably 45 or 50 different causes of burning feet," says John McCrea, D.P.M., a podiatrist in private practice in Beloit, Wisconsin. "But the most common causes that don't involve disease are an excess of sweat or friction, or a reaction to nylon stockings."

Some of the potentially serious causes of which you should be aware are diabetes, alcoholism, and circulation problems.

Another fairly common possibility, according to Dr. Ellis, is neuroma—a nerve inflammation often found between the third and fourth toes.

Wear a metatarsal pad. This cushion, which goes under the ball of the foot, is a fast way to cool the burn.

Switch to cotton-blend socks. This will help hold irritation and friction in check.

Slide into a pair of loose-fitting shoes. Or drop a pair of insoles into your shoes, to further reduce friction.

Let your feet breathe. Shoes made of leather, for example, are ideal. Synthetic materials and rubber, on the other hand, don't breathe, notes Marvin Sandler, D.P.M., author of *Your Guide to Foot Care*.

"Many shoes have their tops and sides made of synthetic materials," according to Dr. Sandler. "Golfers, for example, commonly complain of burning feet on hot days. Rubber soles create heat because of the friction involved and also fail to dissipate heat as well as leather does. Even rubber boots for rain and snow can be responsible for hot, burning feet."

CALLUSES: HANDLING THE PRESSURE

A callus is your body's response to excessive pressure or friction—it's actually there to protect you. And often calluses, though rather unsightly, don't hurt.

But sometimes calluses can be painful—especially those found on the balls of your feet.

Soak your feet, then brush them. Use this two-pronged remedy only if calluses aren't very thick and are causing only minor discomfort, suggests Suzanne M. Levine, D.P.M., a podiatrist and author of *My Feet Are Killing Me* and *Walk It Off*. After brushing with an abrasive brush, spread a soothing cream to soften the callus.

Paste your calluses. For really painful calluses, Dr. Levine suggests the following: Take five or six aspirin tablets, crush them into a powder, and mix with 1 tablespoon of water and 1 tablespoon of lemon juice. Make a paste, and apply it all over your calluses. Then put your feet into a plastic bag and wrap them with a warm towel. Sit like this for 10 minutes. Then unwrap your feet, and using a pumice stone (a rough-edged stone for smoothing skin, available in drugstores), vigorously scrub your feet. The dead, callused skin should flake away.

Slip a Spenco insole into your shoes. This is another quick way to relieve discomfort, Dr. Ellis says. These shock-absorbing insoles are made of the same rubberlike material used in skin divers' wet suits.

To get even more benefits from your Spenco insoles, add lipstick. What? Allow Dr. Sandler to explain.

"Mark the callus with lipstick and place your foot carefully in the shoe, trying not to smear the lipstick. After you walk a few feet, remove the shoe and observe the area marked with lipstick. Use rubber cement or glue to place strips of moleskin, foam, or felt around the area. Then, when you walk, you will put more weight on the pads than on the calluses."

HOW TO COPE WITH CORNS

These hard growths on the toes are usually caused by—you guessed it—friction from your shoes.

Cushion your corns. Insert small, cushioned pads or apply moleskin at the sore spots. While you're at it, tape the toes down. This combined strategy reduces friction with the shoe.

Give your toes some room. Switch to a style of shoe with wide toes. As with most foot problems, this is a natural option to try, according to Dr. Ellis.

Try the four-day wine soak. Glenn Copeland, D.P.M., author of *The Foot Doctor*, details a more unusual remedy introduced to him by one of his patients: Soak your foot in warm water. At the same time, soak a corn pad in red wine, then in a 10 percent solution of salicylic acid. Next apply the corn pad to the corn and leave it on for four days. After four days, soak the foot in warm water again, and this time the corn should be ready to come out. Dr. Copeland says this isn't a permanent solution, but if it provides temporary relief, why not?

Be wary of over-the-counter solutions "guaranteed" to make the corns go away, says Clare Starrett, D.P.M., a podiatrist with the Foot and Ankle Institute of the Pennsylvania College of Podiatric Medicine in Philadelphia. "If it's strong enough to remove a corn, it's strong enough to burn skin. We see a lot of people with chemical burns."

Opt for minor surgery. It's safer than playing around with acid solutions, and according to Dr. Ellis, it only takes about 15 minutes to remove the source of the problem. The result is long-lasting relief.

QUICK CONTROL MEASURES FOR ATHLETE'S FOOT

Those television commercials about athlete's foot—the ones where feet appear literally afire—aren't too far from the truth. Athlete's foot, a skin disease caused by a fungus, can leave your feet burning. And itching. And cracking. And blistering.

Do nothing and you can expect chronic discomfort. Spend just a little time and you can expect relief.

Slip on a pair of thongs. It only takes a few seconds to put them on, and you'll have more protection, especially in high foot-traffic areas such as the showers and locker rooms in health clubs. If somebody else is walking around with athlete's foot, you won't be inviting your own personal foot fire.

Dry between your toesies. Take a moment to thoroughly dry between the toes after bathing, Dr. McCrea advises. Drying is important because athlete's foot usually gains its toehold (literally) on the skin between your toes. And moisture makes it possible. Shoes, unfortunately, create an almost junglelike atmosphere—warm, dark, humid. That's the ideal environment for fostering fungus. So you'll also want to expose your feet to sunlight in your fight against fungus.

Change your socks two or three times a day. This is a good idea because it prevents moisture from building up, Dr. McCrea says. "You can also use Odor-Eaters insoles to absorb perspiration in the shoes," Dr. McCrea adds.

Change your shoes regularly. Sitting out a day or two gives shoes time to dry out, especially if you wear light and airy shoes whenever possible, to reduce perspiration and discourage fungus growth.

Soak your feet in a solution of salt and warm water. That's the advice from Dr. Copeland. The saline solution provides an unattractive environment for the fungus, while at the same time softening the affected skin.

Apply an antifungal over-the-counter cream or powder. Dr. McCrea recommends antifungal products for mild cases of athlete's foot. Tinactin is an effective, non-prescription antifungal medication worth trying. Applying it after soaking your feet helps the medication penetrate more deeply.

Powder both your feet and your shoes. Podiatrists say this maximizes the powder's effectiveness.

Apply a hydrocortisone cream. Hydrocortisone is medicine, and using it is considered aggressive action, warranted if the itching just won't stop, Dr. McCrea says. "Within a day or two, you'll see the itching start to subside." But be careful: More than a week of use can cause "rebound" itching and a rash.

TAKING THE SORENESS OUT OF BLISTERS

Excess friction and perspiration are the twin culprits here. "And because the fluid that builds up inside a blister is a perfect growth medium for bacteria, infection is a real possibility," Dr. Ellis says.

Carry tape. Prevention is much easier and faster than healing, says Frederic Haberman, M.D., a sports dermatologist and clinical instructor of medicine at Albert Einstein College of Medicine in New York City. That's why he takes a roll of adhesive tape to any marathon where he's serving as a doctor. Runners who feel a blister threatening to form should simply cut a small piece of tape and gently place it directly over the sore spot. The same trick, he says, will work on any part of the body where your skin starts to feel irritated from friction.

Give yourself a second skin. If you have to repeat

the action that caused the blister and you can't wait for it to heal, try Spenco's 2nd Skin dressing. This clear, jellylike, spongy substance that comes in sheets or small patches will absorb pressure and reduce friction against your already troubled skin. Rub a little petroleum jelly on the blister, cover it with the 2nd Skin, then tape it in place.

Yield to temptation—pop the blister. "If you pop the blister promptly, within the first couple of hours, the skin layer will adhere back quickly," Dr. Ellis says. "I recommend popping them right after you get them."

Here's how to do it: Clean the area with alcohol, heat a clean needle or pin in a flame, and then pop the blister. "Afterward, be sure to leave the skin on" so it can heal over, Dr. Ellis says. As an added precaution, you may want to cover the remaining skin with a bandage or sterile piece of gauze or tape.

Soap your socks. If blisters are a frequent problem, here's what to do: Turn your socks inside out. Then take a bar of soap and rub it over them. Put the socks back on your feet with the soaped side next to your skin. "That's a little trick I learned from professional basketball players," Dr. McCrea says. It's a great idea for avid tennis and racquetball players, too.

Cushion your feet with drop-in shoe insoles. The extra padding can further reduce friction and perspiration.

Put some moleskin at the point of pressure. Moleskin helps to head off future trouble. "But if you already have a blister, don't use moleskin, because when you take it off it could rip off the blister," Dr. Starrett says. In such situations, Dr. Starrett recommends, use 2nd Skin.

A FRESH PERSPECTIVE ON FOOT ODOR

Just about everybody has at least occasional problems with foot odor—just ask ten people in a crowded room to take off their shoes and see, or smell, what happens.

The breakdown of bacteria on your skin typically causes foot odor. And bacteria love sweat, so if your feet perspire a lot, you can expect foot odor to be worse.

Wash your feet daily. This is a good first step, so to speak, but you probably do that already.

Change your socks and shoes. Frequent changes

don't take much time and don't cost anything. It's a good way to reduce perspiration.

Wash walking or running shoes. If footwear is washable, wash it.

Line your shoes with Odor-Eaters insoles. These inexpensive devices are another easy way to fight the foul foot. Also, replace old insoles.

Roll on some deodorant. "The best thing is to use the same antiperspirant you use under your arms on your feet," Dr. McCrea says. "After all, sweat ducts are sweat ducts." If you want to minimize the risk of skin irritation, use a roll-on, he suggests.

Give your feet some tea time. Soak your feet in a strong solution of tea for 15 minutes twice a day. This is another good way to reduce perspiration.

Or bathe your feet in vinegar. For chronic foot odor, wash your feet three or four times a week in warm water and vinegar. About a half-cup of the latter will do.

HALTING HEEL PAIN

Most of the time, if your heel hurts, it's because you have a heel spur, according to Dr. Levine.

"This is a bony protrusion on the bottom of your foot caused by a growth of calcium that has begun to project downward and is touching your plantar fascia . . . that thick piece of tissue underneath the skin on the sole of your foot that extends from your heel to the ball of your foot," she says.

How do you know if that's what your problem is? You'll need to see a doctor to be sure, "but the key is what it feels like first thing in the morning," Dr. Ellis advises. "If it hurts worse when you first get up, but then warms up," you've probably got a spur.

What to do?

Take aspirin or acetaminophen. An over-the-counter analgesic, such as aspirin or acetaminophen, can alleviate acute pain.

Rest. Even a couple of days of limited movement will help reduce the inflammation around a bone spur.

Prop up your feet and ice them. Twenty minutes of ice and elevation at a stretch should help.

Pad your heels with cushions. A variety of heel pads is available at drugstores.

Protect your feet with arch supports. If your heel pain is associated with a weak arch, this is a good, quick measure to take. Or start wearing running shoes, which usually come with good arch support, Dr. Ellis advises.

Ask your doctor about a nerve block. "This is the most dramatic treatment," Dr. Sandler notes. "It blocks the tibial nerve at the ankle using a local anesthetic. After the bottom portion of the foot is anesthetized, an anti-inflammatory steroid can be injected directly into the area of the spur." This procedure, performed by a podiatrist, provides immediate pain relief.

FIRST-AID FOR INGROWN TOENAILS

The side of your nail is poking—no, make that digging—into your skin. Ouch!

Simply cutting the nail improperly—at a curve or too short—could have started the problem, according to Dr. Levine. "Nails should always be cut straight across," she notes.

Give your toes elbow room. Change to a looser-fitting shoe. "Or cut out the portion of your shoe that presses on the toes, or wear toeless sandals if you live in a warm climate," Dr. Levine suggests. These strategies avoid putting pressure on the painful spot.

Slather on an antibiotic cream. Doing so can reduce inflammation, Dr. McCrea adds.

Soak your toes in a solution of Epsom salts. An Epsom salt footbath can help draw out infection.

ON-THE-BALL RELIEF FOR METATARSAL PAIN

This is pain in the ball of the foot. Any pain in this area could originate in nerves, muscles, blood vessels, bones, joints, ligaments, tendons, or bursae.

Often, Dr. McCrea says, it's a matter of joints, or the tendons covering the joints, becoming inflamed. "For some people, it's an architectural problem," Dr. Starrett adds. "Usually a high-arched foot gets more of this kind of pain."

Ice your feet for 20 minutes. Applying ice is a fast, safe way to reduce that inflammation, Dr. Ellis says.

Take an over-the-counter pain reliever. Analgesics provide quick, temporary relief, but you'll also want to make other, more long-lasting—though still easy to implement—changes.

Kick off your shoes. As with other foot problems, shoes often are partly to blame. So try wearing shoes less, perhaps wearing slippers instead.

Plunk in insoles or pads. Adding cushioned insoles or metatarsal pads to your shoes may be all the help you need.

Take a 5-minute break every hour or so. Don't rule out the possibility that you have simply overused your feet. If that proves to be the case, take a load off for a short while, and you probably can prevent having to stay off your feet longer later.

GETTING RID OF PLANTAR WARTS

These warts usually grow on the bottom of the foot, but they can also occur on the top and sides. They are caused by a virus, which typically enters the skin through a cut or other opening.

There are over-the-counter solutions designed for treating plantar warts, but Dr. McCrea doesn't recommend them because they can easily spread the virus and just produce more warts.

Phone a pro. Freezing or burning plantar warts (a procedure easily done in a doctor's office) "usually is a one-shot deal," Dr. McCrea says. But it will take several weeks for the affected areas on the foot to completely heal. Another possible option is laser surgery, which takes only a few minutes, Dr. Ellis says. "The wart is gone, and in a few days the skin is healed."

SOOTHE THOSE SWOLLEN FEET

Everyone's feet tend to swell a little as the day goes on—that's why it's best to buy shoes later in the day—but major swelling could be sign of a significant health problem.

Swollen feet could be associated with kidney disease,

congestive heart problems, or varicose veins, Dr. Starrett says. For this reason, you need to be checked by a doctor if there is severe swelling.

Of course an injury, such as an ankle sprain, could cause your foot to swell. So could an infection from a splinter or mosquito bite.

Elevate your feet and give them a rest. This is easy enough and can bring surprisingly fast results.

Put your feet on ice. Another time-tested treatment for bringing down swelling is to ice your feet for 20 minutes. As with heel pain, you should elevate your feet while icing, Dr. Ellis says.

Give your feet a quick massage. A few minutes of gentle kneading can both bring down swelling and make feet feel better, Dr. Levine advises. "Massage is especially useful after surgery on the foot," she explains. It increases circulation to the injured area, and that helps speed recovery.

Best of all, you can massage your own feet. Dr. Levine recommends warming your feet first. This is easily done by running a bath and dangling your feet in the water.

"Try starting with warm water, slowly increase the temperature and then decrease it again . . . to make your feet feel tingly and fresh," she suggests.

To begin the massage, sit with one leg crossed over the other with the sole of the foot facing up, Dr. Levine explains. "Your thumbs are your massage tools; use both of them in deep, circular motions, concentrating on very small areas at a time."

Slowly work your way from the tips of your toes to your heel. All movement, and the greatest pressure, should be exerted in the direction of the heart, she says, to help get "stagnated" circulation moving again. Continue working in this direction with your thumbs from toes to ankle to calf.

TIRED, ACHING FEET NEED A LIFT

"Your feet shouldn't hurt at the end of the day," Dr. Starrett says, "even if they have been holding up a body waiting on tables all day. If there is a problem, usually structural causes, such as flat feet, are to blame," she says.

Lace up a pair of running shoes. And wear them whenever possible, Dr. Starrett advises. "They are one of the best cure-alls we have now. Look around, and you'll see a lot of 70-year-old women wearing running shoes. They provide both support and cushioning."

Soak your feet in warm water. Sound familiar? This quick tip is a fast, albeit temporary, fix. Certainly, there's no disputing how good a warm foot soak feels.

Exercise to make your feet stronger. In some cases, tired feet may just be not-well-conditioned feet. These exercises, recommended by experts, take just a few seconds to do. But they may reward you with long-lasting relief.

First, point your toes outward for a few seconds, then flex them inward. Alternate standing on tiptoe for a few seconds with normal standing. Repeat each exercise ten times.

To strengthen heel and calf muscles, sit on the floor with your legs straight ahead, then bend your feet toward you as far as possible.

To alleviate arch strain and pain, rest your weight on the outer sides of your feet, then roll them inward.

Finally, strengthen your toes and the muscles on top of the foot by sitting in a relaxed position with your bare feet on the floor. Attempt to pick up an object, such as a towel or pencil, with your toes.

HABITS

. . . .

Habits are nature's built-in efficiency engineers. We all have habitual ways of speaking, driving, writing, eating, thinking, dressing, solving problems, and carrying out many other daily tasks. They free us up for life's more interesting and enjoyable aspects. Habits enable us not only to walk and chew gum at the same time, but to smell the roses along the way.

That's the good news. The bad news is that sometimes our habits can turn on us, when they have outlived their original purpose or reveal a compulsive dark side. None of us develops a hurtful habit on purpose. If you look closely enough, you'll always discover a positive purpose behind every habit.

Take the guy, for example, who took up cigarette smoking years ago as a way to relax at work. Now, however, he realizes that smoking could "relax" him right out of a long and healthy life.

Knowing that you have a harmful habit is one thing. Putting a stop to it is quite another. We humans *are* creatures of habit. But compare the few weeks of discomfort you might go through in order to quit smoking, for example, to the painful years you could end up suffering from emphysema or other diseases linked to cigarettes. A little effort goes a long way.

For example, you can:

- Make yourself sick of smoking in just 15 minutes.
- Learn how habituated you are to alcohol in two weeks.
- Wean yourself from caffeine in only three weeks.

If you aim to change several habits, start with the one that you find least addictive or troublesome. Give yourself at least eight weeks to get that habit under control before you move on to the next one.

NIPPING THE NICOTINE HABIT

Cigarette smoking, in case you haven't heard, kills an estimated 390,000 Americans each year. Cigarette smoking is a leading risk factor for death from cardiovascular disease. It is responsible for 83 percent of all lung cancer cases and accounts for almost one-third of all cancer deaths. Smoking is also the leading cause of bronchitis and emphysema, diseases in which the lungs lose their ability to function.

Your risk of heart disease starts decreasing the instant you quit smoking. Your risk for lung cancer decreases until, after about 13 years, it's almost as low as that of the person who never smoked. Problems with chronic bronchitis usually disappear. Even people already suffering from emphysema start feeling better and can live longer.

But quitting tobacco is tough. "Nicotine strikes you with a double-edged sword of addiction," says Frank Etscorn, Ph.D., a smoking researcher, professor of psychology, and dean of students at the New Mexico Institute of Mining and Technology.

"First, you smoke in order to feel good or because of peer pressure." Cigarettes give you something to do when you're feeling restless or artificially calm you down during times of stress. But once you're hooked on cigarettes "you smoke in order to avoid withdrawal symptoms," he says.

"Nicotine is a very addictive drug, more addictive than heroin or cocaine or crack," says Charlotte Kosek, director of the smoking cessation program at Hinsdale Hospital near Chicago. "It's hard to quit because a smoker is accustomed to having some level of nicotine in his system all the time."

Difficult though quitting may be, one survey showed that almost half of those who reported ever smoking are now ex-smokers. Plan to join their ranks without delay. Here's how.

Set a date. Name the specific day when you intend to quit, advises Dee Burton, Ph.D., a former consultant on smoking to the American Cancer Society and author of *Fresh Start: 21 Days to Stop Smoking.* "Make it no more than three weeks from today. And start psyching yourself up in advance," Dr. Burton recommends.

Quit on your own. Most quitters do, according to a report from the University of Wisconsin at Madison, and they are almost twice as likely to succeed as those who seek help from a smoking cessation program. But self-quitters may succeed because they are relatively lighter smokers in the first place (less than 25 cigarettes a day). Heavier smokers, the researchers say, may still benefit from professional help.

Count down to Q-Day. "If you generally do your best work by taking small, incremental steps toward a goal," Dr. Burton says, "you may want to do the same with the goal of becoming an ex-smoker." So start tapering off a

HIGH TECH • DEVELOPING A HEALTHY NEGATIVE ATTITUDE

A group of aspiring ex-smokers hold their cigarettes awkwardly between the last two fingers of the hand they normally do *not* smoke with, puffing but not inhaling. At the same time, they watch a slide show that juxtaposes cigarette advertisements with pictures of organs diseased by smoking. Meanwhile, an irritating "white noise" tape plays in the background, and an instructor reads a script informing them that they're not receiving any enjoyment from cigarettes but are in fact feeling a growing ability to control the habit. As the room grows thick with smoke, the whole scene is looking pretty darn ridiculous.

Even die-hard smokers find it impossible to enjoy a cigarette during this "negative smoking" technique, says Don R. Powell, Ph.D., president of the American Institute for Preventive Medicine and creator of the Smokeless Program.

Conducted during the last 10 minutes of each of four 1½-hour quit-smoking classes, negative smoking helps smokers develop negative associations to the habit that affect all five senses—sight, smell, taste, touch, and sound. Additional aversive techniques include fast digit-dragging, in which a person puffs very rapidly on a cigarette, and smoke-holding, in which he takes smoke in his mouth, swishes it around without inhaling, and blows it out.

Participants are also taught to imaginatively reexperience the sickening experience later should a craving for a cigarette strike, effectively short-circuiting the urge.

A self-help version of the Smokeless Program, including a cassette tape and visual aids, is available from the American Institute for Preventive Medicine, 24450 Evergreen, Suite 200, Southfield, MI 48075-5518.

few cigarettes a day for a week or so before quitting day, and then on Q-Day, stop totally.

Join a program for puffers. If you'd like professional help, sign up with a local smoking cessation program. There, over a period of several weeks and in the company of fellow aspiring ex-smokers, you'll receive valuable guidance and group support to see you through any physical or psychological trauma that quitting can bring on.

Get sick of smoking. Aversion therapy helps break strong habits. Your therapist might, for instance, have you take a puff on a cigarette every 6 seconds, something that makes most smokers sick of smoking in about 15 minutes. Research has shown that this technique, when used in conjunction with other antismoking therapies, is helpful to about half the smokers who want to quit.

Chew gum. Popping a wad of nicotine gum (available by prescription) into your mouth, bitter though it may taste, can help relieve withdrawal symptoms and reduce temporary weight gain, especially for heavy smokers. For best results, chew the gum very slowly until you sense a peppery taste or slight tingling in your mouth. This is usually after about 15 chews, but the number of chews varies from person to person. Then "park" the gum between the cheek and gums and don't chew it again until the taste and tingling are almost gone (about a minute). Then chew slowly again until the taste or tingling returns. Then stop chewing and "park" the gum again, using a different location in the mouth. Ten to 12 pieces per day of 1-milligram gum during the early stages of quitting should suffice. Not more than 30 pieces of 2-milligram gum should be chewed in any one day. The gum immediately frees your system of tar and carbon monoxide, two of the deadliest substances in tobacco. It also releases lower levels of nicotine than cigarettes. As you get accustomed to being a nonsmoker, gradually cut back on chewing the gum, stopping altogether within three to six months.

Put on a patch. Offering the benefits of nicotine gum but in more consistent dosages and without the icky taste is a new patch containing nicotine, developed by Dr. Etscorn. Over a period of 6 to 8 hours, nicotine contained in the small, bandagelike patch is gradually absorbed through the skin at just about any place you attach it. Most quitters, says Dr. Etscorn, will want to put one on first thing in the morning when they'd normally be having their first and most satisfying cigarette of the day. Shortly, nicotine starts flowing through the bloodstream. Heavy smokers will probably need to put a fresh patch on later in the day. A one-month supply of the patches, available by prescription from your doctor, should help make a nonsmoker of you within a matter of weeks.

Be ready for withdrawal. Just knowing that you'll probably feel physical withdrawal symptoms may help you get through them. And realize that the symptoms show you're getting healthier immediately. They will probably be worst during the first two days after you quit smoking, Dr. Burton says. After that, all the nicotine is gone from your system.

You might feel light-headed, dizzy, or faint while your brain gets used to receiving a healthy supply of oxygen. Your arms and legs may tingle as your circulation improves. Frequent coughing is a sign that your lungs are doing their job in clearing out smoking debris. You might have a headache or feel nervous. Bear with these symptoms, remembering that they are temporary and are sure signs that your body is rebounding toward health.

Counter cravings. You may experience intense cravings for nicotine, especially during your first week as an ex-smoker (they tend to disappear after two or three weeks). Endless though they may seem, each craving actually lasts no more than 20 seconds, Dr. Burton says, and they always go away on their own, no matter what you do.

Distract yourself during a craving with one or more of these proven methods. By the time you've finished any of them, the craving will have passed.

- Touch your toes ten times.
- Jog in place while you count to 30.
- Practice deep breathing, which can help the craving pass and diminish its intensity. Inhale strongly, expanding your abdomen fully. Then exhale, taking at least twice as long as you did inhaling. Repeat this for 2 to 3 minutes to feel totally relaxed.

Cut caffeine. Caffeine worsens the symptoms of tobacco withdrawal during the stressful first few days after you quit. As a smoker, you're probably not as stimulated by coffee as a nonsmoker because your body metabolizes caffeine faster. Within four days after your last cigarette, however, your metabolism slows down and you end up with "coffee jitters" on top of smoke-quitting tensions. Two cups of coffee to an ex-smoker can feel more like five. Drink less.

Work out. For starters, take a brisk 30-minute walk every day. Exercise not only burns up calories but can help relieve stress and improve your mood. Many smokers,

Dr. Burton says, use cigarettes to comfort themselves in a "self-destructive approach to stress management." Deal with tension more effectively, she advises, by immediately engaging in some form of moderately intense exercise, from a long walk to a game of tennis. Exercise can also counteract feelings of depression, give you more energy, and help you feel better about yourself overall.

"Many people, women especially, are afraid to quit because they don't want to gain weight," Kosek says. "Regular exercise can solve that problem." Actually, she says, an ex-smoker gains an average of no more than 5 pounds, and that only temporarily, so fear of weight gain is a flimsy excuse to keep risking cancer and heart disease.

Drink lots of water. Water speeds nicotine out of your system, Dr. Burton says, so drink lots of it. All that liquid will make you temporarily bloated, which also counteracts cravings for tobacco. And, perhaps surprisingly, water acts as a natural diuretic, prompting your body to dump excess water, which helps you control or even lose weight.

Perk up with breakfast. Your slowed-down metabolism can make you awfully sluggish in the morning, Kosek says. Get going with a hearty breakfast of fresh fruit, whole wheat bread, and a glass of low-fat milk.

Suck on a cinnamon stick. The perfect oral substitute, Dr. Burton says, during your first week or two off cigarettes, cinnamon sticks resemble cigarettes in shape and size but have a refreshing flavor that makes smoking tasteless by comparison. One or two boxes from your grocery store spice rack should suffice.

Fill up on fruits and vegetables. "Tobacco is a taste bud toxin," Dr. Etscorn says. "Seven days after quitting smoking, your deadened taste buds are renewed." Food not only tastes better when you quit smoking, but you might want more of it because nicotine tended to suppress your appetite. Satisfy your hunger, Dr. Etscorn advises, by adding a variety of raw vegetables and fruits to your already balanced diet.

Choose sour over sweet. Many ex-smokers develop a craving for sweets. Interestingly, Dr. Burton says, eating something sour like plain yogurt or a dill pickle often satisfies the urge.

Treat yourself without calories. Avoid using food as

● FLOATING FREE OF TOBACCO

Relaxation can eliminate cravings while you withdraw from nicotine and can rid you of nervousness you might feel during your first couple of weeks as an ex-smoker, says Dr. Dee Burton. Following is her "Floating Exercise," which she suggests you practice in 15-minute sessions twice a day.

Seated comfortably in a chair, look straight up toward your eyebrows, then higher toward the top of your head. Slowly close your eyes all the way, and relax your eyeballs. Take a deep breath and hold it for a second. Slowly exhale until your body feels very limp and relaxed.

Close out all the sounds around you. Think only of your body and this experience. Imagine that you have an infinite amount of time available to concentrate on getting your body more comfortable and relaxed. Relax your body slowly, feeling a pleasant, tingling sensation flow through you from the top of your head to the tips of your toes.

Breathe deeply, slowly, and regularly. Notice as your breathing becomes easier and deeper, you feel more and more relaxed. Notice a feeling of lightness spreading throughout your body. You are becoming so light that you feel like you're floating. See yourself floating through space, feeling very light, very easy, very peaceful, and very secure. Use your imagination to become more and more involved in the fantasy of floating through space, being totally surrounded by space, floating farther and farther away from the world, lightly and happily floating.

And now, with your eyes still closed, roll your eyeballs up toward the top of your head. Open your eyes slowly. You will feel totally relaxed and alert.

a reward for quitting smoking. Stick to calorie-free indulgences like buying some new clothing or sleeping late on Saturday.

Shed a tear. Getting over cigarettes can be a very emotional experience, because smoking is as psychologically addictive as it is physically addictive—sometimes even more so.

To some people, letting go of cigarettes, Kosek says, is like losing a close friend. Others turn to cigarettes to experience feelings of pleasure and become frustrated in their sudden absence.

So go ahead and express your emotions. "If you feel like crying, cry," Dr. Burton says. "If you're angry, let out a good yell." The more you release these feelings, she says, the sooner they will be out of your system—usually within a couple of weeks.

Take it easy. "If you have surgery, you don't expect to get off the table and go right on to normal activity," Kosek says. "Quitting smoking is the same thing. You've let go of a big addiction and need time to recover."

Take a day off, she advises, or a week. Get more shut-eye. "If you need to sleep 12 hours a day, do it," she says. "Whatever it takes to heal, do it."

Pick yourself up if you slip. Quitting smoking sometimes doesn't stick the first time. If you slip, which many people do, be easy on yourself. "It's like a child learning to walk," Kosek says. "If he takes a few steps and then falls, his mother doesn't grab him and yell, 'Forget it, kid, you'll never make it!' If you slip, try again. Give yourself another chance at a healthier way of life."

POURING DRINKING DOWN THE DRAIN

A couple of beers or an occasional glass of wine is a truly enjoyable activity for many people. But when it comes to overindulgence, there's a high price to pay, from the actual cost of the drinks to the loss of precious hours that could have been spent in more positive, creative activity. And if you've been drinking away from home, you could face the life-threatening (and illegal) danger of driving while drunk. If you survive that, you may still have a head-splitting hangover and a full day of fuzzy thinking to look forward to, as well as possible ill effects on your health and relationships. And as if all this weren't bad enough, perhaps you have a growing—and healthy—sense that there's more to life than spending every evening engaged in less-than-intelligible conversations with total strangers at the local pub.

Some people have serious addictive problems with alcohol. (See "Abstaining from Alcoholism" on the opposite page). But not everyone does. "The reality is that there will always be some people who are drinking abusively in reaction to temporary situations of stress, and others who drink heavily but have not yet lost control over their ability to stop drinking after two or three drinks," says alcoholism expert Lawrence Metzger, Ph.D., author of *From Denial to Recovery.*

Even if your drinking is less advanced, quitting may lead to some withdrawal symptoms, among them anxiety, upset stomach, diarrhea, weakness, sweating, irritability, sleeping difficulties, and an indifference to food. But don't worry. These discomforts are likely to last no more than 36 hours after your last drink, Dr. Metzger says.

Here are fast and effective ways to handle a habit that's manhandling you.

Start a drinking diary. Carry a pen or pencil and a pocket-size notebook with you at all times. For at least two weeks, keep an immediate and accurate written record of your drinking, including the type of drink you had, the time and place you had it, your reason for drinking, your thoughts and feelings about 20 minutes after each drink, and the consequences of drinking, including actions by yourself and reactions by others. Simply keeping track of your drinking can help you cut back, says psychologist John S. Crandell, Ph.D. Old habits die hard, often because the stimuli that set them into motion will always be there. If you always drank on Friday nights or while watching sports on television, chances are good that despite your best intentions, when Friday night rolls around or the football game goes on, you'll want to drink.

Your drinking diary, Dr. Crandell says, helps you "identify the situations in which abuse is a particular risk." You can then make plans to avoid such situations, from not walking past your favorite old bar to not making a beer your answer to feeling lonely. The mere act of having to keep a record helps some drinkers cut back, Dr. Crandell says. And seeing this improvement, they can

ABSTAINING FROM ALCOHOLISM

One-third of all Americans say that alcohol causes problems in their families, according to psychologist Dr. Lawrence Metzger. At least ten million Americans, or one out of every ten drinkers, are problem drinkers or alcoholics.

Most alcoholics have an inherited, genetic predisposition to the problem. About half the alcoholics in the United States come from families where alcoholism was prevalent. If one of your parents has a drinking problem, your chances of becoming an alcoholic are 30 percent higher than those of a person whose parent doesn't have a problem. Your risk is five times higher if both your parents are alcoholics.

Though sometimes viewed as a weakness of will or lack of moral fiber, alcoholism is actually a disease, much like diabetes. Both are *chronic* and *progressive.* Chronic means that there is no cure, that the physical sensitivity to alcohol will last as long as the person remains alive. And progressive means the symptoms will increase in number and seriousness as long as the disease is untreated.

For alcoholics, what began as an enjoyable activity eventually, over a period of years, starts causing problems, from bouts of uncontrollable drinking to serious and life-threatening health problems that can include gastric ulcers, liver disorders, heart disease, dysfunctions in the immune system, sexual dysfunctions, and destruction of brain tissue.

If you think that you or someone you know has a drinking problem, contact a local hospital or alcoholism treatment program for professional assessment. The next step may be Alcoholics Anonymous, the highly successful (and free) 12-step program that combines self-responsibility with a strong support group.

Depending on how advanced the drinking is, checking into a three- to four-week inpatient hospital or private recovery program might also be beneficial. Such a program, Dr. Metzger notes, provides medical support in the event of serious withdrawal symptoms like seizures, puts space between the drinker and the people and places that may have promoted the drinking, and offers valuable education and counseling. However, the cost of such a program can be as much as $ 10,000 a month.

become even more motivated in their efforts to drink less.

Replace alcohol with exercise. Exercise is a basic human need, Dr. Metzger says. And it's a great substitute for sitting around drinking. If you're not getting any exercise, a 20- or 30-minute walk is a good daily regimen. Run, dance, work out in a gym, or otherwise get physically active if you're feeling stronger or more energetic. These activities can quickly help you sleep better, reduce depression, and improve your self-esteem.

Go someplace new. In your first few months of cutting back or cutting out alcohol, declare all the places where you used to drink off-limits, Dr. Metzger advises. If every night was big-league drinking night at the bowling alley down the block, put your ball in storage for a while and take up another sport. If you imbibed at home, mixing drinks at your fully stocked wet bar, remove all alcohol from the premises. Get up and go someplace you've never been before. Try out a new restaurant that doesn't push drinks. Take a bike ride. Sit on a shoreline and watch a sunset.

Make new friends. Drinkers' friends are usually other drinkers and should be avoided, Dr. Metzger says. When you cut down on or quit drinking, you'll probably need to acquaint yourself with a new crowd. Join a club. Get to know your nondrinking neighbors and your co-workers.

Nourish yourself. Alcohol can interfere with the efficient absorption, transport, and storage of nutrients from your food. When you cut back or quit, do yourself the favor of eating a well-balanced diet. You may also want to take a vitamin supplement, Dr. Metzger suggests. This will start repairing tissues that might have been damaged by drinking.

Ease away anxiety. Many people drink as a way of handling stress. Develop healthier alternatives. When stress strikes, sink into a warm bath for half an hour. Immerse yourself for hours in a captivating book. Lose yourself in music. Practice a relaxation exercise. Eventually you'll feel calmer and will be glad you're relaxing in a way that's good for you.

Set goals. Set two goals, one that you can attain in three to six months, and one that may take several years. You may decide you want to take a vacation in three months. You also want to attend and graduate from college.

Next, break each goal down into a series of manageable steps. Put money aside each week for your vacation. Plan your college schedule one class or one semester at a time. While you're at it, identify possible obstacles and devise ways to overcome them. Then get a move on, thoroughly enjoying what promises to be what Dr. Crandell calls a new sense of mission in life. Moving on to new challenges can take your mind off old habits, give you self-confidence, and make you feel positive about the future.

QUITTING CAFFEINE

Coffee and other forms of caffeine aren't necessarily bad for you. A potent stimulant, caffeine triggers the release of adrenaline into your bloodstream and raises your blood sugar levels, energizing your brain and your body. One or two cups of coffee can reduce fatigue or drowsiness, increase your alertness, and quicken your reaction time. The effects peak about 30 minutes after you swallowed the last drop, and the caffeine stays in your system for 5 to 7 hours.

Caffeine drives your body to burn more fat for energy. Runners in one study were able to go for 15 minutes longer after taking the equivalent of two cups of strong coffee. In another study, caffeine-drinking bicyclists were able to pedal harder.

Contrary to what you may have heard, moderate coffee drinking has not been definitively linked in research studies to heart disease, and connections with cancer have been refuted. The key word here is "moderate," which means two or three 8-ounce cups per day. Drink more than that, though, and problems could start showing up.

A caffeine-drinking habit doesn't usually rank with such serious addictions as nicotine or certain drugs, says Manfred Kroger, Ph.D., a food science professor at Pennsylvania State University. "A person probably isn't going to walk a mile barefoot for a cup of coffee," he says. "At least not in the snow," he adds.

So far, so good, right? Energy, fat-burning, doesn't

cause cancer. But who's in control here, you or a little bitty bean? Do you feel miserable, physically and emotionally, without a bottomless cup of the brew? Are you pretty darn irritated at your apparent dependence on the stuff? If you've had it with wearing a hole in the carpet between you and the coffee machine, these tips may help you make some changes quickly.

Decaffeinate yourself. Gradually weaning yourself from caffeine over a period of three or four weeks will let your body adjust to the change and help you stick with it. Switch to low-caffeine or decaffeinated beverages to ease the transition. Or buy one can of caffeinated coffee and one can of decaf and mix your brew half-and-half. Fancy gourmet coffees often contain about one-third less caffeine than regular brands. Instant coffee's freeze-drying process reduces its caffeine to 30 to 120 milligrams per cup, compared with 50 to 150 milligrams in brewed regular coffee. Lowest of all is decaf, which contains only 2 to 5 milligrams of caffeine per cup and is also free of compounds that can give you a case of "acid stomach."

Beware of caffeine's other disguises. Tea, chocolate, and cola drinks all contain caffeine, so cut down on them, too.

Keep it to two cups. You, like many others, may feel an urgent need for caffeine first thing in the morning, says brain researcher Judith Wurtman, Ph.D., author of *Managing Your Mind and Mood through Food*. After a whole night without caffeine, your brain cells are more sensitive to the stuff when you wake up. The day's first cup of coffee will kick in within a matter of minutes, keeping you alert and on your toes for hours. Have one or at the most two cups in the morning. Have another cup if you feel the need for a pick-me-up in the late afternoon.

Outlast your withdrawal symptoms. Perhaps you prefer to part company with caffeine altogether. Go ahead —but prepare for withdrawal. (You'll feel withdrawal when you cut back, too, but not as severely.) Within 18 hours after you quit, you may feel fatigued and irritable, so soothe yourself with a long soak in a tub, a brisk walk, a nap. You may also have a throbbing headache. Caffeine makes your blood vessels contract, and when you quit cold turkey, they swell, giving you a headache. Treat it with your favorite headache remedy, but beware of headache pills containing caffeine.

Not everyone suffers from withdrawal. "Some people can go in and out of coffee drinking for weeks at a time without any effect," Dr. Kroger says. "Others who habitually drink coffee are all aflutter when they don't have it." Any withdrawal symptoms you experience may feel severe but are temporary, lasting only a few days.

Eat for alertness. If you use coffee to wake up your brain, adjust your diet to include foods that serve the same purpose. Foods containing very high protein, low amounts of fat, and almost no carbohydrates help keep your mind energized and alert, Dr. Wurtman says. Psych yourself up for a busy afternoon, for instance, by lunching on shellfish, fish, chicken without the skin, veal, very lean beef, or low-fat, high-protein dairy products. Stay away from fatty meats, hard cheeses, whole milk, and regular yogurt.

Take a break. People who feel in desperate need of a 3 o'clock coffee break probably don't need the coffee as much as they need that break, Dr. Kroger says. "Their mood has changed, their energy has gone down, and they just need a rest." When midafternoon rolls around for you, try a skim milk break or a water break or a walk around the block instead. You don't need a cup of coffee to get refreshed.

CHAPTER 21

HAIR

elilah made a big deal out of it. Rapunzel's boy-friend wanted to climb all over it. And the ancient Egyptians buried their dead with it.

Hair. Throughout the centuries, it's been a potent symbol associated with beauty, power, sensuality, and youth. In the 1960s, refusing to cut your hair meant you were part of the counter-culture. A thousand years earlier, shaving off your hair meant you were part of the church. But now, unless you're headed for the monastery, chances are pretty good that you want a whole head of it.

How fast does hair grow? Don't hold your breath. It won't win any races. Generally speaking, your head's 100,000 strands of hair crawl along at less than half an inch a month.

All hair goes through three phases throughout its growth cycle. The first phase, lasting four to five years, is the growth stage. At any given time, 85 to 90 percent of your hair is in this phase, which is followed by a short transitional period (phase two). The other 10 to 15 percent is resting (phase three) for two to three months, after which time those hairs fall out, making you feel perhaps like a shedding dog. But don't be alarmed by the fallout. Everyone loses hair every day. And according to Douglas Altchek, M.D., professor of dermatology at Mount Sinai School of Medicine in New York City, losing up to 100 strands a day is a normal part of the growth process.

If you hate watching the scary part in horror films, then close your eyes to this frightful fact: You are walking around with a headful of the living dead. The only place where your hair is actually alive is at its source, the scalp.

All the rest of your tresses, no matter how gorgeous, are strictly dead material. So although you can apply shampoos, conditioners, and rinses—which will help improve the *look* and *feel* of your hair—what you do to your scalp is crucial, says Richard Stein, Manhattan hair-care professional and author of *Set Free*. Stein likens hair to a plant. If you nourish and care for the soil (the scalp), your plant (the hair) will flourish. Makes sense, doesn't it?

So the question is, how do you get your hair in tip-top shape as fast as possible? How about:

- A 1-minute injection to stop hair loss in women?
- A 5-minute way to increase the effectiveness of your dandruff shampoo?
- A 20-minute treatment for your dry hair?

These and other timesaving, hair-saving tips are now at your fingertips.

THE CARE AND FEEDING OF YOUR HAIR

If you lived in a perfect, pollution-free environment, were in optimal physical and emotional shape, and could boast a family tree full of ancestors with thick, beautiful hair, the odds are that you'd have a gorgeous head of hair yourself. But let's face it: Thanks to the sun, pollution, harsh chemicals, daily stress, and heredity, most of us have some kind of problem. So to keep your mane mainly magnificent, here are some quick fixes for the overall health of your hair.

Hop into the shower. You wash your face every day, don't you? Why? Because your skin gets dirty and the pores get clogged. Same with your hair and scalp. Unless you're living in the middle of a crystal-clear glacier (and that presents its own problems), you have to wash the dirt, dust, cigarette smoke, and other everyday debris from your hair. Wash your hair every day with a gentle or diluted shampoo. In most cases, a single lathering will do it. A minute or two of sudsing beats a day's worth of damage from dirt.

Do the fingertip boogie. A great night of jitterbugging brings a healthy pink to your cheeks. Why not give your scalp the same good time? It needs stimulation, too.

Most hair-care professionals advise massaging the scalp with your fingertips, not your nails. Scalp massage is great for relieving tension and accelerating the removal of hair that's ready to be shed. Start at the nape of your neck with your fingers spread like starfish. Using the pads of your fingers, work forward slowly, going against the direction of your hair. Remember to maintain constant pressure while massaging. Keep it as brief as 60 seconds or as long as 10 minutes. (And if you do this while your hair is drying, it adds body, too.)

Grab a jug of distilled water. If you live in a big city, there's a good possibility that the water you're washing and rinsing your hair in is full of minerals that can dull and dry your hair. Occasionally, they even turn the hair colors that only rebellious teenagers appreciate. So a quick and easy solution is to rinse your hair with softened or distilled water. The next time you're at the supermarket, add a few gallons of this mineral-free water to your cart. Then give your locks a 60-second rinse with it after every shampoo. Your hair should appear shinier and fluffier.

Put down the brush. Believe it or not, hair-care experts and dermatologists debunk the brushing myth. Contrary to what your grandmother told you, 100 strokes a night with your favorite boar-bristle brush is not the route to shiny hair. Remember, in the days when this routine was popular, people just didn't wash their hair as often as we do. Nor did they subject it to overly drying appliances or chemicals. The "glossiness" they achieved from vigorous brushing was probably due to a combination of dust removal and the distribution of built-up scalp oils. Today, experts caution that heavy-handed brushing is apt to tear or break hair. If you feel you must brush your hair, be gentle and limit the sessions to a few minutes a couple of times a week.

Give wet hair the brush-off. Whatever you do, advise the hair-care specialists, never brush wet hair. Hair is at its most vulnerable when wet, and brushing can do real damage. If you need to detangle damp tresses, use a wide-toothed comb. Or simply spread your fingers apart and work them gently from the roots to the tips. In either case, 2 minutes of nice-and-easy untangling can save you from breaking off strands that will require months to grow back.

Double-check your diet. Vitamin and mineral deficiencies can contribute to hair problems, including dryness, brittleness, and even hair loss. "Since hair is 97 percent protein, a diet rich in protein is essential," says Howard Donsky, M.D., associate professor of medicine at the University of Toronto. "Lean meats provide protein, and most vegetables and leafy greens give you the vitamins you need for healthy hair." So take a few minutes to honestly review your eating habits. If you find they're not up to snuff, consult a doctor or nutritionist. And remember that as you get older, your ability to absorb vital nutrients may decrease, so a healthy diet is even more critical. Keep in mind that even a radical improvement in diet won't show up in your hair for several months.

RESCUE REMEDIES FOR DRY AND DAMAGED HAIR

If you're constantly complaining of hair that's flyaway or brittle and split at the ends, you've got a problem with dry hair. And it may be due to too much chemical processing (coloring, bleaching, highlighting), too much direct heat (sun, electric curlers, blow dryers), too much indoor heat in winter, or a combination of these factors. But take heart. There are lots of quickie solutions to revive those traumatized tresses.

Pour on the vinegar. Here's a super-fast way to add beautiful shine to your hair: Dilute apple-cider vinegar in water (1 part vinegar to 7 parts water) and rinse with it after your shampoo. A vinegar rinse is also great for overprocessed hair. And it livens up a tired perm, too.

Cream and steam. Creams and oils are great for your skin, and the truth is, they're wonderful for your hair and scalp, too. The general consensus among salon owners and hairstylists is that an occasional cream/wrap/steam routine works wonders for dry, lackluster hair. Start with a cream-based conditioner, says Jack Myers, director of the National Cosmetology Association. Massage it into your scalp and hair, then wrap your head in a hot towel. Sit tight for 20 to 30 minutes. The heat acts as a catalyst for deep penetration. When the towel cools, rinse your hair with diluted vinegar (see above) and get ready for some shine!

Dress your hair. Since many hair-care experts say that mayonnaise makes a good overall conditioner, try leaving it on your hair for anywhere from 5 minutes to an hour. Just make sure to shampoo it out thoroughly.

Pull the plug. Electricity did wonders for Frankenstein and his bride, but did you ever notice their hair? For your crowning glory, pack away your electric appliances, or at least use them less often. You'll save both time and hair wear-and-tear. Overuse of electric curlers—as well as blow dryers and curling irons—damages and dries out hair. "If you're using electric curlers every day," says Steven Docherty of Vidal Sassoon, "then your haircut isn't working for you. Try a different cut or even a loose perm." If you must use a blow dryer, Docherty recommends that you use one with no more than 1,000 watts, and reduce the temperature and power level as your hair dries.

Let your fingers do the walking. Whenever possible, just let your hair air dry. But with this simple, body-building technique, you can get the same fullness a blow dryer would help achieve: Gently fluff and style the hair with your fingers as it dries, always lifting the hair up off the scalp. Bending over as you work lets gravity help contribute extra fullness. Finger drying is especially advisable if you have split ends, which are so vulnerable to further damage from heat.

Attach and diffuse. If you must use a blow dryer, protect your hair with a diffuser, a device available in drugstores and beauty supply shops. It takes but a second to snap this attachment on to your blow dryer. And it does exactly what the name implies: It diffuses the heat so it's not blasting directly on your hair.

Don't be power hungry. Furthermore, turn off your blow dryer—with or without a diffuser—*before* your hair is completely dry. Letting your slightly damp hair dry on its own for those final few minutes minimizes any damage the blow dryer might inflict.

Crank up the humidifier. Nothing is worse for dry hair than dry indoor air. So when winter rolls around, counteract the standard low-moisture environment with a humidifier. The few minutes it takes to fill and clean the appliance as needed pay great dividends in hair health. And if the humidifier is located in your bedroom, your hair can benefit from 8 hours of added moisture every night.

Use sun sense. Don't think you're home free when summer arrives. Humidity may be high, but so's the sun. And too much sun is as damaging to your hair as it is to your skin, making your locks dry, brittle, and dull. If you can't limit sun exposure, make it a point to apply a conditioner that contains sunscreen after shampooing. In a pinch, you can even rub some of your regular sunscreen on your hair.

Keep it under your hat. Chic chapeaus and smart sunbonnets are back in style. And they're an ultra-quick alternative to sunscreen application—it takes just a second to don a protective hat before venturing out in the summer sun.

Baby your hair. To protect your hair from chlorine damage when swimming, set aside a few seconds to apply baby oil before taking the plunge. Use about ½ teaspoon—more if your hair is long—and work it in. The oil coats hair shafts and prevents them from absorbing the harsh chlorine. After your dip, shampoo the oil out.

SPLIT ENDS: TIMESAVING TIPS FOR YOUR TIPS

Contrary to the popular oldie "Breaking Up Is Hard to Do," when it comes to split ends, breaking up is much too easy. You suffer from split ends when the hair sheath literally splits up toward the scalp. Almost everybody who has hair has to deal with the problem. Split ends can be due to everything from chemical abuse (dyes and bleaching) and excessive heat to tearing your hair with a brush or comb when it's wet. Here are some quick fixes for this universal problem.

Apply a light dressing. If you have curly hair and you absolutely must look fabulous in minutes, try spraying some baby oil lightly on the ends of your hair. It temporarily closes the split ends by coating them. But take it easy—you don't want to smell like a baby or have greasy-looking hair.

Protect the tips. If you simply insist on curling your hair, at least give up your electric curler habit — which no doubt contributed to your problem in the first place. Instead, try this ends-saving tip: Wrap the very ends of your hair in rags or the old-fashioned spongy rods. That will keep the hair from coming in direct contact with the curler and protect it from potentially damaging direct heat.

Dial a cure. Of course, the quickest *cure* for split ends is to pick up the phone and call your favorite salon to schedule a good old-fashioned haircut. The split ends get snipped off in seconds. And if you take proper care from then on, you can discourage their return. (But don't play barber at home. Too often you'll do a cockeyed job. Schedule frequent trims to keep your hair looking its best over the long haul.)

RAPID RECOVERY FOR OILY HAIR

If you have oily hair, you know it. And it's generally due to overactive sebaceous glands in your scalp. Don't fret, though. There are lots of speedy ways to deal with that excess and transform your problem hair into a beautiful mane.

Flip on the faucet. It's simple advice but the most potent. Wash your hair as often as necessary — twice a day if you must. Your goal is a clean, oil-free scalp, and if a 10-minute wash does the trick, it's time well spent.

Use the right products. Choose a shampoo formulated especially for oily hair. Then increase its effectiveness by lathering up and leaving the shampoo on your hair and scalp for about 5 minutes. That gives the product extra time to cut through the oil. If your problem's really bad, lather a second time. And either forgo conditioners — which often contain oil — or reach for a brand that's oil-free.

Squeeze a lemon. A fast way to brighten up your hair and remove the excess oils and any shampoo buildup is with a homemade lemon rinse. Just squeeze the juice of two whole lemons into half a gallon of warm water. (For variety, you can use one grapefruit instead.) After shampooing thoroughly, rinse with this great-smelling water. It's that easy.

Play the piano. Or twiddle your thumbs. Or file your

nails. In other words, keep your hands away from your hair. The best thing you can do is cut down on brushing, combing, and touching your locks. Blow your hair dry and let it be. The trick is to keep the hair up and off your oil-producing scalp. Brushing and combing not only flatten the hair onto the scalp but also distribute oil from the scalp onto the hair shafts. And playing with your hair can transfer oil from your palms onto your tresses.

Change your style. If your hair is long and exceedingly oily, hairstylists agree that a good trim is in order. Why? With a fresh haircut you'll eliminate the weight of your hair and keep it from coming in contact with the oily scalp. A quick trip to the hairdresser for a layered cut on top keeps the hair fluffier and off the scalp. And your hair will have more style and versatility.

Doff your hat. Simple common sense says that if your scalp is oily, you need to let it breathe as well as keep it clean. So stop hiding your hair with a hat unless it's needed for protection from the sun. Headgear will just promote sweating and flatten your hair onto your oily scalp—double trouble. Besides, think of all the time and money you'll save *not* trying to find your hat.

DANDRUFF: HOW TO CONTROL IT . . . FAST

Unfortunately, we all know what dandruff is. Those annoying TV commercials have made it perfectly clear how embarrassing those snowy white flakes can be. Dandruff is an accelerated form of your scalp's regular cell-shedding process. A normal scalp sloughs off its dead skin, in tiny bits, every 28 days or so. Someone suffering from dandruff, on the other hand, produces oversized flakes and sheds them every 4 or 5 days. If dandruff is excessive, however, it might be a form of seborrhea or psoriasis. A dermatologist will be able to tell you if such is the case. But for normal dandruff, here are some ways to slow the snow.

Dry up. Contrary to popular belief, dandruff comes from an oily scalp. Those white flakes decorating your black sweater are not dry flakes but actually greasy scales. "Too often people think dandruff signals a dry scalp," says New Orleans dermatologist Patricia Farris, M.D., "so they start rubbing creams and moisturizers into their scalps." Your first step is to toss out those oily products.

Take five. Over-the-counter dandruff shampoos are tremendously effective, dermatologists agree. Within a few days you should see results. But for these special products to really work, says Thomas Goodman, Jr., M.D., assistant professor of dermatology at the University of Tennessee, "leave the dandruff shampoo on your scalp for a full 5 minutes. With anything less, you're undermining the shampoo's effectiveness."

Change partners. Different dandruff shampoos have different active ingredients, says Diana Bihova, M.D., clinical instructor of dermatology at New York University Medical Center. Some brands contain tar or zinc pyrithione; others have selenium sulfide, salicylic acid, sulfur, or a combination of ingredients. To get the most from their varied formulas as quickly as possible, regularly alternate among two or three products. (And because dandruff shampoos can be harsh, add a gentle baby shampoo to your rotation schedule.) One caution: Most dandruff shampoos aren't made for hair that's bleached, blonde, or gray — these ingredients can discolor light hair. But some are specially formulated for this type of hair: Check the label.

Turn on the light. The quickest way to deal with your flakes — while waiting for other remedies to work — is with camouflage, say fashion experts. Simply wear light-colored outfits so the flakes don't show. Prints and patterns are preferable to solid colors. Whatever you do, avoid dark clothes — they'll only showcase those unsightly flakes.

Say no to synthetics. Another quick way to give dandruff the brush-off is to wear natural-fiber clothing, recommends New York fashion consultant Aliceanna Brooks. "Cotton and wool release particles, such as dandruff, from their fibers more quickly than synthetic materials do." That means many of the flakes are apt to dislodge themselves as you go about your business. And they'll be easily swept away by a minute's worth of contact with a lint brush. (Carry one in your bag or briefcase for periodic dustings.)

BALDNESS — NEW HELP

If you're a man, if your hairline is receding, and if you have bald relatives on both sides of your family, then you share the genetic legacy called male pattern baldness (MPB). This condition—which results in the characteristic horseshoe pattern of a bald crown with hair on the sides and back of the head—strikes as many as 40 percent of all men in their forties, 50 percent of men in their fifties, and 60 percent of men in their sixties.

Remedies run the gamut from simple cover-ups all the way to extensive operations such as hair lifts and scalp reductions, in which sections of bald scalp are actually removed and replaced with still-viable hair. Before you opt for a big-deal treatment, try these less-exotic options.

Keep it short and sweet. Resist the urge to grow your remaining hair long and comb it over the balding area. Short hair all around looks neater and is more apt to be in proportion with your face. Further, short hair makes it easier for you to keep both your hair and your scalp clean. That's important for two reasons: First, clean hair generally looks fuller. Second, "a hormone called DHT seems to be largely responsible for MPB," says Karen Burke, M.D., a dermatologist and adjunct clinical member of The Scripps Clinic and Research Foundation in La Jolla, California. "Frequent shampooing reduces surface sebum, which contains high levels of testosterone. Testosterone converts to DHT, which may reenter the skin and accelerate hair loss in people from families with a history of male pattern baldness."

Try moving your part. After a shower, pat—don't rub—your hair dry. While it's still damp, try moving your customary part, says George Roberson, a Manhattan hairstylist and author of *Men's Hair.* Flip your part to the other side, for instance. Your hair will automatically have more lift because you're changing the root direction of the hair. So just raising or lowering your part can make your receding hairline less noticeable.

Grow a beard. You may also want to grow some facial hair to draw attention away from the top of your head and onto your face, says Roberson. Try a neat beard, a moustache, or even a goatee—whatever suits your face.

Dab on some liquid hair. Hollywood makeup artists are famous for doing wonders with large noses, bad complexions, and even balding heads. And a scalp colorant is the "instant" secret solution that dozens of well-known celebrities have been using. You simply dab some on the top of your head with a sponge and then comb the remaining hair right over. It comes in five colors (light, medium, dark brown, black, and gray), costs relatively little, and will last for at least 60 applications. Order a kit from Cinema Secrets, 4400 Riverside Drive, Burbank, CA 91505; (818-846-0579).

Buy a bowler. Instead of fretting about your naked crown, adorn it with a stylish hat. "There are many options open today for balding men," says image consultant Barbara Bonetti. "The type of hat a man chooses depends entirely on his personal style. There are peaked caps for the casual look, fedoras for business, and berets for the more eccentric streak. A Stetson on the weekend with jeans and a leather jacket is very popular. And even the English bowler, with a walking stick or umbrella, can look spectacular on the right man."

Get a rug. Another instant solution to the waning mane is a hairpiece. For between $600 and $2,000, you can get a custom-made piece that matches your existing hair to a tee. Synthetic pieces are preferable for active, sports-minded men because they hold up to weather and water better and are easier to keep clean.

Natural pieces do tend to look slightly better at first, but the harsh processing done to some hair can make it break down sooner. Often, a combination of the two types is ideal. Just remember that you get what you pay for, so don't buy a hairpiece that's going to draw more attention than your baldness. And always keep it as clean and well-groomed as your own hair.

Try a weave. It may be worth your while to try a hair weave. Natural or synthetic extensions are attached to existing hairs. Although the extensions must be repositioned every four to six weeks as the hair grows out, you may find it's less trouble then dealing with a hairpiece every day.

Flaunt it. You've paid your male dues by losing your hair. So now, pay your dues to the Bald-Headed Men of America. Shine that noble crown and strut your stuff. Baldness and virility are firmly linked in the minds of many women. Look at retired-007 Sean Connery, once voted the Sexiest Man Alive (balding head and all) by *People* magazine. Or the world-famous Kojak, Telly Savalas. And let's not forget *Time* magazine's 1989 Man of the Year, Mikhail Gorbachev. For your $10 fee, you get a lapel pin, a membership certificate, and an open invitation to celebrate your sexy head with over 20,000 men across the country. Write BHMA, 3819 Bridges Street, Morehead City, NC 28557.

Plug in your own. If flaunting it is not your style and you still have some hair, you can get a hair transplant. Dermatology professor Dr. Altchek says transplants are "100 percent successful" and are faster and more cost effective than drugs. Transplants have been around for decades and involve taking plugs of hair from one area of your head and surgically embedding them into a bald section. About $3,000 will take you through two or three sessions—and that's a substantial amount of hair (150 plugs consisting of 15 hairs each). Sessions take about 2 hours each and are repeated at four-month intervals.

Grow more of your own. If you're in your twenties or early thirties, if your hair loss started within the past five years, or if your bald spot measures only about 2 inches in diameter, you may benefit from minoxidil, the wonder drug that can help fight MPB. Minoxidil (brand name Rogaine) dilates blood vessels in the scalp, stimulating hair follicles to grow thicker hair. But it doesn't work miracles, regardless of what you've heard. It won't do a thing for a receding hairline or grow new hair in a completely bald location. Some experts say it's better at slowing loss than growing new hair—it stimulates existing follicles to become more active. Success depends on the number of follicles still there and how well they respond to minoxidil. You must apply minoxidil twice a day (it takes about 30 to 60 seconds a shot), and a year's supply can cost over $700. And if you quit, you'll lose whatever hair you gained within six months.

HAIR LOSS: THE WOMAN'S VIEW

It's an unfortunate fact of life that women, too, often face hair thinning and loss. That's in part because hair naturally thins as people age. Then, too, heredity, menopause, medications, illness, stress, or physical trauma can conspire to wreak havoc on women's hair. So the first thing you have to do is pinpoint the cause. That means a quick phone call to your doctor to schedule an appointment. A change in medication or lifestyle factors may be all that's needed to prevent further damage.

Be advised that although women don't generally suffer from male pattern baldness, many of the options described above for men are equally effective for the softer sex. Hair transplants or minoxidil, for instance, may very well be the answer; again, consult with your doctor. A different hairdo may render your thinning hair less noticeable. And remember that wigs have always been a nifty fashion accessory, even for women without hair problems. Here are some other ways to either minimize your losses or camouflage the damage.

Loosen up. Rapunzel's Prince Charming had the right idea when he begged her to let down her hair. Dermatologists and hair-care professionals agree that traumatizing thinning hair compounds the problem. So ease up on tight, pulled-back ponytails. Avoid vigorous brushing, teasing, curlers, caustic bleaches, dyes, and perms. "And don't use curlers on a wet head of hair," Dr. Goodman stresses. "When your hair dries, it shrinks, so the curlers can damage your scalp and cause you to lose more hair." Your motto should be: Do less—give your hair a rest. And conveniently, *not* doing all these things can save a lot of time.

Hit the bottle. A great natural thickening agent for thinning hair can be found near the TV in the middle of a Sunday afternoon football game. Gerry Leddy, hairstylist from David Daines Salon in New York, says beer can do wonders for your hair because of its high malt content. "Malt is the main ingredient in most hair-thickening products," he explains. "And beer actually has less drying alcohol than those products. Imported beer is the best because it's got the purest ingredients." What about smelling like a taproom after the game? Nothing to worry about. The odor evaporates completely when dry. Just pour the beer into a spray bottle mixed with water, spritz it on your wet head, and style normally. Your hair will look thicker and have great body—with just a minute's worth of effort.

IMAGING UP BEAUTIFUL HAIR

Close your eyes . . . and imagine. How often have you wished your hair was longer, thicker, and more beautiful? According to Gerald Epstein, M.D., a private psychiatrist and assistant clinical professor of psychiatry at Mount Sinai Medical Center in New York City, author of *Healing Visualizations,* imaging can work—if you do it actively.

He calls it "imaginal medicine" and has more than 16 years of clinical experience proving its effectiveness with everything from cancer to speeding the healing of broken bones. Recently, he had some success with a female patient who had been totally bald for eight years. Her hair loss was connected with psychological factors, including reactions to changes of environment. Nothing worked for her—until she began practicing the visualizations regularly. Within three months, her hair began to grow.

Here's how to practice Dr. Epstein's form of imaging.

Close your eyes and relax. Breathe in and out three times. See, sense, and feel yourself as a gardener planting new seeds for your hair growth. See your scalp as the garden. Picture yourself walking through this garden with a bag of seeds made of growth hormones for the hair. The seeds are in the form of balls of golden light. See yourself seeding the garden. See each seed being received by a hair follicle.

Water the whole area with a can of golden water. See, sense, and feel the water being absorbed through the follicles—forming a golden network of fluid through the scalp, nourishing all the follicles, and causing hair to grow. Breathe out. See the hair sprouting throughout the scalp, growing up toward the top. Breathe out and open your eyes, knowing your hair is growing.

For optimal results, do this twice a day, once in the early morning and once at twilight. Spend up to 3 minutes each time. Repeat for 21 days, then stop for 7 days. Continue that 21-to-7 cycle until your hair grows.

Condition yourself. Commercial hair conditioners—which can be applied in a minute to damp, freshly shampooed hair—often contain body-building ingredients that coat and thicken hair shafts, giving them a fuller appearance, says Roberson. Some hair thickeners use a special wax formula that does the job but doesn't provide the natural shine and manageability that protein-based conditioners do. The protein formulas tend to be absorbed right into the hair shafts for a more natural, healthy-shine look. Ask your hairdresser about the various brands available.

Create a distraction. If your hair is excessively thin, Bonetti suggests that you put on an attention-getting accessory—perhaps a stunning brooch. "A beautiful scarf around the neck or a spectacular bag will draw people's eyes away from the head," she says. "Don't wear big, noticeable earrings. And keep your makeup simple and natural."

Make an appointment. If the thinning is due to hereditary factors, progesterone injections into the scalp are the best way to stop further hair loss in women, says Ronald Sherman, M.D., senior clinical instructor in dermatology at Mount Sinai Medical Center. The injections take but a minute. "There are no side effects and the cost is the price of an office visit," he says. "Going once a week, for ten weeks, will reduce hair loss." (Progesterone injections can also work for men, Dr. Sherman says.)

CHAPTER 22

HEAD AND NECK PAIN

re you having an "Excedrin moment"? Are "plop" and "fizz" two words you frequently repeat? And is there a stunningly sharp pain accompanying the crackling noise you hear when you look over your shoulder?

If your answer is yes, you don't stand head and shoulders above the crowd—you are in the crowd of people suffering from head and neck pain.

Fortunately, there are timely measures that can help you beat many of these problems. Read on to discover how:

- In just 1 minute, ladies, you can remove a common source of neck pain (no, it's not your husband).
- In just a minute a day, you can boost your neck's resistance to injury.
- In just one month, you can cut in half the number of headaches you usually get.

Here's how.

CALLING A HALT TO HEADACHES

There are essentially three different categories of headaches—tension, vascular, and those caused by underlying disease. Tension headaches afflict 90 percent of us, according to Seymour Diamond, M.D., director of the Diamond Headache Clinic in Chicago and author of *Hope for Your Headache Problem*. Less common are vascular headaches, such as migraines, and those caused by an underlying disease (see "Headache Danger Signals" on page 288). The so-called mixed headache combines features of both tension and vascular. In fact, some experts think that vascular and chronic tension headaches may have more in common physiologically than previously thought.

Headaches and their remedies are very individualistic: What works for someone else may or may not work for you. So check your symptoms, choose your headache, and pick your fix.

HEADACHE DANGER SIGNALS

Sometimes a headache is more than just a headache. It can be a sign something is seriously wrong—a burst blood vessel, an underlying disease. When you or someone you know has headaches in any of the following situations, see a doctor or go to a hospital emergency room immediately.

- A sudden, severe, unexpected headache
- A headache accompanied by convulsions
- A headache accompanied by fever
- A headache accompanied by mental confusion, or a drop in awareness or alertness
- A headache accompanied by specific pain in an eye, ear, or other localized area of the head
- A headache following a severe head injury
- Sudden headaches in someone who's never been bothered by headaches before
- Recurring headaches in children
- Daily or frequent headaches.
- Headaches you've had for a long time that suddenly change in character or pattern
- A headache that results from exercise

TACKLING TENSION HEADACHES

If you have a tension headache, the culprit is probably readily identifiable. Spat with your mate? Under a tight deadline at work? A long drive? Stuck in traffic? The muscles around your skull ball up, as if someone gradually pulled a drawstring. You feel a dull, aching sensation in a narrow band around your entire head. What can you do to quickly relieve the pain?

Heat it up. A hot-water bottle or heating pad applied at the first sign of a tension headache can help the tightened muscles relax.

Battle your headache with biofeedback. Have your doctor recommend an instructor in biofeedback. In six to ten sessions you can learn to relax the muscles that are squeezing your head into an ache. Biofeedback works wonders for 80 percent of those who learn it, and Dr. Diamond says he uses it on all of his hospital patients with great success.

Find an acupuncturist. Acupuncture is usually used as a last resort for chronic headaches, but consider trying it as a first resort. Improvement rates of 55 to 85 percent have been reported, according to Alexander Mauskop, M.D., director of the Downstate Headache Center in Brooklyn Heights, New York.

Take the tension out with TENS. In about 10 minutes, transcutaneous electrical nerve stimulation (TENS) can short-circuit headaches caused by shoulder area stiffness, says Gary W. Jay, M.D. He gave 50 patients at his Beverly Hills Pain Control Center portable TENS units to use at home for 10 minutes twice a day. The device emits electrical current that relaxes muscle spasms in the neck and upper back. About half the patients were also given massages, ultrasound, and special exercises in addition to the TENS. After six months, all of the TENS users were almost headache-free, regardless of whether they had supplemented the treatment with other therapies.

Electrify your cranium. Cranial electrotherapy stimulation (CES) may reduce the pain in as little as 20 minutes' time, according to a six-week study of 100 headache sufferers at the Headache Unit of Montefiore Medical Center in the Bronx. The doctors found that those who used the Pain Suppressor unit for 20 minutes reported that their pain decreased by an average of 35 percent. Those who used a nonactive device reported that their pain decreased by an average of 18 percent. About 3 percent of the people who used the device reported slight skin irritation.

The Pain Suppressor C.E.S. (made by Pain Suppression Labs in Wayne, New Jersey) comes with sponge electrodes that you attach to your temples with the accom-

• MIGRA-LIEF COOLS OUT HEADACHES

If you suffer from migraine, tension, or cluster-style headaches and are the type who enjoys trying the latest technology, ask your doctor about testing out the new Migra-lief helmet. The fiberglass softpack helmet has a cooling compartment that encircles the head and extends down the neck and a separate warming compartment for the top of the head. It attaches to a mobile refrigeration and heating unit and has an adjustable timer.

In an Australian study, the device was found to reduce severity of migraine headaches in 15 of 20 migraine sufferers; tension headaches in 6 of 7 tension-headache sufferers and a cluster headache in the 1 cluster-headache sufferer in the study. It also reduced the duration of the headache pain to less than a quarter of its usual length for 10 people in the study. Putting the headgear on at the first sign of a headache was also found helpful.

Not everyone in the study liked the helmet. Several complained that the headgear made them feel claustrophobic and one complained about the humming noise of the refrigeration unit. Three others became nauseated when heat was applied to the head.

This patented product is built so that the heating component can be detached and placed on other areas of the body, like the shoulders or stomach. Several participants in the study liked that feature.

The device is being marketed by Medi-therm of Australia.

panying Velcro strap. The unit delivers an adjustable amount of high-frequency, low-voltage current, and automatically shuts itself off after 20 minutes. The device is available only by prescription.

Gulp your analgesic. Aspirin, ibuprofen, and acetaminophen are proven headache pain relievers—they usually work within half an hour. But they should be used only for the occasional headache. Modern headache therapy is turning more and more to nondrug remedies because chronic use of analgesics can be dangerous: Aspirin and ibuprofen can harm your stomach, and acetaminophen can cause liver damage. And if you've been taking two or more tablets daily for three months or more, you could set yourself up for a rebound headache whenever you *don't* take them. If you're taking an analgesic every day for a chronic headache, ask your doctor for another pain-relief method.

MANAGING MIGRAINES

At some time in their lives, up to 17 percent of young men and 30 percent of young women will get a migraine. No one knows why some people get these vascular headaches, but age and heredity play roles. Migraines usually begin during puberty and dwindle after age 45, and they run in families.

The headache can range in intensity from moderate to excruciating and usually occurs on one side of the head. Nausea and vomiting are common accompaniments, along with hypersensitivity to light and sound. A classic migraine is preceded by an "aura," visions of lights, blind spots, weird sensations, and/or other symptoms. The common migraine—80 to 90 percent of migraines—may hit you without warning.

Something usually triggers the headache—certain foods, stress, light, and too much or too little sleep. What-ever the trigger, it sets off a cascade of physiological changes. A complex and particularly devilish interaction of blood components, hormones, and brain chemicals first constricts the blood vessels in the head and reduces blood flow. The blood vessels react by dilating fiercely. This, combined with all those chemicals and hormones, makes the arteries extremely sensitive to pain and pro-duces the intense, throbbing agony of migraine. When the initial constriction and drop in blood flow is severe, a classic migraine results.

Migraines are tough cookies. The standard drug, ergotamine, can quickly relieve the pain, but adds dis-tressing symptoms of its own. Fortunately, there are other fast ways to beat back a migraine.

Ice your head . . . At the very first sign of a migraine, try an ice pack or one of the commercial gel packs. Strap it around your head with elastic for 20 to 30 minutes. This is an old remedy that works by constricting those swollen blood vessels. And it's been proven in studies at the Diamond Headache Center. A cold compress made from a commercially available ice pack provided almost instantaneous pain relief for 52 percent of 89 people suffering from migraine, cluster, and mixed-type headaches.

. . . and heat your hands. Lie down, relax, and concentrate on directing blood to flow from the swollen arteries in your head down into your hands. Feel your hands getting warmer and warmer with the increased blood flow. The blood vessels in your hands are expanding while the vessels in your head are shrinking. As they shrink, the pain lessens, and soon is gone. You can learn this method on your own, but biofeedback training is easier and faster and gives an immediate report on how you're doing. This technique has been tested thoroughly, and Dr. Diamond says you can learn to hike the temperature of your hands by 10 to 15 degrees—and that's a lot of blood that's no longer throbbing through your head. So ask your doctor to refer you to an instructor in biofeedback.

Make love. Or not. You may think that sex and migraines don't mix, and for many people, they don't. But you may be surprised to learn that men, not women, make up the majority of people for whom sex begets migraines. These sex migraines run in the families of many of those unfortunate men, most of whom are middle-aged, overweight, out of shape, and have mildly high blood pressure. Drug therapy is the usual treatment— and getting fit and less fat couldn't hurt.

But a minority of people can actually make their migraines milder or even help them disappear by having sex when a migraine strikes. James R. Couch, M.D., professor of medicine at Southern Illinois University School of Medicine, interviewed 46 migraine sufferers. Of those, 17 percent told him that sex brought moderate to complete relief. He also found that the better the orgasm, the better the relief. Dr. Couch theorized that nervous system activity or the release of painkilling endorphins might be the key to relief. Masturbation and sex without orgasm provided no respite, however.

Snort salmon. Italian researchers have found that a nasal spray containing a hormone derived from salmon reduced both the intensity and duration of headaches in 22 people they studied. The hormone, calcitonin, is normally produced by the thyroid gland in humans and regulates bone loss—in fact, it's also used to treat osteoporosis. The researchers aren't sure why it works for migraines, but theorize that it interferes with brain chemicals that may be involved in the attacks. The spray, available only in Italy, appears to have no side effects. In previous studies, calcitonin had been effective, but only when given by injection.

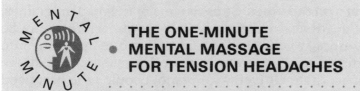

THE ONE-MINUTE MENTAL MASSAGE FOR TENSION HEADACHES

You can head off a tension headache before it gets under way if you can remain aware of the body sensations that occur just as the face, neck, and jaw muscles begin to tighten. Once you learn to observe this, you can reverse the trend toward tightness by mentally relaxing the muscles.

First, follow the relaxation technique described on page 376. Now, see light filling the tense area. Breathe in the light and see the muscle fibers expanding. Breathe out and feel the muscle fibers relaxing. Now imagine that fingers made of light are massaging the area and loosening it up. (You can imagine as many pairs of hands as you want.) See the blood returning to the area, flowing freely, and carrying the dark tension away from the area.

STOPPING HEADACHES BEFORE THEY START

Migraine or tension or mixed, many headaches can be prevented or lessened in severity and frequency by one or more strategies. Take some time to go over this checklist and see if any of the suggestions might work for you.

Become more irresponsible. A common cause of migraine is fatigue and lack of rest. Some migraine sufferers are classic examples of the super-conscientious, super-hardworking, never-relaxing stereotype. If this is you, try giving yourself a break—*lots* of breaks, in fact. Exercise 20 minutes a day, four times a week; take time to read, listen to music, play, do your hobby. You may find yourself with half as many headaches in as little as 30 days' time.

That was the outcome for one-quarter of the all-work-and-little-play migraine sufferers in a study at the Northern California Headache Clinic in Mountain View. "Headache symptoms were telling these people to back off," says Alfred Scopp, Ph.D., the study's researcher.

Turn on the tunes. Stress is a major trigger of migraines, and biofeedback a proven way to de-stress. You may be able to amplify your biofeedback technique by tuning into soothing music. In a study done by researchers at the California State University, Fresno, people who practiced biofeedback or relaxation techniques had remarkably good results. Within a year of starting the program, those who listened to music experienced only one-sixth of the migraine headaches they used to have. The intensity and duration of headaches subsided as well, says biofeedback researcher Janet Lapp, Ph.D. Some people even used the music to stop a migraine before it reached full force.

Flatten your feet. High heels force the back muscles to tense in order to keep the body erect. The tension works its way up your spine to your neck and head, and a headache can be the result. Low heels can solve this problem.

Gain without pain. Getting a headache during exercise can be a signal of underlying disease, says Morris Mellion, M.D., associate professor at the University of Nebraska. If you've found that your exercise-related headache is not due to an underlying disease, try taking aspirin or ibuprofen *before* you exercise. It could stop the headache before it gets started. And remember, exercise headaches are more likely to occur if you're not well conditioned, live at a high altitude, or drink alcohol before or during your exercise or play.

Find out about feverfew. British researchers who studied 72 volunteers found that a capsule a day of dried feverfew, an herb, helped reduced the number and severity of attacks and incidents of vomiting, within a two-month period. There were no serious side effects, according to the study's authors.

Cork the red wine. Red wine is not at all cordial when it comes to migraine headaches, British researchers report. Nineteen migraine sufferers were given equal amounts of alcohol in the form of either red wine or vodka mixed with lemonade. The drinks were made indistinguishable in both appearance and taste, but the wine uncorked its wrath nonetheless. Nine of the 11 wine drinkers suffered headache attacks, while none of the 8 vodka drinkers did. Champagne and beer have also been found to set off migraines.

Chop the MSG out of your suey. Monosodium glutamate (MSG), a sodium-loaded flavor enhancer typically found in Chinese food (and many other prepared foods), can cause headaches. Check labels of processed and frozen dinners (be aware that even if the label doesn't say MSG, an additive called hydrolyzed vegetable protein contains as much as 20 percent MSG), and tell the waiter you want your chop suey MSG-free. Also be aware that kombu extract, found in health foods, is nothing more than MSG extracted from seaweed.

Wean yourself from caffeine. Caffeine is a well-known constrictor of blood vessels. That's why it's a common ingredient in headache medications. And that's why cold-turkey withdrawal from five to six cups of coffee a day can quickly dilate the blood vessels in your head, causing intense headaches. So instead of stopping caffeine *today,* gradually wean yourself over two to three weeks. For example, take a week to cut back from three cups of coffee a day to two, then another week to cut down to one, and in your third week—if you want to quit drinking coffee altogether— drop down to none.

Say "baloney" to hot dogs. Luncheon meats, hot dogs, ham, bacon, and other cured meats usually contained nitrates, which are implicated in many people's migraines.

Smile without saying "cheese." Aged and processed cheeses, especially the strong ones like cheddar, are common instigators of migraine.

In other words, diagnose your diet. As you are probably aware, various foods are known migraine triggers. Besides the ones already mentioned, add these to your list of possible culprits: food additives such as meat tenderizers, soy sauce, and yeast extracts; pickled or dried herring and smoked fish; chicken livers; peanuts and peanut butter; homemade yeast bread and yogurt; and chocolate.

Eat. Missing or skipping meals is another way to bring on a migraine.

Belay the B₆. Vitamin B_6 in large doses can cause headaches. So can vitamin A and iron.

Commute without carbon monoxide. Rush hour is loaded with this migraine trigger. Avoid the mob by changing your commuting schedule.

Ask about aspirin . . . An aspirin every other day seems to have helped doctors decrease the number of their own migraines by 20 percent, according to data from the 22,000-doctor Physicians' Health Study. The theory: Aspirin keeps the blood's clotting agents, platelets, from sticking together and releasing headache-causing serotonin. Since aspirin can interfere with other medications, and on its own cause stomach ulcers, check with your doctor before embarking on your own aspirin therapy.

. . . and other drugs. Several prescription drugs are being used to prevent or abort migraines. All must be taken under a doctor's supervision. Among them are the heart disease drugs known as beta-blockers and calcium channel blockers; the antidepressants amitriptyline, nortriptyline, and doxepin; the migraine drug methysergide; and such drugs as naproxen and ergonovine.

NORMALIZING A KINKY NECK

You carry the world on your neck. That column of muscle and fiber and bone is the resting place not only of your head—and the brain that presumably inhabits it—but jewelry, ties, collars, and, for horse thieves in the Wild West, nooses. What do you think keeps your head up and giving the appearance of wakefulness at operas? What swivels your head to follow that slice into the water trap? What lets your chin rest on your chest when you're taking a snooze?

Now that you have reestablished the importance of your neck (and even if you haven't), you'll want to know what to do when something gives you a pain in it. If your neck hurts, chances are good that the pain stems from an injury, old or recent. You may have *sprained* it by partially tearing or excessively stretching a *ligament*. Or maybe you've *strained* it by partly tearing or stretching a *muscle*. Failure to care for your neck promptly may cause the pain to recur and become chronic. Fortunately, neck pain is a common complaint, and the remedies are fast and simple.

Ice it down. Apply an ice pack from the freezer, or a commercial gel pack, for up to 20 minutes at a time over a period of one to two days. The ice will constrict the small blood vessels and reduce pain-causing inflammation.

Heat it up. After two days of icing the injury, apply a heating pad for 10 to 20 minutes at a time. Be careful not to get burned. The ice will have dampened the inflammation, so now you can use heat to bring back healing blood to the area.

Rest it and support it. The best immediate measure to take when you have neck sprain or strain is to rest your neck and support it with a collar. But use the collar only for a short period of time or only at night.

Take it easy. While you're recuperating, follow this plan of gentle neck movements and posture corrections. This will shorten recovery time of acute neck sprains and reduce the likelihood of persistent symptoms. That's the finding of a Northern Ireland study of 247 people treated in emergency rooms for neck pain. The group who received instruction in home care suffered less severe neck pain and were much less likely to have persistent symptoms than those who rested their necks and relied on collars and those who received physiotherapy.

The theory behind the success of home care is that if you're given responsibility for your own treatment, you're more likely to become self-sufficient in managing episodes of minor discomfort. Learning what hurts and what feels good can prevent a vicious cycle—you have a muscle spasm, so you scrunch your neck one way and your shoulder another, and the resulting unnatural posture causes more spasms. Another plus seems to be that you become your own doctor instead of a victim of your symptoms.

Here are the essential components of this easy-to-do program. The exercises may hurt initially, but they won't harm your neck. Repeat the exercises as often as you like, the more the better. And be sure to start your day with these exercises to relieve any overnight neck stiffness.

- Remain aware of your posture when you sit, stand, read, and drive. Avoid slouching with your chin stuck out. Make sure your back is straight and your shoulders are braced.
- Ten times each hour, draw yourself up straight and tuck your chin in to assure yourself of correct posture.
- Straighten your back, then try to touch each ear down on the corresponding shoulder. Then straighten up and try to look over one shoulder, then the other.

Sleep right. That's on your side or back, supporting your neck with a collar or firm roll. The people in the study in Northern Ireland who had the best recovery rates for acute neck sprain were advised not to use too many pillows in bed, but to support the neck with a collar or by firmly rolling a hand towel and placing the roll inside the bottom edge of the pillow case.

Pull the trigger. If you carefully feel your sore neck, you'll find a spot of maximum tenderness called the trigger point. Pressure here may make the pain feel worse immediately, and may cause pain at points distant from the trigger point, but ultimately it will bring relief. Try pressing that sensitive spot for 1 to 2 minutes.

The sensitivity you feel may stem from injury to the area, muscle fatigue, too much cold, chronic bad posture, or emotional stress. These factors can cause the muscles to be easily irritated, overworked, and undersupplied with blood. The muscle fibers respond by banding together and tensing up. By restoring blood flow to the area, with its warmth, you can help "unstick" the muscle fibers and wash away the cellular wastes contributing to the pain. Apply heat and stretch gently afterward.

Ladies, remove your bras. Or at least loosen the shoulder straps, especially if you're "blessed" with large breasts. The trapezius muscles of your shoulders and back were designed to carry no more than an arm or two. Large-breasted women in particular feel the strain when they ask these muscles to also carry their breasts, says Australian physician Edward L. Ryan, M.D. When you wear a bra, the rear bra strap works like a pulley over the shoulders, doubling the downward pull on both shoulders.

Stretch it. You bend your neck forward to read, write, do the dishes, sulk, drive. So much time spent in one position makes your neck muscles tighten and shorten, and so increases your risk of injury when you decide to look up at the stars. Compensate by lying on your back with your knees bent, flattening your neck to the floor by tucking your chin without lifting your head. Hold for 5 to 10 seconds, repeating ten times. Turn your head slowly to either side while the chin is tucked.

TAKING THE BITE OUT OF TMD

If you think "temporomandibular joint" is a toughie to pronounce, suffering from temporomandibular disorder (TMD, formerly called TMJ) is even worse. About 30 percent of all Americans have this condition, but fewer than half of them are troubled enough by it to require treatment, says Owen J. Rogal, D.D.S., executive director of the American Academy of Head, Facial, and Neck Pain and TMJ Orthopedics and author of *Mandibular Whiplash*. For some unfortunate members of the latter group, however, the pain can be a constant, excruciating presence.

While there is no quick fix for TMD discomfort, there are new treatment options that can reduce the pain by half, in just six weeks' time, without drugs or surgery. (Complete resolution of the pain and discomfort may take up to six months.)

What makes TMD so difficult to diagnose is that it often produces pain at sites fairly distant from the joint itself. The most common initial symptom is headache. Other symptoms may include earaches, neck aches, facial pain, difficulty opening and closing the jaw, and popping or clicking sounds when you do move the jaw.

There are two types of TMD problems. In one problem, the pain comes from the temporomandibular joint itself, and in the other, it comes from the jaw muscles. You can locate the joint by placing a finger in front of your ear. With your finger touching the skin in front of your ear, open and close your mouth. The movable structures that you feel beneath your finger are the condyles, the round-tipped ends of the lower jawbone. The condyle sits in the bony temporomandibular joint when the mouth is closed. A cushion of cartilage protects these bones from rubbing against each other. The cartilage allows the condyles "to ride inside the socket like a ball bearing," Dr. Rogal says.

The pain originates in either the joint or the related muscles, Dr. Rogal says. "For many people with TMD, the ball bearing is out of place. So when people try to open their mouths, they feel pain, or their jaws jam," he says.

However, the most common TMD problem that people have is caused by tension in one of the muscles responsible for opening and closing the mouth. "In this case, the pain is not necessarily coming from the joint," Dr. Rogal says. "Rather, it's coming from the muscles, ligaments, and tendons in the face and neck."

If you place your fingers over the temple muscles right behind your eyes and bite down tightly on your teeth, you can actually feel the temple muscles tighten. This demonstrates how the jaw affects the way the muscles of the face and head work. "The temple muscle that you just touched covers most of each side of your head," Dr. Rogal says. "This muscle is so big that when it hurts and feels tender, the whole head hurts. We call that pain a headache." The secret of treating TMD without medication or surgery is simply to relax that muscle.

"I treat these associated muscle problems as you would a backache," he adds. "That's the conservative method of treatment."

His patients wear a clear plastic cover over the bottom teeth, often for 24 hours a day, for the first few months of treatment. "The plastic acts as a cushion when you bite down. As the muscles relax, the pain starts to go away."

Dr. Rogal also uses a combination of ultrasound, various electrotherapies, and manipulation techniques to relax the injured tissue and promote blood flow. The point, he says, is to break the pain-spasm-pain cycle and start the process of healing. Stimulating blood flow to the area ensures that the muscles get the nutrients they need.

Dr. Rogal says that his method can fully resolve the pain of TMD in four to six months and reduce pain by 50 percent within the first six weeks. Surgery is rarely necessary, he says.

Whether the cause of your TMD is the muscle or the ball bearing, you have a permanent injury, Dr. Rogal says. Here are some easy home remedies to use in conjunction with medical treatment.

Ice it. Wrap an ice cube in a paper towel and rotate it over the temporomandibular joint for up to 20 seconds. Remove it as soon as the area feels numb. Next, apply moist heat. (You can use a cloth wrung out in very warm water or a moist heat pack wrapped in a small towel for this.) Leave the moist heat on for just a minute. Rub the area gently. If that doesn't give you the relief you want, wait 5 minutes and begin the process again. You may even need a third round for maximum relief.

"For some people, this helps for a few hours. For others, it brings all-day relief," says Sylvan Lande, D.D.S., a professor of dentistry at the University of Southern California School of Dentistry. "It depends upon how acute the pain is."

Change your sleep position. This is central to gaining control of the pain caused by TMD, Dr. Rogal says. First, while lying on your back, place a pillow underneath your knees. Make sure the pillow raises your legs enough to take the pressure off your back. Next, place a flat towel underneath your midback. Take another towel and roll it so that it's not thicker around than your wrist. This towel goes under your neck and substitutes for your pillows. A rubberband placed around the towel will prevent it from unrolling.

This position will gradually help to relieve your pain, including the headaches and backaches associated with TMD.

Separate your teeth. If you clench your teeth, practice the following technique until it becomes a habit, Dr. Rogal says. Place your tongue behind your front teeth, resting it against the roof of your mouth. This position will help you separate the top and bottom teeth and relax your jaw. Adjust your mouth so that your teeth are "just a hair" apart, but your lips are still touching.

Perfect your posture. If you have a desk job or work that requires you to jut your chin forward, stand up every hour or so and straighten your posture. The muscles of the neck control the muscles of the jaw, Dr. Rogal says.

Misuse of the neck muscles "will cause your jaw to be off" and aggravate any existing problem. He enthusiastically recommends the Alexander Technique, a movement re-education system that stresses proper alignment of the head and neck.

Stop that yawn. One way to break a yawn is to gently bite down. If you have TMD, the likelihood is that your ligaments are already stretched beyond their comfort zone, Dr. Rogal says. A yawn will just put more stress on them.

Eat a soft diet. If you feel jaw fatigue when you're chewing, choose less chewy foods. Pasta, casseroles, and noodles can substitute for meat courses. Baked or steamed vegetables will be easier to eat than raw ones.

HEART HEALTH

T he statistics are impressive: Heart attacks kill more Americans every year than any other single cause of death: more than half a million people—513,700 in a given year. At this moment, there are almost five million people with coronary heart disease.

Okay, you say, nobody lives forever, we all have to die of something. True, but we don't have to die nearly as young as we do. Forty-five percent of all heart attacks strike people under 65. Five percent hit people under 40.

The statistics, however, are not all bad news. As a matter of fact, part of the good news is that heart disease deaths have been steadily declining for several years. From 1977 to 1987, for example, the coronary heart disease death rate dropped 28.7 percent, according to the American Heart Association. This decline in heart disease deaths is not occurring by accident. The tens of millions of dollars in research—$69 million by the American Heart Association in 1988–89—aimed at finding better ways to prevent, diagnose, and treat heart disease have been paying off.

For example, though increasing age is a risk factor, the doctors conducting the massive Framingham Heart Study say that heart disease is not inevitable after age 65. The researchers followed 2,500 Framingham volunteers who sailed past age 65 without heart problems. This doesn't mean all of the 2,500 were doing their best to lower their risk. Not at all. As they got older, those who maintained the bad habits of their younger years were more likely to develop heart disease than those who continued to live in ways that reduced their risk factors.

There are any number of strategies you can employ to lower your risk of heart disease in very short order. Here are a few examples.

- In just three weeks, you can cut your cholesterol by about 20 percent if you add lots of beans to your diet.
- In just one month, you can begin to cut your risk by giving up cigarettes.
- In only three months, you can tip the ratio of good to bad cholesterol in your favor by drinking low-fat milk.
- And you can cut recovery time after a heart attack from six weeks to one week with a special clot-dissolving therapy.

A few weeks is time well spent if it can add years to your life and make those years healthy ones. And once you get started, you'll find those weeks pass quickly.

TOSSING TOBACCO OUT OF YOUR LIFE

Let's begin by taking the most dramatic step in preventing a heart attack.

Quit smoking. Within a year of your last cigarette, your risk of developing heart disease drops by almost half. And it continues to fall until, ten years after quitting, your risk is equal to that of a nonsmoker. Some aspects of your heart disease risk fall even faster. Within 30 days of quitting smoking, levels of beneficial HDL cholesterol rose from an average of 50 to an average of 60 in 18 women studied by Florida State University researchers. This level of HDL cholesterol is comparable to that of nonsmokers.

Cutting back is not enough. You have to quit. For women, anyway, Harvard Medical School researchers found, there may not be a "safe" level of smoking. Just a couple of cigarettes a day still doubles the risk of heart disease.

If you feel you need some extra incentive to quit, wait long enough and you just may get it: A very effective kick in the pants to encourage kicking the habit appears to be a heart attack. Almost half of heart attack victims successfully quit smoking for at least a year.

But you don't have to wait for that tap on the shoulder from Eternity. Ask your doctor about nicotine gum and counseling to get the cigarette monkey off your back. Quitting smoking doesn't have to be a lifetime struggle. (See chapter 20 for more encouraging advice about quitting.)

Danish physicians found a highly effective, speedy program that consisted of chewing gum containing 4 milligrams of nicotine and attending six group counseling sessions spanning four months. Participants were told to stop smoking completely at the first counseling session and instructed to chew from 6 to 14 pieces of gum per day at first, and slowly taper off use of the gum. After six weeks, 81.5 percent had not smoked any cigarettes. After a year, 44.4 percent were still abstinent. The doctors attributed their success not only to the nicotine gum but also to the atmosphere of support, acceptance, and encouragement provided by the group counseling.

CUT YOUR RISK FAST WITH FOOD

Lowering dietary cholesterol significantly lowers your risk of dying from heart disease—and from other causes as well. In one massive study in the United States, lowering daily cholesterol intake by 200 milligrams/1,000 calories led to a 37 percent lower risk of death from any cause and added 3.4 years to total life expectancy. In this same study, the combined effects of having blood cholesterol at 200 or lower, a systolic blood pressure of 120, and not smoking cigarettes added 11.8 years to total life expectancy.

Lowering your heart disease risk by means of your diet does not necessarily mean a long, difficult transition. There are so many quick, simple ways to lower your bad cholesterol (LDLs) and raise your good (HDLs), you'll have no trouble incorporating enough to get you on the fast track to a healthier heart.

FIBER DOES THE JOB

A University of California at San Diego study is among the most recent to demonstrate the protective role of dietary fiber. The researchers measured daily fiber intake and then followed heart disease mortality among 859 men and women aged 50 to 79. The magic number appears to be 16. People whose diets included 16 grams of fiber per day had only about one-third the risk of dying from heart disease as those who ate fewer than 16 grams. You can get a daily dose of fiber with oat bran for breakfast, a sandwich with whole wheat bread for lunch, and ½ cup of lima beans with dinner.

When asked why fiber seems to work so well to reduce heart disease risk, Elizabeth Barrett-Connor, M.D., one of the study's authors, said, "We know that certain types of fiber are more effective in lowering cholesterol than other types, but we think that fiber does more for the heart than just lower cholesterol. It's been suggested, for example, that fiber might hinder the formation of blood clots that can lodge in the arteries, causing heart attacks and strokes."

Sprinkle on the oat bran. Just a few tablespoons of oat bran added to the daily diet of healthy young adults succeeded in lowering cholesterol an average of 5.3 percent in four weeks. LDL cholesterol also dropped by 8.7 percent and triglycerides by 8.3 percent.

Plant some beans in your diet. Beans are as rich in cholesterol-lowering, water-soluble fiber as oat bran. In one study, researchers added 115 grams (about ½ cup) of beans a day to a typical American diet consisting of 43 percent of its calories from carbohydrates, 20 percent from protein, and 37 percent from fat. After only three weeks, cholesterol levels of the 20 men had dropped and stabilized 19 percent lower than the original high levels. LDL cholesterol dropped 24 percent, too.

Count on corn bran. While it's not as widely promoted as oat bran, corn bran can lower cholesterol, too. Georgetown University Hospital researchers tested the ability of corn bran to lower cholesterol levels in people with values over 240. After 12 weeks on a diet containing 17 to 34 grams (about 1 to 2 tablespoons) a day of dietary fiber from corn bran, serum cholesterol was lowered 20 percent and triglycerides 31 percent.

Chow down a soy-fiber cookie or two. Researchers at Washington University's General Clinical Research Center baked a daily dose of 25 grams of soy fiber into cookies and gave them to patients with genetically determined high blood cholesterol. The soy-fiber cookies alone accounted for a 5 percent drop in cholesterol. In combination with a low-cholesterol, low-saturated-fat diet, the soy-fiber cookies lowered cholesterol a total of 15 percent.

Take a teaspoon of psyllium. Psyllium is a water-soluble fiber made from the husks of blond psyllium seeds. As anyone who has taken a bulk-forming laxative containing psyllium knows, when added to water it forms a gel. Some recent studies have demonstrated that when a teaspoon of psyllium is added to your diet three times a day, cholesterol levels can drop substantially. In one study, psyllium lowered by 15 percent the high cholesterol levels of men not following a low-fat diet. In a study to determine what psyllium could do for people eating a somewhat low-fat diet (30 percent calories from fat instead of the typically American 40 percent), 3 teaspoons per day caused cholesterol levels to drop an additional 4.8 percent.

Slice a grapefruit for breakfast. Grains and beans are not the only sources of cholesterol-lowering soluble fiber. Fruit contains soluble fiber, too. And citrus pectin, the soluble fiber in grapefruit, oranges, lemons, and limes, lowers cholesterol as well as anything out of the oat bucket. In a University of Florida study, 15 grams of grapefruit pectin in capsule form per day lowered dangerously high total cholesterol levels by 7.6 percent and LDL cholesterol levels by 10.8 percent.

Cut your cholesterol with a couple of carrots a day. That's all it takes for people with high cholesterol levels to lower their cholesterol by as much as 10 to 20 percent. Carrots contain a form of fiber called pectin, which binds bile acids and thus reduces blood cholesterol. Other favorites of the vegetable bin, broccoli and cabbage, may have the same risk-reducing effect.

GOING BEYOND FIBER

There's much more to food than fiber. There's fat. There's caffeine. There are extra added ingredients that can help or harm. Fast, simple changes in the way you eat can go a long way toward improving the health of your heart.

Consume coffee with caution. The jury is still out on the case of coffee versus your heart. The evidence is conflicting: Some studies show dramatic increases in cholesterol levels and heart disease risk, even from moderate use; others show no effect. Some of the coffee-*might*-be-bad studies say it's moderate-to-heavy consumption that seems to increase risk; other studies say it's high levels of caffeine.

So what can you do now? Play it safe — avoid coffee altogether, drink only one or two cups a day, or switch to decaffeinated coffee or tea.

Add some onions to your meat loaf. In the cholesterol-lowering department, onions (and garlic, too) are as powerful as their aroma. Food has a host of factors besides fiber that can help push your cholesterol levels down. And all are fast and easy additives to your daily diet. For a start, slicing some onion and/or garlic into the frying pan when preparing that high-cholesterol meal could prevent your blood cholesterol levels from skyrocketing, as scientific studies have demonstrated.

And several studies have shown that various daily amounts of garlic can lower cholesterol levels anywhere from 15 percent to 28.5 percent. In one study, low cholesterol levels were closely linked with the amounts of onion and garlic people consumed over the course of a week. Blood levels of cholesterol were lowest (154) among those who ate more than 600 grams of onion (about 3 cups) and 50 grams of garlic (about 17 cloves) every week; higher (172) among those who ate only 200 grams of onion and 10 grams of garlic weekly; and highest (208) among the people who never ate either one.

One large, raw, white onion per day could boost your levels of good HDL cholesterol by 30 percent, according to a recent study at St. Elizabeth's Hospital in Boston.

Onions and garlic can reduce your heart disease risk in another very significant way — by lowering the tendency of your blood to form dangerous, artery-blocking clots, even after a high-fat meal.

Pour a glass of low-fat milk. Hot and spicy foods aren't the only ones that lower your cholesterol. Breath-friendly skim milk does, too. In a Chicago Medical School study, men who drank one quart of 2 percent milk a day increased the ratio of good-to-bad cholesterol, HDL-to-LDL, in their blood by 19.5 percent after only three months.

After six months drinking just a quart a day, their ratio increased by 31 percent.

Splash on some olive oil. A little olive oil added to the low-fat, low-saturated-fat, high-complex-carbohydrate diet that has become the standard diet for lowering cholesterol may improve the diet's ability to reduce heart disease risk. Dutch researchers compared the ability of two diets to lower blood cholesterol. One diet was a standard low-fat, high-complex-carbohydrate diet, with 22 percent of its calories from fat. The other diet was relatively high in fat, 40 percent, but most of the fat was in the form of olive oil. After five weeks on the diets, the results of blood tests were compared. Both diets lowered cholesterol. The olive oil diet lowered total cholesterol by 46 points, compared with the low-fat diet's 44. However, whereas the low-fat diet lowered good HDL cholesterol by 19 points, the olive oil diet raised HDL by 3 points.

Make a meal with mackerel. Eating deep-sea fish rich in omega-3 fatty acids, fish such as tuna, mackerel, and salmon, can reduce your risk of heart disease. Eating fish can drop your cholesterol, LDL cholesterol, and triglyceride levels. It can reduce the tendency of your blood to clot, improve oxygen supply to tissues nourished by narrow vessels, encourage relaxation of the coronary arteries, and slow plaque deposits on the artery walls.

Do all these effects add up to anything? Yes: longer life. Swedish researchers started keeping records on people they classified as either low, moderate, or high consumers of fish. After 14 years they tallied the records and found that the more fish people ate, the lower their risk of heart disease death. A similar study performed by the Dutch found that over a 20-year period, men who ate fish had about half the chance of dying from heart disease as men who did not eat fish—despite the fact that some of the fish eaters also ate more saturated fat and cholesterol than those who did not eat fish. Apparently, eating only one or two fish dishes per week was enough to make the difference. The American Heart Association recommends that while you should add fish to your diet, you should limit your shellfish entrées to no more than one a week.

Evaluate your diet for vitamin E. If you're eating
(continued on page 312)

LET PRITIKIN PUT YOU
ON THE FAST TRACK TO HEALTH

Would you like to change all your risk factors for the better in only four weeks? Would you be interested in a program that could possibly reduce or eliminate your dependence on drugs, help you bypass a bypass operation, and shave several pounds in the same short period of time?

For more than a decade the Pritikin Longevity Center (there are two—in Santa Monica, California, and Miami, Florida) has been helping thousands of people to do just that—and more. The program is not billed as a diet or a spa but as an education in a new way of life. If that's starting to sound like a lengthy commitment, think of it this way: In less than four weeks—in two weeks if you have no symptoms of heart disease—you can turn around your entire risk factor profile so that if it's not solidly on the low-risk side of the line, then it's well on its way there. And you will leave with all you need to know to keep it heading toward the healthier, longer-life side of the chart.

You'll get results, and fast. The center has performed and published more than 20 studies, all of which demonstrate the benefits of the program. These studies have shown, for example, that the program can help participants:

- Lower cholesterol and triglycerides by an average of 25 percent.
- Reduce high blood pressure: In one study of over 800 Pritikin participants, 83 percent who entered the program on high blood pressure medication were able to leave their drugs behind when they left.
- Decrease angina pain: In one study, 62 percent left their heart medications behind them when they left the center.
- Avoid bypass surgery: In one year alone, out of 64 patients who went through the program instead of getting the surgery, 80 percent still did not need the operation five years later.
- Lose weight: Overweight people have lost an average of 13 pounds during the 26-day program.
- Reduce dependence on insulin: In one study, more than 50 percent of diabetics on insulin left the program free of the drug and over 90 percent on oral drugs left drug-free.

- Quit smoking: In one study, 85 percent of the smokers stopped by the end of the program.
- Increase exercise ability: In one study, angina patients who could walk only an average of ½ mile a day were walking an average of 5½ miles each day when they left.

How does the Pritikin Center do it in just 26 days?

By totally immersing you in the diet and lifestyle that will heal you and reduce your risk factors.

The staff acknowledges that changing years of bad habits is one of the toughest challenges to accomplish on your own. So they make sure you're never on your own at the center. You are led through the entire education process.

The program begins with a complete medical and fitness evaluation that results in an "exercise prescription." A daily exercise class will get you over the bumps and grinds of finding muscles you never knew you had—and learning to enjoy using them.

You'll spend several hours a day getting an education in your new lifestyle: weight control workshops, stress management classes, smoking cessation workshops, lifestyle management workshops, and nutrition classes.

Then there's the food. Although many participants go in afraid they'll be calling on friends to sneak in "real food," they usually wind up inviting their friends to the center for dinner. The Pritikin Diet is composed of 75 to 80 percent complex carbohydrates, less than 10 percent fat, and 10 to 15 percent protein. A chef creates meals out of basic, natural ingredients such as pasta, fresh fruits and vegetables, whole grains, corn, rice, lean poultry, fish . . . and potatoes.

And you're never hungry, the staff guarantees, because you're fed five times a day—your basic three squares, plus a midmorning and a midafternoon snack.

Make that six times a day. You can get a sample plate of more goodies at the end of the daily cooking classes. Some participants are known to show up for two classes per day.

Along the way, if you need any individual counseling or medical attention, the staff is always available.

When you graduate, you're sent home with a diploma, a cookbook of fabulous recipes, a "source book" containing all the facts you've been taught in classes—and a new you, minus several percentage points off your heart disease risk.

polyunsaturated vegetable oils like safflower, sunflower, or soybean oil, you're probably getting enough vitamin E. Another good source is wheat germ. Recent research has revealed that vitamin E can raise levels of good HDL cholesterol and reduce the likelihood of artery-blocking blood clots by making the blood platelets less "sticky."

French and Israeli researchers gave 500 international units per day of vitamin E to 30 people with high cholesterol levels. After 90 days, all 30 had significantly higher levels of HDL than a similar group who were not given vitamin E. The people taking vitamin E also had reduced ratios of total cholesterol to HDL. "These results support the use of vitamin E supplementation for people with high blood-fat levels," said the researchers.

In another study, ten people were given 400 to 1,200 international units of vitamin E daily for six weeks. Manfred Steiner, M.D., Ph.D., of Brown University, said that after six weeks, the volunteers' blood platelets were definitely "less sticky." Dr. Steiner says that further research will be needed before it's certain that vitamin E will have a similar effect in people with clotting abnormalities that increase heart attack risk.

Get knowledgeable about niacin. Do that by asking your doctor, because when it's used in high doses, the B vitamin niacin acts more like a drug—and a very effective one for lowering heart disease risk. In one very long-term study called the Coronary Drug Project, niacin was tested against other therapies for heart disease. The initial results of the study indicated that people who took 3 grams a day of niacin had 27 percent fewer nonfatal heart attacks than people taking other drugs. Many years later, on follow-up, it was discovered that this group also suffered from 9 to 13 percent fewer deaths from all causes than the other groups. In another study, 1 gram of niacin taken three times a day for a month lowered cholesterol 22 percent and reduced triglyceride levels 52 percent. Niacin also is an effective drug for raising levels of good HDL cholesterol.

TARGETING HEART ATTACKS BY SEX

When Adam and Eve realized they were different, they probably couldn't have guessed they'd have to be treated differently to prevent heart attacks. But as long as these two remedies work, *vive la différence!*

Men: Ask for aspirin. In the landmark five-year study conducted by Harvard Medical School and involving more than 22,000 middle-aged male physicians, researchers found aspirin could cut their risk of fatal and nonfatal heart attacks nearly in half. According to Charles Hennekens, M.D., the study's director, "The mechanism involved seems to be aspirin's effect on reducing the adhesiveness of blood platelets and hence the propensity for the type of clotting that can lead to heart attacks." The current wisdom is that an aspirin a day will do the trick. Just be sure to consult your doctor before you begin this regimen.

Women: Ask about ERT. Aspirin's anti-blood-clotting, anti-heart-attack effects do not seem to be as effective for women. But postmenopausal women have a weapon not available to men: They may now be able to turn to postmenopausal estrogen replacement therapy (ERT) for a protective effect rivaling aspirin's effect for men. After menopause, a woman's heart disease risk factor profile is known to get worse: Her total cholesterol, LDLs, and triglycerides tend to rise. The administration of estrogen not only may protect against rising LDL levels, it also seems to deliver an overall protective effect. In several studies, the risk of cardiovascular death for women receiving ERT appeared to be reduced anywhere from 34 to 59 percent of that of women not receiving estrogen.

EXERCISING FOR A HEALTHIER HEART

The evidence is in: Physical activity is an ingredient of a longer life. Sedentary people are at greater risk not only for heart disease death but for death from other causes as well. This really should come as no surprise, since other studies have also established that exercise has a favorable effect on so many risk factors for heart disease.

Physical exercise lowers LDL cholesterol and triglycerides, gives good HDLs a healthy boost, tends to help with weight reduction, and lowers the percentage of body fat. Exercise also has a favorable effect on blood pressure, glucose tolerance, and heart rate.

Being physically fit even helps protect the heart against mental stress. A University of Toronto study revealed that in people who are less physically fit, the heart tends to overreact to hormones that are released during periods of psychological stress.

But does this mean you have to become a world-class cyclist, run marathons, or spend most of your leisure time sweating at the gym? Do you have to dedicate major portions of your life to exercise to get the beneficial effects? Not according to the most recent research.

Take a fitness vacation. A study of more than 17,000 people found that people who exercised only infrequently—such as when they were on vacation—were still only one-third as likely to have heart disease as people who never exercised.

Go rake the lawn. Gain doesn't have to mean pain. Research named, aptly enough, MRFIT (Multiple Risk Factor Intervention Trial), involving more than 12,000 men, has revealed that the amount and the intensity of exercise necessary to substantially lower heart disease risk is considerably less than had been believed. The latest results of the MRFIT study show that men who regularly engage in light to moderate physical activity enjoy the same protection from heart disease as men whose activity levels are considerably higher.

Men who expended only 224 calories a day in leisure-time activities were as well protected from fatal heart attacks as men who expended more than 600 calories. It took the men an average of only about 48 minutes a day to gain that protection. And they didn't have to come anywhere near a running shoe or a gym to do it. As a matter of fact, the most common activities were things like working around the yard, gardening, walking, and home repairs.

Take a walk. A British study has found that brisk walking can slightly lower total cholesterol and significantly raise HDL cholesterol levels in previously sedentary women. The walking was decidedly low-intensity, as the women raised their heart rate to only 60 percent of their maximum aerobic rate. Other studies of the impact of exercise on cholesterol show that women can lower their heart disease risk by 42 to 50 percent.

Just nod off. You may not need to exercise at all to

lower your heart disease risk. In fact, quite the opposite. Taking a siesta may lower your risk, too. You can't get any lower intensity than that! According to researchers at the University of Athens Medical School, that afternoon nap may be the difference between heart disease and health. In their study, which compared heart patients with people who had no heart problems, those who took an afternoon nap of at least 30 minutes daily had only 71 percent the heart disease risk as those who did not. The longer the siesta, the more heart disease risk declined. These results may help explain why the heart disease risk is greater in countries that do not take naps (like the United States, Canada, northern Europe, and Scandinavia) and lower in countries where the siesta is common and accepted (like tropical and Mediterranean countries).

HAPPY HEART, HEALTHY HEART

A happy heart is a healthy heart, according to the latest research. Until recently, it was generally believed that so-called Type A behavior such as impatience, talking fast, and working long hours were at the core of the emotional or psychosomatic risk factors for heart disease. But recent studies suggest that suspicion and hostility toward others is what puts the Type A person at risk. Redford B. Williams, Jr., M.D., professor of psychiatry at Duke University Medical Center in North Carolina, led a study that looked at the health records of 118 attorneys who took a standard personality test 25 years ago. Those who scored high in hostility were more than 4 times more likely to die than those who scored low. When Dr. Williams further narrowed the field by focusing only on those who scored high in portions of the hostility scale involving cynical mistrust, anger, and aggression, he found that those who scored high had a death rate 5½ times that of low scorers. Other studies have confirmed this link.

What is it about mistrust, anger, and aggression that appears to be so toxic? Dr. Williams, the author of *The Trusting Heart: Great News about Type A Behavior,* believes that hostile people may simply have a shorter fuse before firing off stress hormones that can damage the heart and blood vessels. Trusting people may have a reduced risk because situations and events that trigger a stress explosion in angry people do not cost them nearly as much physiologically.

Consider counseling or group therapy. Research has shown that this is an effective way to lengthen your Type A fuse and extend your life. Meyer Friedman, M.D., one of the physicians who originally described Type A behavior and its effects on the heart, put almost 600 cardiac patients through a course of Type A behavioral counseling. At the end of 4½ years, those who went through the counseling had a cardiac recurrence rate that was less than half the rate of those who received no counseling and was still substantially less than those who received cardiac counseling but no behavioral therapy.

Such therapy is becoming more and more available, according to Dr. Williams. Medical schools and hospitals often have rehabilitation programs for heart patients which include group counseling.

Add exercise to your life. Not all the news about Type A's is bad. For one thing, a Type A person benefits more from exercise than his mellower, more laid-back counterparts. And, contrary to A-type expectations, the most effective exercise is *mild* exercise, such as walking. It appears to clear the blood of excess stress hormones better than strenuous activities — which can actually stimulate more of the hormones.

MAKING THE DIFFERENCE WITH A FASTER DIAGNOSIS

Nothing absorbs time, energy, and money like a less-than-accurate diagnosis. The good news is that diagnostic techniques for heart disease are becoming more and more sophisticated. The bad news is that this increased sophistication doesn't always filter down quickly enough to be of use when you need it.

Forget the fast test for cholesterol. Here's a case where fast isn't best. Not all cholesterol tests are created equal. In fact, those finger-prick tests that are popping up in malls and in our workplaces may be sending a lot of people into an anxiety-filled, time-consuming round of further diagnostic tests. And perhaps all for nothing — because one in ten finger-prick cholesterol tests gives a false high reading. Phillip Greenland, M.D., of the University of Rochester School of Medicine and Dentistry, says that blood samples from fingers are consistently higher in cholesterol than those drawn from veins. Tests performed on blood which is drawn from the arm after a 12-hour fast are more accurate.

Investigate echocardiography. Your doctor can tell you about this faster, safer, and less costly picture of the heart. It's a relatively new use for ultrasound that's making it easier on both physicians and heart patients to take a look at ailing hearts. In the recent past, the only methods that could be used to visualize the working heart were X-rays and angiography, which involves snaking a catheter through the blood vessels—a long, arduous procedure that must be performed in the hospital. Echocardiography is changing all that. According to Edgar C. Schick, Jr., M.D., director of echocardiography at the cardiology section of the Lahey Clinic Medical Center in Burlington, Massachusetts, "Echocardiography is very simple to perform, definitely faster and easier than angiography. Echocardiography is noninvasive and really carries no risk whatsoever to the patient—in contrast to angiography, which does."

Echocardiography operates on the same basic principles used to obtain ultrasound pictures of unborn fetuses. An ultrasound beam is aimed at the heart and related structures. Like sonar, the sound waves are reflected back and transferred into images. "With the echo we're actually able to see the walls and valves of the heart in action," Dr. Schick says. "Its primary use is to diagnose abnormalities in the valves and in the chambers of the heart, to assess cardiac function, and to measure the velocity of blood flow in the heart. It's potentially applicable to all heart patients.

"A patient might have a heart murmur heard during a physical examination or there may be some question about heart function that can't be evaluated from the physical exam alone," he continues. "Before the echo was available there might have been some uncertainty about the next step because that step would probably have involved catheterization. Now, the echo can be ordered to further follow through on the physician's suspicion. Not only is there no risk in an echo, but it costs far less than catheterization."

Consider getting a PET. Not the kind with fur or feathers. If you're a heart patient and your doctor is thinking of having you take a stress test or undergo cardiac catheterization, ask about the possibility that you can choose, instead, a new high-tech option called positron emission tomography (PET) scanning. These scans were once confined to the brain, but now they're being adapted to the heart, where they appear to offer some advantages.

A PET scan is painless, simple, and fast. A radioactive tracer is injected intravenously. The scanner detects gamma rays emitted by the tracer as blood carries it through the heart. Instead of actually stressing you on a treadmill, the tester will simulate exercise stress conditions by giving you a vasodilating drug. The three-dimensional color image given by the scanner allows doctors to spot inadequate blood flow.

PET scans are as safe as treadmill tests—but more accurate (95 percent versus 60 percent). They give fewer false positives and can detect artery blockage at an earlier stage (40 percent blockage versus 75 percent on treadmill tests).

According to Donald G. Gordon, M.D., medical director of Memorial PETscan Center in Jacksonville, Florida, PET scanning is much safer than cardiac catheterization, which until now has been the standard method of gauging the severity of artery blockage and the success of treatment. "I think it has such distinct advantages it will become standard practice," Dr. Gordon says.

NEW TREATMENTS PAVE A FASTER ROAD TO RECOVERY

Nothing is static when it comes to treating heart disease. There is so much research on heart disease that new treatments are always being developed, as are new ways of looking at the few old standards that remain. A lot of this new research is aimed at saving time and effort as well as lives.

Think about thrombolysis. If your doctor is willing and able to follow the most up-to-date strategy after your heart attack, you may be able to avoid costly and potentially dangerous procedures like catheterization or angioplasty—as well as get out of the hospital and back to your life sooner. Thrombolytic therapy, which involves administering a clot-dissolving drug within hours after a heart attack, may be enough to restore your circulation to the point where you can go home within one week. The first large study sponsored by the National Heart, Lung, and Blood Institute (NHLBI) of the National Institutes of Health in Bethesda, Maryland, has demonstrated that a conservative approach using thrombolysis alone is as effective as thrombolysis followed by the more invasive and riskier angioplasty (in which blockages in the heart arteries are mechanically opened by special catheter, or slender tube, with a balloon on the end of it inserted into the artery).

"The management of the heart attack has evolved quite a bit," says George Sopko, M.D., physician scientist-medical officer at the Division of Heart and Vascular Diseases of the NHLBI: "A decade or two ago a patient was put in a bed for about five or six weeks, given some anticoagulation, and told to rest. Today patients who have undergone thrombolysis may leave within one week after the heart attack if it is uncomplicated and everything else is fine."

Thrombolysis, according to Dr. Sopko, "has provided us with the ability to modify the natural history of the heart attack. The majority of heart attacks are caused by a clot in the blood vessel. The area of the heart muscle supplied by the blocked blood vessel will die unless blood flow is promptly restored. So if you can dissolve the clot quickly with thrombolysis, you can minimize the injury."

The NHLBI study compared the conservative strategy to the more aggressive, invasive strategy of routinely performing the angioplasty after the thrombolysis. In the conservative course, the angioplasty was still a treatment option but was limited to patients who still suffered restricted blood flow to the heart.

Did the patients who did not automatically receive coronary angiography (and possibly angioplasty) experience any greater risk? No, according to the results of the study. They suffered no greater risk of further heart attacks or heart damage.

According to Dr. Sopko, elimination of the automatic second step of angioplasty results in a significant savings in resources as well as time. But he advises that you talk to your personal physician to find out what is the most appropriate approach for you.

See about checking out early. From the hospital, that is. Twenty-five years ago, your heart attack was likely to grant you an automatic eight-week hospital stay. Nowadays, the conventional hospital stay after a heart attack is more like seven to ten days, but even three days may be enough. A group of doctors decided to test the relative value or risk of early release from the hospital—as long as the heart attack was "uncomplicated." (They defined "uncomplicated" as meaning that there was no lingering angina pain, no heart failure, and no arrhythmia 72 hours after admission to the hospital.) They compared 80 heart attack patients who were assigned either to conventional (seven to ten days) or early (three days) discharge. The early-discharge patients suffered no more complications or readmissions than the group that stayed in the hospital—unless you consider saving more than $5,000 in medical charges and going back to work more than two weeks earlier "complications."

Find out about a fast return to work. Whether your doctor lets you out of the hospital in three days or eight, ask about the possibility that you might get back to work sooner. In a Stanford University study, men who returned to work 51 days after their heart attack experienced no more complications than men who were required to wait a full 75 days. The men who went back to work faster gained an average of more than $2,000 in salary.

Get a second opinion on bypass surgery. Nothing will save you more time than avoiding unnecessary bypass surgery. A recent study took a long, hard second look at almost 400 cases in which coronary bypass surgery was performed. It compared the records of the surgeries with a nationally compiled list of 488 possible legitimate indications for bypass surgery. Fully 14 percent of the surgeries were performed for inappropriate reasons, 30 percent were performed for debatable reasons, and only 56 percent were judged to have been performed for appropriate reasons.

Ask about aspirin for angina. A 325-milligram tablet of aspirin per day has been found to both relieve and prevent attacks of unstable angina by thinning the blood and making dangerous and painful clots less likely, thus also lowering your risk of a heart attack.

Make sure your nitroglycerin is fresh. Researchers analyzed nitroglycerin tablets carried by 150 heart patients and found that one quarter of them were carrying around nitro that had lost its punch. Nitroglycerin should be stored in the small amber glass container in which it comes. Cotton should not be stored in the same container, nor should any other drugs, because nitroglycerin can vaporize and be absorbed by foreign materials. For that reason, the amber container should be kept tightly closed and away from heat. And you should replace your old supply of pills with fresh ones after about six months.

Moisten your mouth. If your nitroglycerin tablets aren't dissolving your angina like they should, the problem may be in your mouth, not in the pills. The pills themselves may not be dissolving, according to Frank E. Rasler, M.D., of Winnipeg, Manitoba. Dr. Rasler says that it's not uncommon for patients with dry mucous membranes to find no relief even after taking several doses of nitroglycerin. A person's mouth may become dry during an angina attack because he or she will switch to mouth breathing. The increased flow of air can quickly dry oral tissues. Angina pain can also decrease saliva secretion.

Dr. Rasler recommends moistening the membranes under the tongue with a squirt of salt solution, which should moisten the tissues enough to allow the pill to dissolve and be absorbed.

Another answer may be to use a new spray form of nitroglycerin, which has been shown to be just as effective as nitroglycerin tablets.

After a heart attack, turn to your spouse. For many people, life takes a turn for the worse after a heart attack— even after they've been told by their doctor that everything is going to be all right. Psychologist Herb Budnick, Ph.D., says that once a patient is released from the protective confines of the hospital, his problems are often just beginning. Suicidal thoughts, guilt, stress, depression, fear, anxiety, anger, frustration, feelings of inadequacy and dependency, and sexual dysfunction are often strong enough to send a man right back to the hospital, says Dr.

Budnick, who has treated heart attack survivors for more than 12 years.

Where should you go for help? The person who can best help, Dr. Budnick says, is often the last one turned to for support—the spouse. Studies have demonstrated that the spouse is the person who can most positively affect the emotional recovery of a heart patient. Dr. Budnick advises heart attack survivors to "increase your quality of life by communicating more, by addressing your emotions, by reaching out to your spouse—and by allowing her to reach out to you. Do that, and you will create a feeling of emotional closeness and intimacy."

Share the stress. Does Dr. Budnick's prescription for togetherness extend to a treadmill stress test built for two? Not quite, but some Stanford University researchers decided to try to boost wives' confidence in their husbands' ability to come back from a heart attack. Overprotective wives are often able to delay their husbands' recovery. So the researchers divided 30 couples of heart attack survivors and their wives into three groups. The first group was split up during the men's stress tests. The wives waited outside. The second group was brought in together and the wives watched the stress tests. The third group of wives, however, not only watched but were required to walk on the treadmill for a full 3 minutes at their husband's maximum workload. Later, all three groups were asked about their confidence in their husbands' recovery. Sure enough, the group of wives that shared the treadmill experience were significantly more confident than the other two groups.

Make love as soon as you can. "It's easy for men to feel emasculated by a heart attack—and we physicians are often guilty of fostering that kind of feeling," says Paul Thompson, M.D., medical director of cardiac rehabilitation at Brown University's Miriam Hospital. "We tell them to be careful, take it easy, don't get into any arguments. Pretty soon the wife won't even let the poor guy sign a check! I take the opposite tack. I tell couples, for example, that if they want to have sex on the day the guy gets home from the hospital, go ahead! In 11 years of practice I haven't lost one patient yet on that first day home. And I think that my telling them this is a powerful indication that things are going to be okay."

• FIRST DENY—THEN ACCEPT

You're in the hospital. You've just had a heart attack, or you're about to have bypass surgery. What do you do? Deny that you're seriously ill? According to some recent research, that attitude might get you out of the hospital faster. That's the good news.

The bad news is that it might also put you back in faster if you don't change your attitude the minute you get out.

The researchers gave a psychological test to a group of heart patients in the hospital for heart attacks or for bypass surgery, then followed them for one year. At the beginning, "high deniers" spent less time in intensive care and had less cardiac dysfunction than "low deniers."

But once they got out of the hospital, the high deniers did not do so well. They didn't follow their doctors' orders as well as the low deniers, who apparently were better convinced of the seriousness of their illness. As a result, the high deniers landed back in the hospital more often than the low deniers.

The researchers concluded that denial of illness was a good way to adapt during the initial hospital stay—but a bad way to adapt in the long run.

Although it's always a good idea to consult your personal physician on a matter such as this, there are other statistics to help you make up your mind. In 1963, a study was made of over 5,000 cases of sudden death in males. Thirty-four of those men had died during sex, only 18 of them from heart attacks.

But stick to your spouse. Wives are a good thing to have close by after a heart attack, sharing your treadmill and your bed. But don't get the idea that if one is good, then two must be better. Not in this case. In the previously mentioned study of sudden death, most of those men who died of heart attacks during sex were not with their wives. Only 5 of the 18 died in their marital beds.

Two doctors from New York reported cases of men whose philandering may have cost them the ultimate price. One 53-year-old man who had had bypass surgery 11 years earlier was admitted to the hospital with chest pains. The next morning he was visited in the coronary care unit by his wife. A short while after she left, he received another visitor: his fiancée. Not too long after she left, he died.

Another patient, who was younger, 34, but was also having a heart attack, was treated to the same scenario: a visit by one fiancée followed rapidly by the visit of another. He survived. But the doctors were compelled to conclude that having two women might have presented such severe psychological stress that it greatly accelerated the course of heart disease—and that perhaps it should be listed as a new risk factor.

IMMUNITY

. . . .

Your blood is red and white. The red blood cells carry oxygen and food; your white cells are an army of defenders—organized ranks of sentries, soldiers, and scavengers. These troops move with the speed of a blitzkrieg. For example, in times of infection, one minuscule battalion, the microbe-fighting neutrophils, can be produced in the bone marrow at the astonishing rate of about 694,000 cells per second.

The components of your immune system spend life in the fast lane. These billions of cells live hard and die young—in only a few days. Then your body has to replace them with fresh troops that are just as strong and viable.

Building your immune system would seem a long-term project, but it's made up of many short-term parts. Some you're already using, others you probably don't know about. Here are tips so you can pick and choose your own program. Each takes a small fraction of time.

- You can get lifelong immunity to a disease with a 1-second vaccination.
- You can arm yourself against disease in the time it takes to have a good belly laugh.
- You can build a mental shield with a few minutes of daily meditation.
- You can boost your resistance in 45 minutes by walking that long, five days each week.

FEEDING YOUR IMMUNE SYSTEM

Napoleon once observed that a good army travels on its stomach. Your inner troops, too, need good food and top-

THE ABSOLUTELY FASTEST WAY POSSIBLE
TO BOOST YOUR IMMUNITY

When you get a vaccination, you hand your immune system a picture of a disease. In fewer than 60 seconds, you buy long-term protection from a disease that could kill.

The memory cells in your immune system keep a file on viruses they have encountered and conquered so they can react faster during a reinvasion. And they also keep a dossier on potential diseases. That's what a vaccination is—a file that not only tells them what the disease looks like, but starts a small brood of antibodies that can multiply like gangbusters if the body comes in contact with the germ.

Some diseases stay permanently on file with the memory cells. Others fade in time, like a poorly developed photograph. That's one reason people need booster shots for some diseases, such as tetanus, diphtheria, pertussis, and polio.

Also, as you age, your immune system changes its filing system. Older people, for instance, may not develop as strong an antibody level against a disease, and the reaction may not last as long as it does in a younger person. This means you may need more frequent vaccinations. Those who live in groups, such as a nursing home, may need special shots—especially flu—on a regular basis because they're exposed to more germs from more sources than people who live separately.

This is the recommended schedule for immunization for people who were not immunized during childhood.

WHEN	VACCINE
First visit	Tetanus, diphtheria Measles, mumps, rubella Polio (live oral vaccine if younger than 18; injection if older than 18)
1 to 2 months after first inoculation	Tetanus, diphtheria, polio
6 to 12 months after second inoculation	Tetanus, diphtheria, polio
Every 10 years	Tetanus, diphtheria

notch nutrition to fight off bodily invaders. Specific nutrients, in fact, play distinct roles in this inner body-building. "Food is not just fuel. It's not simply gas in the car," says

James O'Leary, M.D., Ph.D., associate professor of laboratory medicine and pathology at the University of Minnesota Medical School in Minneapolis. "It's the building blocks for the system. You can get what you need if you eat sensibly."

THE NUTRIENT-DENSE DIET

Preliminary evidence suggests that a "nutrient-dense" diet may help slow the natural decline in immunity that comes with age, according to Jeffrey Blumberg, Ph.D., of the USDA Human Nutrition Research Center on Aging.

You tend to absorb some nutrients less efficiently as you get older, he says, so focusing on foods high in these nutrients will load your body with vitamins, minerals, and fiber, while keeping your diet low in fat and calories.

- Vitamins A and C can boost the immune response, according to registered dietitian Michele M. Gottschlich, Ph.D., at the Shriners Burn Institute in Cincinnati, Ohio. When those vitamins were combined with zinc and fish oil in a formula fed to burn patients, the survival and recovery rate of those people went up. They had fewer infections and got well more quickly.
- Beta-carotene, a substance from which your body makes vitamin A, is thought to spark the antitumor activity of macrophages, the white blood cells that engulf and destroy bacteria, among other invaders, adding protection from diseases. Some researchers think beta-carotene can also protect your macrophages from deteriorating and enhance your T- and B-lymphocytes.
- Vitamin E can actually make your immune system "more vigorous" according to Dr. Blumberg. He and a colleague studied the role of vitamin E in animals, measuring the vitamin's effect on immune functions. They noted that immune cells need a special chemical, called prostaglandin E_2, to turn them off after they've finished fighting a specific threat to the body. As animals got older, they produced more and more of this "shut-off" chemical, which meant it began to inhibit the immune system.

A vitamin E supplement reduced the production of prostaglandin E_2, so that the immune system could stay turned on.

The scientists also discovered that vitamin E increases interleukin-2, a naturally occurring substance that is necessary for a healthy, fighting immune system.

- Zinc is best known as an activator of the thymus gland, which develops the T-cells of your immune system. The average American may not be getting enough zinc from his diet to meet the Recommended Dietary Allowance (RDA). Zinc deficiency is especially common in people with AIDS, and can be found even before the diagnosis has been made, according to Susanna Cunningham-Rundles, Ph.D., of New York Hospital–Cornell Medical Center.
- Iron, selenium, folate, and vitamin B_6 are important, too. A deficiency of vitamin B_6, for instance, depresses your overall immune function. A deficiency of iron may increase your susceptibility to infections. Selenium is important as a fuel for antibodies responding to infection. Folate boosts the immune function.

So how do you go about getting a nutrient-dense diet? Where do you get these immune-boosting nutrients? It's surprisingly fast and easy.

Lettuce eat Romaine. When you survey your choices at the green grocer's, take an extra minute to choose foods that offer lots and lots of nutrition. By selecting Romaine lettuce, for instance, instead of iceberg, you'll get eight times more vitamin A and double the iron. A half cup of cooked broccoli has more than double the vitamin A and eight times the vitamin C as the same amount of lighter green beans. Other good sources of vitamin A and beta-carotene are deep yellow, orange, or green vegetables (such as beet, mustard, or turnip greens; carrots; chili peppers; pumpkins; spinach; and winter squash) and fruits (like apricots, cantaloupes, mangoes, papayas, and peaches).

Just say "Aw, nuts" for vitamin E. Nuts, sunflower seeds, and wheat germ can increase your vitamin E intake by the bite if you want to boost your immune function. Vegetable oils are also excellent sources—soybean is one of the richest.

Stew up some iron. Animal meats and fish are some of the best sources because their iron is readily absorbed by the body, but be sure to choose lean cuts. Dried beans are one of the best vegetable sources of iron. Iron-enriched cereals are also good sources.

Have a piece of fruit. Bananas, cantaloupes, lemons, oranges, and strawberries are good fruit sources of folate, a B vitamin known to strengthen the immune system. Good vegetable sources are asparagus, broccoli, lima beans, and spinach.

Play chicken. Play it up in your diet, that is. White meats (chicken, fish) are one of the richest sources of vitamin B_6, a nutrient that's key to smooth immune function. Whole grains and potatoes are also good sources.

Go pearl diving. And while you're seeking this gem, *eat* all the oysters that you open. They are the richest source of zinc—a mineral that motivates your thymus gland to produce fighting immune cells. Other seafoods and meats are also good sources.

Prospect for selenium. This mineral fuels your antibodies. The best sources are usually foods high in protein—meats, cereals, and dairy products.

MAKE YOUR ARMY LEAN AND MEAN

Your immune system is just like the rest of you when it comes to fat: A certain amount is necessary for life, but beyond that it's just . . . well, *fat.* Keeping your diet lean will help make your immune system mean, according to research reported in the *American Journal of Clinical Nutrition.* The activity of the natural killer (NK) cells increased as the consumption of fat decreased in the men being studied. For each percent decrease in calories from dietary fat, the NK cells' activity increased by a half percent, researchers reported. Ideally, you should get no more than 30 percent of your calories from fat, and no more than 10 percent of your calories from saturated fat, the kind found in meat, dairy products, and hydrogenated vegetable oils.

You can reduce your fat intake simply and quickly.

Drain your oil. Use one-half to three-quarters less oil or margarine than a recipe calls for.

Fake fry your fish. Simulate the crunch of panfrying by oven-frying. Fish, for instance, can be dipped in egg whites and cracker crumbs, then baked on a nonstick baking sheet until done.

Buy a nonstick frying pan. Or use a nonstick vegetable spray. That means you don't have to fry in oil.

Sprinkle on fat-free flavor. Low-calorie flavor enhancers include mustard, horseradish, chopped green and red pepper, tarragon, dill, and curry powder.

Chill out the fat. Refrigerate foods such as soups, sauces, gravies, and stews, then remove the hardened fat from the surface.

Fish around for help. Here's where you may actually want to *add* fat to your diet. Dr. Blumberg's family eats fish at least twice a week because, he says, there's evidence that the special polyunsaturated oils in fish and shellfish—the omega-3 fatty acids—may improve immune system function.

Think of fish as a fast food because cooking takes only about 10 minutes per inch of thickness on the grill, under the broiler, or in an oven preheated to 450°F.

TAKE THE RIGHT DOSE

In the right amounts, vitamins and minerals can power your best defense against infection—your immune system. In too large quantities, however, they can weaken immunity and boost your risk of infection. That's why you should rely first on your diet for these nutrients, and take supplements only after consulting with your doctor.

"I suggest eating a diet low in fats and rich in complex carbohydrates like whole grains, fruits, and vegetables. I suggest eating lean meat in moderate amounts," says Adria Rothman-Sherman, Ph.D., chair of nutritional sciences at Rutgers University.

"I wouldn't suggest taking supplements unless there's reason to believe you're at risk for deficiency. That is, if you're on a very low-calorie diet, on medication, pregnant or lactating, or recovering from severe illness.

"If someone chooses to take a supplement, my caution would be to supplement moderately, right around the RDA, particularly with iron," Dr. Rothman-Sherman says.

TURN ON YOUR DISEASE RESISTANCE

Click. It's on. Click. It's off. Can you turn your immune system on and off that easily? The answer is maybe. And all it takes is less than an hour of exercise.

Studies show exercise affects some hormone and hormonelike substances in the body called neurohormones or neurotransmitters. Scientists know that these chemicals, produced by the brain and the nervous and endocrine systems, are responsible for communications in the brain and nervous system. Now, preliminary studies show these substances may also have the ability to turn on and turn off the cells in your immune system.

So how much exercise and what kind will keep the immune system in good repair?

Take a 45-minute walk to immune power. In just six weeks of walking 45 minutes a day for five days a week, mildly obese, normally sedentary women raised the number of immunoglobulins in their immune systems, according to a study by David C. Nieman, D.H.Sc., formerly at Loma Linda University in California.

Run it off. Intense running can raise your core body temperature, much like a fever. Fever is Mother Nature's way of making protective lymphocytes more responsive, limiting some viral infections and decreasing iron concentrations in the blood, making it harder for some bacteria to survive.

Pedal yourself around town. A study in Denmark showed higher NK cell activity in bicycle racers compared with untrained men who did not play sports regularly.

Take a swim. It's easier on our joints but produces the same immune benefits. Exercise triggers endorphins, a type of neurotransmitter that aids the activity of some immune cells. It temporarily increases the level of interleukin-1, a protein that stimulates the activity of helper T-cells, which are the white blood cells or lymphocytes that identify threats and call other immune cells for help. And exercise stimulates B-cells, which produce the proteins called antibodies that destroy the invaders.

Sweat smart. Too much exercise, however, can impair your immune system because the overload of activity acts like stress. Scientists at Loma Linda University surveyed runners in the 1987 Los Angeles Marathon and found that 13 percent of 2,300 race participants who responded became sick with a cold, the flu, or an upper respiratory infection soon afterward. Only 2 percent who applied for the race but did not run got sick. Runners who trained for 60-plus miles a week were twice as likely to be sick as those who trained for less than 20 miles per week.

What happened? Exercising to exhaustion produces large amounts of hormones and neurotransmitters like cortisol and epinephrine, chemicals that are classic components of a stress response, according to Loma Linda's Lee Berk, D.H.Sc. Those chemicals impair the activity of immune cells such as the NK cells. Those NK cell levels, according to the marathon study, were depressed 6 hours after competition, leaving a large window for illness to strike.

YOU'VE GOT TO SMILE A LITTLE . . .

And laugh a little . . . or so the old song goes. When you do, you're adding muscle to your immune system. When you're stressed or feeling miserable, your immune system sags, too.

Studies show a link between depression and a drop in the ability of your lymphocytes to fight off disease. In a group of 15 widowers studied at Mount Sinai School of Medicine in New York, for instance, researchers found a link between depression and a drop in their lymphocyte levels. In San Diego, a Navy psychologist found depressed recruits were more likely to get a cold during basic training than those who felt positive about their experience.

At Ohio State University, the immunologist/ psychologist team of Janice Kiecolt-Glaser, Ph.D., and Ronald Glaser, Ph.D., found that chronic stress can retard the immune system. They studied people caring for relatives with Alzheimer's disease and found the stressed-out caregivers had lower percentages of T-cells. They discovered women who are separated or divorced and depressed had lower percentages of NK cells, less immune stimulation, and higher antibody levels to latent viruses.

The Glaser team also demonstrated that a reduction of stress or building positive feelings can boost immunity.

Relaxation training just three times a week significantly increased NK and T-cell activity, they said.

Positive feelings can be as important as exercise to keeping your body in tip-top health. Well-known Yale University cancer surgeon Bernie Siegel, M.D., says "positive emotions like love, acceptance, and forgiveness stimulate the immune system."

Have a good laugh. If your immune system slumps when you're sad, does it surge when you're happy? Several psychologists wanted to know, so they made people laugh, then measured their immunoglobulin A (IgA), an immune system soldier on the front lines of respiratory defense. They found that when people laughed, their IgA increased. Immediately. No waiting.

"A certain amount of IgA is always flowing around in our blood," says Herbert Lefcourt, Ph.D., a psychology professor at the University of Waterloo in Ontario, Canada. "When you laugh, there's a rapid transfer of IgA to your saliva, where it will have a more protective effect."

Laughter can increase your production of lymphocyte warriors or block immunosuppressive chemicals trying to rub out your T-cells, according to a joint study by a psychologist at Stanford University and an immunologist at Loma Linda University Medical Center.

One group of people watched a 60-minute comedy videotape while a second group sat twiddling their thumbs. Blood samples showed that laughter had increased the production of lymphocytes by 39 percent and decreased by 46 percent the amount of cortisol, a stress hormone that suppresses the immune system. Laughter, said the researchers, can cut the effects of everyday stress on your immune system almost in half.

Build your own Laughmobile. The Laughmobile is one of the tools used at the Duke University Comprehensive Cancer Center to get people feeling better. It's a cart filled to overflowing with things that make people laugh, including movies, books, audio tapes, and games, says recreation therapist Louise Bost, who is director of the oncology/recreation therapy program.

Save Laurel, be Hardy. You can use those same items stocked on the Laughmobile in just moments. Mobile mirth includes: books by Erma Bombeck, Phyllis Diller,

Lewis Grizzard, and Garrison Keillor; movies featuring The Three Stooges, the Marx brothers, and Laurel and Hardy; and audio tapes by Bill Cosby, Lewis Grizzard, and Garrison Keillor.

Lighten up. It's not just a laugh but a good sense of humor that boosts your protection.

"People with a sense of humor are more likely to take life in a light way," Dr. Lefcourt says. "If a waiter drops a glass of water on you in a restaurant, do you get angry or do you laugh that the world is a random, capricious place? If you can realize that the sun doesn't rise and set with any of our personal problems or concerns, you have a sense of humor."

Find love. "If I told patients to raise their blood levels of immune globulins or killer T-cells, no one would know how. But if I can teach them to love themselves and others fully, the same changes happen automatically. The truth is: Love heals," says Dr. Siegel, author of *Love, Medicine, and Miracles.*

The ability to love and care about others seems to result in lower levels of the stress hormones and a higher ratio of helper T-cells, notes Blair Justice, Ph.D., in *Who Gets Sick.* A study at the Menninger Foundation clinic in Topeka, Kansas, showed that people who are romantically in love have fewer colds and their white blood cells fight infections better.

Give a care. Other evidence shows that caring for someone or something besides yourself is potent medicine. People who have pets, for example, seem to recover faster from illness. People who do things that help others seem to be healthier and live longer lives.

Write it out. Spend 15 or 20 minutes a day for four days putting your problems down on paper and you could boost your immune power for as much as five months, says James W. Pennebaker, Ph.D., a professor of psychology at Southern Methodist University in Dallas, Texas. He is the author of *Opening Up: The Healing Power of Confiding in Others.* Write your deepest thoughts, he says, with the understanding that you'll throw the paper away afterward and no one is going to read what you write. Write continuously for that short time, paying no attention to grammar or sentence structure.

TAKE A MEDITATION BREAK AND BOOST YOUR STRENGTH

Someday coffee breaks may give way to brief, deep relaxation breaks. And perhaps doctors will hand out prescriptions for meditation instead of medication. Teachers will encourage schoolchildren to daydream in class.

Relaxation can give your immune system a boost, according to researchers at Ohio State University. Scientists found that senior citizens who were taught relaxation techniques and guided imagery showed a significant boost in natural killer (NK) cells, the white blood cells that fight the growth of tumors.

Relaxing by meditating just a few minutes each day can give long-term tranquillity to your life, according to Albert Marchetti, M.D., a pathologist and author of *Beating the Odds: Alternative Treatments That Have Worked Miracles against Cancer.* He recommends you find a quiet time and place free from all distractions to do your meditating.

Sit for a few minutes quietly in a straight-back chair, your head in line with your hips, ears in line with shoulders, and nose in line with navel. If you need to, wiggle in small circles until you find the correct posture that will allow energy to flow up and down your spine.

Place your hands in your lap, touching but not clasped. Leave your thumbs and palms pointed upward and your fingers slightly bent.

Take a couple of slow, deep breaths through your nose. Pace your breathing. Close your eyes.

Clear your mind. Now use the words "ham" and "so," a universal mantra recommended by the Siddha Yoga Foundation to erase distractions. As you inhale, repeat the word "ham," and as you exhale, "so." Think only this mantra, repeating it over and over. If thoughts come, just repeat your "ham so," letting images come and go.

Find time to renew your inner self with meditation for 15 minutes several times a day.

In a study, Dr. Pennebaker found that people who pour out their thoughts on a traumatic, upsetting, or unresolved event in their lives are less likely to get sick and seek medical help than those who keep their feelings unspoken. This exercise, he found, enhances the immune system's T-cells.

Dr. Pennebaker isn't talking about a daily journal. People who keep daily journals are no healthier than those who don't, he says. Those people tend to write about superficial happenings in their lives and never quite let go emotionally.

Talk about it. If you can't bring yourself to put on paper the things that trouble you, confiding in someone should be your second choice. "It works best if you can find someone you are completely trusting in, who accepts you no matter what you say, so that you don't distort what you want to say," Dr. Pennebaker says. "That takes a certain kind of friendship."

Get into the swing. Music as a part of medical therapy has been around since ancient times. Today, healing with sound, rhythm, and chanting is widely accepted in many cultures. Music can alter your brain's electrical rhythms and influence the level of stress hormones circulating in the blood. Slow, quiet, nonvocal music can lower your bodily reaction to stress, while a faster tempo heightens alertness and arousal.

Music therapy also can help some people cope with the emotional and physical effects of illness, according to Helen Bonny, Ph.D., a music therapist and cofounder of the Bonny Foundation, an institute for music-centered therapy in Salina, Kansas. She used music therapy to help heal herself, she says, when she developed heart disease. She launched a hospital project that used quiet music successfully to reduce heart rate, lower blood pressure, increase pain tolerance, and lessen anxiety and depression.

Music can be a preventive measure in illness, too, as a booster for your immune function. Music therapist and researcher Mark Rider asked night- and rotating-shift hospital nurses with health problems due to stress to listen to a 20-minute tape of relaxation exercises, guided imagery, and mellow music.

As the days passed, the nurses' stress-hormone levels rose less steeply than they did before the study.

Trek to the mountaintop. You need to experience a sense of hopefulness, according to Carl Hammerschlag, M.D., a Phoenix psychiatrist and lecturer at the University of Arizona School of Medicine in Tucson.

To find hopefulness requires only a brief trip, Dr. Hammerschlag says. Go to a beautiful place where you can be reminded that from darkness comes light. Camp out on a mountaintop or a beach and awaken before sunrise so you can watch the day dawn.

Dr. Hammerschlag spent 20 years practicing medicine in the American Southwest and learned of the connections among mind, body, and spirit in Native American traditional medicine. Native American medicine men, he explains, tell their patients that they must have faith in themselves and that they must call up inner strength—a concept similar to what western scientists now call psychoneuroimmunology—a link among the mind, emotions, and immune system.

Defy the verdict. Research shows that "belief can become biology," according to the late Norman Cousins, adjunct professor in the School of Medicine at UCLA. He was the author of several books on using emotions to combat disease, including *Anatomy of an Illness* and *Head First: The Biology of Hope.*

Positive attitudes and adaptive coping can bolster components of the immune system, Cousins said. According to one study, this may be what is helping to offset the devastation of certain helper cells in six AIDS patients who have survived far longer than expected.

The findings of George Solomon, M.D., professor of psychiatry at UCLA, Cousins explained, don't mean you *deny* the diagnosis of cancer or AIDS or any other disease or health problem. It just means you *defy* the verdict. If you meet the problem with a positive attitude and emotional strength and pay attention to your own needs, you'll gain in immune strength. Emotional distress, on the other hand, depressed the immune system in people with AIDS.

LEG PAIN

Pay a visit to Dr. Kneebone's Leg Pain Clinic, and you'd meet lots of intriguing people with equally intriguing complaints about their legs: weak knees, legs as heavy as stone, midnight charley horses. Dr. Kneebone might have to do some canny detective work to figure out what's causing these individuals' leg pains. Take Jake, for instance. His symptoms remind Dr. Kneebone of a letter to the editor that appeared in the *New England Journal of Medicine* just a few months earlier. A man about Jake's age went to his general practitioner complaining of dull pain and tenderness deep in his right calf muscle. The doctor told him to go home and take some aspirin. Two nights later, the man had just fallen asleep when he was awakened by a sharp pain in his right calf, caused by a kick from his wife.

"Don't kick me there!" said the man. "There's where my leg hurts."

His wife replied, "That's where I always kick you. You were snoring again, and that's how I get you to stop."

When his wife stopped kicking him, the man's pain disappeared. (He still snored. But that's another story.)

The case of the mysterious leg pain reported in the medical journal is real. And so are the leg aches and pains experienced by millions of people. Sometimes the causes— and treatments—for leg pain are simple, and sometimes they're not. But many may be managed. For example:

- Wiggling your toes for a minute or two can relieve the pain of varicose veins.
- A half-hour of alternate walking and resting can ease the discomfort of intermittent claudication.

- Massage manages a charley horse faster than any pill.

Now it's time to get a leg up on leg pain.

DETOUR PAST LEG CRAMPS

You say you have writer's cramp in your *legs?* That's not so strange. Sudden, exaggerated, unprovoked leg cramps plague all sorts of people—athletes, cashiers, pregnant women, people on certain medications (like diuretics), and many older individuals.

"As you get older, your leg muscles lose their tone, so when you participate in a physical activity, your muscles become more susceptible to cramping," explains Stanley Silverberg, M.D., a cardiologist and peripheral vascular specialist in Chevy Chase, Maryland.

Leg cramps hurt like the dickens! So when they strike, you'll want relief *fast*. Here's how to find it.

Rein in your charley horse. You can massage away a calf cramp in a few minutes by grasping your toes and gently pulling them toward you. Use the other hand to rub lengthwise along the calf, from the back of the knee to the ankle. And always rub up and down the muscle, not across it.

"Massaging out the cramp works faster than any medication possibly could," Dr. Silverberg says. (A heating pad or hot-water bottle would also help. "But in the time it takes to find the thing and heat it up, you could have massaged away your pain," Dr. Silverberg says.)

Quell those cramps with Q-Vel. This is an over-the-counter quinine caplet designed to relieve nighttime leg cramps. Quinine has been used to prevent and relieve nocturnal leg cramps since the 1930s. Fifty years later, doctors at the University of Utah School of Medicine decided to run a scientific test on the drug. They recruited eight men and women between the ages of 47 and 81 (the most susceptible age for nocturnal leg cramps) who'd been suffering cramps on the average of two nights a week for a year or more. When they took quinine, they experienced fewer, less severe cramps. What's more, when they took a placebo (inactive pills), the cramps lasted longer—anywhere from 6 minutes to more than *4 hours*.

But when they took quinine, the cramps either disappeared completely or didn't last long—14 minutes at the most. Don't bother with tonic water, however—it's a poor source of quinine.

Try Benadryl. This over-the-counter antihistamine seems to prevent leg cramps in some people. "Using Benadryl hasn't been proven effective in scientific tests," Dr. Silverberg says, "but a lot of patients and doctors find it works."

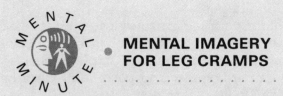

MENTAL IMAGERY FOR LEG CRAMPS

As you massage your leg's contracted muscle, you can further speed relief by using mental imagery.

"If you measure a leg cramp—and we can do this in the lab—the instruments detect a shower of nerve impulses triggering repetitive, sustained muscle contractions," says peripheral vascular specialist Dr. Stanley Silverberg. If you can mentally visualize the muscle relaxing or the nerve impulses slowing, you may get rid of the cramp a lot faster.

Begin your visualization by totally relaxing. (Use the progressive relaxation exercise on page 376.) Then, using Dr. Silverberg's description of a shower of nerve impulses, develop your own scenario. You can, for example, picture a narrow pathway running from your brain to your cramping leg. The pathway is crowded with messengers, each running toward the contracted muscle, each carrying a long spear. As they approach the muscle, they toss their spears at it, causing it to spasm with pain.

Now imagine that you have erected a stone wall across the pathway, a wall so high that no messenger can breach it. Picture the protective wall. No sharp lance can go over or through it.

Your muscle, now safe, begins to relax. Feel it become warm as you massage it. Feel the knotted fibers loosen and spread. Feel the relief.

INTERMITTENT CLAUDICATION: A LEG ATTACK

Sometimes calf muscles cramp up in the midst of a leisurely stroll. When you rest for a few minutes, the pain subsides, but then your muscles knot up again after walking another few yards.

Intermittent claudication is the technical term for this "occasional lameness," a special brand of cramp caused by partially blocked arteries in the legs (and sometimes in the foot, thigh, hip, or buttock, depending on where the blockage develops). When you walk, your leg muscles don't get enough blood. Starved for oxygen, they cramp up.

"You can only walk so far—half a block, two blocks, half a mile—before pain stops you in your tracks," says Guylaine Lanctot, M.D., a specialist in varicose veins. "And it happens at the same distance every time."

Intermittent claudication is caused by the same problem that causes heart attacks: atherosclerosis, in which plaques, or fatty deposits, form inside blood vessels. (High cholesterol, high blood pressure, and diabetes contribute to the problem.)

A total leg transplant might cure the problem. But so far, that's only been done in rats. Luckily, there's plenty you can do right now to stop intermittent claudication from getting worse, to increase the distance you can walk without pain, and perhaps even to reverse the damage. Here's the game plan.

Toss all your cigarettes in the trash. If you smoke, quit at once. Doctors aren't sure how smoking causes atherosclerosis, but they do know that it's the number one risk factor for claudication.

"Patients who claudicate are almost universally cigarette smokers," says Robert Ginsburg, M.D., director of the Center for Advanced Cardiovascular Therapy in Palo Alto, California. "I don't think I've ever seen a claudication patient in my life (except for those with diabetes) who did not smoke at some time. The most crucial thing is for them to stop smoking. It helps dramatically."

Walk, rest, then walk some more. Despite the fact that walking often triggers cramps for people with intermittent claudication, regular walks are one of the best *remedies* for the problem.

How can something that hurts help?

"When you walk until the skeletal muscles in the legs become oxygen deprived, it stimulates an automatic process in the body that regulates blood flow. This auto-regulatory process sends more blood to the legs," Dr. Ginsburg explains. "The body releases hormones and other agents (in the area of the cramp) that open up the small 'collateral' leg-muscle vessels that have been dormant."

These newly opened blood vessels take over some of the job of the clogged ones. The trick is to walk to the point of discomfort, rest, then resume your walk, says Mark Creager, M.D., director of the Noninvasive Vascular Laboratory at Brigham and Women's Hospital in Boston, and assistant professor of medicine at Harvard Medical School. Continue this stop-and-start walking for half an hour, one to three times a day. In fact, almost any kind of exercise—swimming, bicycling, or whatever—can be good for people with intermittent claudication, Dr. Creager adds. Over a period of three to six months, pain will lessen, and you'll be able to walk further without lameness.

"You probably won't be able to run a marathon," Dr. Ginsburg says. "But many people [who walk regularly] go from being housebound to being able to shop." (By the way, this recommendation will work only if you don't smoke. Nicotine constricts the blood vessels.)

Go lite. In fact, if you are overweight, begin a sensible weight-loss diet. The more excess weight your legs have to carry around, the more they are taxed. Lose weight, and you take the strain off your vascular system.

Ask your doctor about aspirin. While there's no drug to improve blood flow to your leg muscles and stop intermittent claudication, aspirin may help some people. "We recommend that our patients take one aspirin tablet a day," Dr. Ginsburg says. "It's based on experience with carotid-artery disease [in the neck] and heart disease, not any solid data on the legs, per se. But it probably prevents further deposits of platelets [elements of plaque] and therefore the progression of the disease."

Note: Don't try aspirin or any of these remedies for intermittent claudication without your doctor's permission. Claudication is a symptom of underlying artery disease, and if not managed properly, it can lead to serious problems, such as amputation or stroke. So it's imperative that anyone who experiences leg cramps when walking (or sitting) see a doctor for proper diagnosis and treatment.

REVERSING VARICOSE VEINS

People with varicose veins typically complain that their legs feel painful, tired, achy, or heavy, especially toward evening or after hours of shopping or sightseeing. Or they experience a burning or jerking sensation in an isolated area of a leg. The underlying problem is failure of the saphenous veins, just underneath the skin surface—they don't pump blood in the legs back toward the heart the way they should. Either the one-way valves designed for this job disintegrate or they don't close completely, leaking blood "like an overflowing toilet," as Dr. Lanctot describes it. Or the blood vessel walls weaken and bulge. (Spider veins are simply varicose veins in the capillaries, the smallest branches of your blood vessel system.)

Whether you have leaky valves, weak walls, or both, blood stagnates, leading to swelling and discomfort.

"Anything that increases blood pressure in your legs increases pain, so your legs hurt more at the end of the day, especially if you've been standing or if you force a bowel movement," Dr. Lanctot says. "Or a woman may find her legs ache more just before her period."

Conversely, anything you can do to reduce the pressure will relieve pain. Lying in bed with your feet propped up can help counteract gravity and get the blood flowing back toward your heart. But you can't spend the rest of your life on your back. Luckily, there are a few fast ways to counteract gravity and get blood pumping the way nature intended. Dr. Lanctot offers the following measures.

Wiggle your toes. Long periods of sitting stymie blood flow back through your veins. So if your job has you anchored at a cash register, word processor, or desk for hours on end, spend a minute or two every half hour or so wiggling your toes inside your shoes. Also, flex your leg muscles and lift yourself on tiptoe as often as you can.

Take a short, brisk walk. If it's practical, leave your work station and take a 5-minute walk around the block

SCLEROTHERAPY: HIGH-TECH HEALING FOR VARICOSE VEINS

The preferred treatment for damaged veins is to destroy them with injections, called sclerotherapy," says varicose vein specialist Dr. Guylaine Lanctot.

A doctor well trained in sclerotherapy can obliterate varicose veins in just two or three office visits. Most problems develop in the superficial venous system between the groin and the ankle. These veins lie close to the surface and are dispensable. They circulate only about 10 percent of the blood in your feet and legs. The deep veins below the muscles carry the rest of the burden.

Sclerotherapy also can be used to treat varicosities in the branches of the long vein running from ankle to groin.

Surgery is reserved for varicosities in the long vein itself. Even when surgery is called for, treatment is high-speed. The doctor needs to make only two tiny incisions, one at each end of the problem. "The vein can be removed under local anesthesia, on an outpatient basis," Dr. Lanctot says. "You can schedule surgery for Friday afternoon and be back to work on Monday."

(or down to the coffee machine and back) every hour or so. As you walk, your calf muscles contract around the blood vessels, taking over for the faulty valves and helping pump blood up through your veins.

Sign up for volleyball. Or dust off your stationary bike. Or swim a few laps in your neighborhood pool. Since rhythmic, muscular exercise compresses the veins and forces blood up toward your heart, daily exercise of some kind can help counteract varicose veins. Walking, jogging, skiing, and skating are good, too.

Wear elastic support stockings. "I highly recommend wearing support stockings," Dr. Lanctot says. "They force the blood back up through your veins." And you don't necessarily need the heavy, unsightly compression stockings prescribed for people with phlebitis or other special circulatory problems. Dr. Lanctot recommends medium weight, department store support hose. "High-grade support hose exert pressure of between 8 and 20 milliliters of mercury [a measure of compression]—enough to relieve discomfort," she says. Good stockings might cost $6 or $8, but your legs will say, "Ahhh, thank you . . ." (Hint: Exercising regularly *and* wearing elastic stockings maximizes pain control.)

Let your fingers do the walking. Walking through the yellow pages, that is. Dr. Lanctot encourages anyone with varicose veins to locate a doctor specializing in vascular problems, even if your only symptom is small, painless spider veins. "Troublesome veins are more than just a cosmetic problem—they can sometimes lead to serious complications," she says. So you want to treat the underlying problem, not just the symptoms. Also, if you have a history of phlebitis, varicose eczema or ulcers, or other serious vein-related problems, always consult a doctor before attempting to manage pain on your own.

SHORTCUTS FOR SHINSPLINTS AND STRESS FRACTURES

Shinsplints is a catchall term for a variety of problems that cause pain and aching between the knee and ankle, especially up and down the front of the shin bone, or tibia. The most common type of shinsplints is medial tibial stress syndrome—inflammation of the muscle on the inner side of the leg, behind the shinbone, about midpoint or lower. Pain usually occurs after a couple of weeks of rhythmic, repetitive activities like aerobic dance or long-distance running. Training errors such as increasing intensity or distance too quickly or changing running surface or shoes also may often bring on pain.

Here's a checklist of fast remedies to heal shinsplints— and keep them healed.

Sit it out. Shinsplints won't heal without rest. So don't try to exercise through pain. "We're not talking about lying-in-bed rest, though," says William W. Briner, Jr., M.D., of the Parkside Sports Medicine Center in Park Ridge, Illinois. "I prescribe 'relative rest.' That is, abstain from any activity that causes pain—running, aerobics, whatever. Instead, do something else—biking, for instance. Just make sure you stay seated while peddling, to keep pressure off the legs."

Listen to your legs. After a week or two, you can gradually resume running. "But you if start to feel pain, ease back," Dr. Briner says. Cut your distance or intensity.

Ice the pain. An ice massage can help reduce inflammation after activity. Ice is also helpful if walking itself triggers pain. "Freeze water in a paper cup," Dr. Briner says. "Then as the ice melts, peel off the paper and rub it up and down your shin. Massage your leg with ice for 20 minutes after activity, or three or four times a day for 15 or 20 minutes at a time."

Take your medicine. "I often advise people to take an anti-inflammatory medicine, like aspirin or ibuprofen, for up to two weeks, when the pain is most acute," Dr. Briner says. "Continuing the dosage around the clock helps maintain blood levels of the medicine, helping to keep inflammation down." (Two cautions: Read the label for possible side effects and contraindications, and don't try this if you have ulcers.)

Cushion the blow. To prevent repeat episodes of shin pain, buy a well-cushioned pair of shoes and replace them every six months or so. "Look for supportive shoes with shock-absorbing materials like air pockets or gel," Dr. Briner says. You might also want to slip Sorbothane insoles (available in sporting goods stores) into your shoes. "It's the most shock-absorbent material I know of, and it lasts for years," he says.

Seek and ye shall find. Seek out an unpaved running track and find relief for shinsplints. "Running on soft surfaces like crushed gravel is easier on your shins than asphalt or hard pavement," Dr. Briner says. "Even if you have to drive there, it's worth the inconvenience."

Stretch before you strut. "You should stretch the heel cord before and after activities like running or aerobics," he says. "Lean forward with the palms of your hands pressed against a wall, with one foot forward and one back, heels flat on the floor," he explains. "Stretch each leg, first with your knee straight, then with your knee bent, for a total of 3 to 5 minutes."

Have little impact. Surprisingly, shinsplints are more common among aerobic dancers than runners, Dr. Briner says. Many aerobic classes involve a lot of high-impact jumping around. "Instead, go for low-impact or non-weight-bearing routines if you have trouble with shinsplints," he says.

About pace. Alternate hard days with easy days, or cross-train, alternating running or aerobics with biking, swimming, or walking. Pace yourself and your workouts to reduce stress on your shins.

Repeated jarring may also cause stress fractures in the shinbone or in the fibula (the smaller bone running alongside the shinbone, the outside of the leg.) A special X-ray called a bone scan may be the only way to distinguish between shin pain caused by stress fractures or soft tissue inflammation.

If you do in fact have stress fractures, *rest* is the order of the day. Stay off the leg for three or four weeks, until it heals. (Doing nothing may sound easy. But for exercise enthusiasts, this may be the hardest advice to follow. Nevertheless, continuing to work out with fractured shins only prolongs the agony.)

KNOCK OUT KNEE PAIN

Most people think of the knee as a simple hinge. But knees are complex joints of niftily engineered cartilage, ligaments, tendons, muscles, and bones that give you mobility and support.

"When you run, for example, you're reproducing three times your body weight on ankles and knees," says Dennis Phelps, athletic trainer with the Athletic Rehab Care clinic in Anaheim, California. Yet most people, especially weekend athletes, runners, and aerobic dancers, take their knees for granted, rendering them very susceptible to injury. Abuse your knees and you'll know it!

"Recreational athletes are no different from competitive athletes," Phelps says "They still have to condition their bodies to minimize trauma."

Many of the same remedies for shinsplints can help bypass knee pain. Here are some assorted measures to relieve knee pain—or prevent relapses that keep exercise enthusiasts sidelined.

Vary your running course. "Most streets and roadways are crowned, so as you run, one leg strikes the pavement at a different distance than the other, creating an imbalance. Changing direction keeps you from irritating one spot," Phelps says. "For example, if you always

KNEE-BRACING EXERCISES

The best way to keep your knee properly hinged and prevent another injury is to strengthen the muscles that keep all those bones, ligaments, and tendons together and moving. These exercises don't take much time, and that minimal investment pays off handsomely.

First get your doctor's okay. Some of these exercises could aggravate your injury, especially if you do them too soon after your injury or with too much weight. *If the exercise hurts, stop immediately.* Try less weight, or no weight at all. You want to feel muscle "burn," not joint pain—that's the signal to back off. Always perform the motion smoothly and slowly. Do the exercises daily or as directed by your doctor.

You can do most of these exercises on the kind of weight machines found in a gym, or you can buy ankle weights for home use. Even cheaper: Put penny rolls (about three to a pound) or lead fishing sinkers in a sock, knot the end securely, distribute the weight equally between both ends of the sock, and drape it over your ankle. When it's time to add weight, put your pennies in an old purse and hang the strap over your ankle.

Straight-leg raise. Lie on your back on a hard surface. Bend one leg up at the knee, keeping the foot down flat. Gently lock the knee of the other leg in an extended position and lift from the hip. Raise your foot no more than 6 to 8 inches and hold for about 6 seconds. Slowly lower your leg and rest for 6 seconds. Do ten repetitions with each leg.

You may want to begin this exercise without weights. Gradually add weight as you gain strength—up to 5 pounds maximum. Then, rather than add more weight, try to keep your leg up for 10 seconds instead of 6—without shaking. You can eventually build up to three sets of ten repetitions each.

Seated quadriceps extensions. Home version: Sit in a chair with your feet resting on a box that is far enough in front of you that when your knees are bent, your lower legs form a 45-degree angle with the floor. Begin with light weight or no weight. Raise your leg until it's horizontal, or as close as you can get it, and hold it for 6 seconds. Then lower it slowly and rest for 6 seconds. Repeat ten times with each leg.

For the next exercise, begin with your legs hanging straight down. Then raise one leg to a 45-degree angle, hold it, and lower it. Alternate legs. These two exercises work different muscle groups and protect the knee from strain. If either exercise hurts, just do the other.

Gym version: This exercise can be duplicated on a leg-extension machine. Have the gym instructor show you how to adjust the machine so it allows you to lift the weight from the 45-degree angle.

Whatever version you use, gradually work up in weight as you grow stronger, and aim for three sets of ten repetitions each. When you reach 10 pounds, instead of adding more weight, try to hold it for 10 seconds instead of 6.

Hamstring strengthener. Home version: Stand facing a wall, with your hands braced against it for stability. With your ankle weight secured, raise your foot behind you and slowly bring your shin parallel to the floor. Hold for 6 seconds, then slowly lower your foot to the floor, and rest 6 seconds. Repeat ten times with each leg.

Gym version: This exercise can be duplicated on a hamstring or thigh and knee machine where you lie on your stomach and pull the weight up until your feet are straight up. On the machine you can exercise just one leg, or both legs at once.

Again, as your doctor advises, gradually work up in weight as you grow stronger, and aim for three sets of ten repetitions each.

. . . .

start your run heading north, and return heading south, reverse directions every other run. That is, head out going south and return going north."

Nudge up your distance. Add to your mileage slowly. Sudden changes in training appear to be a major culprit in certain forms of knee pain, especially among people training for competition. "Don't increase your mileage by more than 10 percent a week," advises Douglas W. Jackson, M.D., an orthopedist practicing in Long Beach, California.

Cut your aerobics class in half. Phelps treats a lot of people who plunge back into exercise full force before an injury is completely healed, delaying the healing process and risking reinjury. "If you insist on testing your knee, take it easy," Phelps says. "If you're itching to get back to aerobics, take half the class instead of a full hour, to see how it feels. If you feel pain, you know you're not ready. Stop and apply ice."

Stick close to home. By the same token, rehabilitated runners who've been nursing a knee injury should run on a track or around their neighborhood, so they don't get stranded in the middle of nowhere, crippled with pain. "Mark off a ½-mile length, then run back and forth, so if you develop pain, you don't have to hobble a couple of miles to get home," Phelps recommends.

Abandon your running course. If your knees have been through the mill, consider using a treadmill—no hills, no potholes, no surprises, no pain. "I've had knee surgery three times," Phelps volunteers. "Now, I jog on a treadmill. If you've had any kind of knee trouble—iliotibial band syndrome, tendinitis, bursitis, or arthritis of the knee—you should run on as flat a surface as possible."

Take the no-pain train. By planning your training program, you may be able to avoid knee pain altogether. "If you're going to ski in winter, start your conditioning program in July," Phelps says. "If you're going to water ski next summer, get on a treadmill and pump iron in February. The idea is to spend a couple of days a week doing some kind of moderate exercise to get your knees (and heart and lungs) in shape ahead of time, so when the time comes to exert yourself, your body will be accustomed to the extra work." The same applies to golfers, tennis players, softball players, and other weekend warrior athletes, especially if you sit around at a suit-and-tie job all week, Phelps says.

While walkers and day hikers are less susceptible to knee injury than runners or aerobic dancers (they don't tend to travel at the blistering pace that runners do, Phelps says), they, too, can overdo it. Here are some quick, out-on-the trail fixes for knee pain.

Throw in the towel. "If you're going to be hiking near a stream or other cold waterway, carry a small towel or facecloth with you," Phelps suggests. "When you stop to take a break, plunge the cloth into the cold water, wring it out, and wrap it around your knee."

Backpack some aspirin. As with shinsplints, aspirin (or other anti-inflammatory medicine) and rest are time-honored remedies for knee pains and strains. As with any medication, check with your doctor for a recommendation.

Say "uncle." "If rest, ice, and other home treatments don't reduce pain within a week to ten days, get professional advice," Phelps says. "If you don't know whom to consult, call the sports medicine department of your nearest university or junior college, and ask who treats their athletes." Your problem may call for strength training exercises, knee braces, or other measures specifically tailored to your needs.

MEN'S HEALTH

en and women may be equal under the law, but at least where health problems are concerned, there's inequality above and below the belt. Though women are catching up to men in many of the health problems of modern civilization, such as heart disease and cancer, there are a few problems women will never share because . . . well, because they don't have the same equipment. No woman will ever have a prostate problem, for instance, despite the fact that this pesky gland eventually causes some grief to almost every man.

Another difference between men and women is that men are notorious for avoiding doctors as if they had the plague (see "Overcoming the Fear of Doctors" on the opposite page). But all of the particularly male health problems described in this chapter can be healed faster once they are properly diagnosed and examined by a physician.

- In an instant, an ultrasound scan may diagnose a prostate problem—including early detection of a tumor—at the speed of sound.
- A 10-minute sitz bath, two or three times daily, may relieve symptoms of seminal vesiculitis, a painful inflammation.
- In half an hour, a modern surgical procedure can repair a hernia—and no overnight hospital stay is required.

Speaking of hernias, now's the time to take a few minutes to learn about this mostly male malady.

OVERCOMING THE FEAR OF DOCTORS

American men go to the doctor 20 percent less often than American women. Does that mean that men get sick less than women? No, the truth is that men are afraid of doctors. In writing her book, *Male Stress Syndrome,* Georgia Witkin, Ph.D., asked men what they are most afraid of. "Doctors of all kinds scored very high," says Dr. Witkin, assistant clinical professor in the departments of Psychiatry and Obstetrics and Gynecology at Mount Sinai Medical Center in New York. Men are also more afraid of illness than of death, she says.

It's not only fear that keeps a man from going to the doctor, however. Often, men don't realize they need a doctor's care. "Men are absolutely unaware of the most blatant body signals," says Francis Baumli, Ph.D., a medical health consultant in Columbia, Missouri, and a representative of the Coalition of Free Men, a national men's rights organization. "Their perceptive faculties have been so numbed by the masculinizing factors of our society that their bodies could be screaming to them for help and they wouldn't notice."

Men avoid the doctor because they don't like to be vulnerable or dependent, according to Dr. Witkin. "Going to a doctor, for men, is putting themselves in someone else's hands," she says. "This is very frightening for men, because they are trained to maintain control over every aspect of their lives."

As you might expect, avoiding the doctor does not, in reality, strengthen a man's control over his health. In fact, putting off going to the doctor can often result in a man's losing not only control of his health but also precious time that he could put to better use.

So the first rule for speedy healing for men's health problems is: *Go to the doctor.* As Dr. Witkin says, "When men see the risk/reward ratio, they see the risk of not getting care is much higher than the risk of losing control or changing their lifestyles. And the reward for taking care of themselves is much higher than the reward of kidding themselves that nothing is wrong for a few months until it gets too bad to ignore."

More often than not, a visit to the doctor is the shortest, fastest route to healing.

HELPING A HERNIA

The vast majority of hernias are inguinal, and the vast majority of people who get them are men. Heavy lifting, coughing, or accident makes a loop of the small intestine protrude downward through a weak spot in the abdominal wall, or push into the scrotum through the inguinal canal, the path the testes follow when they descend into the scrotum before birth. There are usually no symptoms except a bulge or swelling. The hernia may stay small, but often it gets bigger with time. When it's small, a doctor can usually push the intestine back where it belongs. A truss is usually only a temporary solution. Larger hernias may need surgery—a half million such operations are performed in America yearly.

Try the new, improved hernia surgery. A high-speed, modern surgical technique and use of local rather than general anesthetics have made hospital stays for hernia repair almost obsolete. "It's highly unusual today, in any metropolitan area where there are physicians who concentrate on hernia surgery, for a patient to need to be hospitalized for a routine hernia operation," says Arthur Gilbert, M.D., founder of the Hernia Institute of Florida, in Miami, and past president of the medical staff at South Miami Hospital. In fact, only about 1 out of 20 people, or even fewer, need to spend a night in the hospital.

You go in the first thing in the morning, the surgery takes about half an hour, and you're home and walking around by 11:00 A.M. "It's not unusual for people to be playing golf in a week and tennis in two weeks," Dr. Gilbert says. "People who do office work are usually back in the office the next day or the day after. People who do heavier work are usually back within a week or two."

Those who are not eligible for walk-in hernia repair with local anesthetics include obese people, those with complicated recurrent hernias that have a lot of scar tissue, and underage patients, according to Dr. Gilbert.

Patch up. In the old days of hernia repair, surgeons repaired the muscle tear by sewing the abdominal wall back together. Dr. Gilbert, and many other contemporary surgeons, now prefer to repair the hernia with a prosthetic mesh made of polypropylene. "We use prosthetic materials almost all the time," Dr. Gilbert says. "I am a strong believer that defective tissues, even though repaired, continue to undergo degeneration. Why not take the opportunity to perform a repair that gives the patient the least chance that he'll ever have to come back to the operating room for another operation because the first repair failed?"

By using the prosthetic mesh, Dr. Gilbert has reduced the hernia recurrence rate to about $\frac{1}{10}$ of 1 percent—compared with national hernia recurrence rates as high as 10 to 25 percent.

REDUCING THE PAIN OF VESICULITIS

This inflammation of the seminal vesicles, two sausage-shaped glands located near the back of the prostate that produce 90 percent of the liquid part of the ejaculate, has been described as the wrath of God visited upon a man's genitourinary system. Symptoms may include painful urination or ejaculation, frequent urination, pain in the lower back or abdomen, pain behind the scrotum, and possibly blood in the semen.

Most likely you didn't do anything wrong to get this problem, says E. Douglas Whitehead, M.D., director of the Association for Male Sexual Dysfunction in New York City. Nevertheless, the first step in a speedy cure is to see a physician. The doctor will want to rule out other problems with similar symptoms, such as prostatitis or cystitis, which require different treatments. If the inflammation seems to be caused by an infection, your physician will prescribe antibiotics.

Dr. Whitehead says there are other strategies you can try which may relieve symptoms if the inflammation is not caused by an infection.

Try a bland diet. Spices that burn your mouth don't lose their sting once you swallow them. They can attack delicate tissue inside your body, too. The seminal vesicles happen to be a prime target for spicy food irritation.

Go on the wagon. Alcohol also can irritate delicate tissue.

Drink plenty of fluids. They will dilute and help remove any irritants in your urinary tract.

Alter your sexual frequency. Have sex less often if you're very active, more often if you're not so active, Dr. Whitehead advises.

Try a sitz bath. Simply sitting in a tub of warm water for 10 to 20 minutes at a time two or three times a day may relieve symptoms.

QUICK RELIEF FOR EPIDIDYMITIS

Maybe you didn't even know you have an epididymis. It's kind of tucked away in your scrotum, all 13 to 20 feet of it, a long, convoluted, cordlike tube that stores and carries sperm and provides a place for them to mature. Epididymitis is the term for an inflammation of the epididymis, and it's a fairly common condition, says Seattle urologist Richard E. Berger, M.D. The exact cause is unknown, but some believe it's the result of a sexually transmitted disease (STD) like chlamydia or gonorrhea, or by a urinary tract infection. Whatever the cause, the symptoms are similar — sudden pain behind the testicle, followed by swelling and tenderness in the scrotum — and so are the treatments, primarily a ten-day course of antibiotics. Any unusual pain should be checked and treated by a physician, Dr. Whitehead cautions, "particularly in men aged 20 to 35 who are at risk for testicular cancer." But there are a few things you can do to ease your pain and speed your recovery.

Rest. Your scrotum is rather free-swinging, and that swinging can increase pain. So take it easy. You probably won't feel much like doing anything anyway.

Use an athletic supporter. If you must be active, a jock strap will support the scrotum and keep it immobile.

Avoid sex. This advice isn't hard to follow, because sex is one of the things you won't feel like doing anyway. Nor would you want to pass along a possible STD or a urinary infection.

Take a painkiller. Aspirin and ibuprofen are anti-inflammatories, so they help relieve pain. Check with your doctor first, though.

Ice it. Applying ice to the area helps reduce swelling.

Take a sitz bath. Soaking your scrotum in warm water can help relieve discomfort.

PRESCRIPTIONS FOR PROSTATE PROBLEMS

Add prostate problems to the list of the inevitable calamities of a man's life. An estimated 12 million American men over the age of 40 suffer from painful disorders of this tiny gland. And cruising through the fifth and sixth decades of life without prostate problems is no guarantee you're home free, because the odds increase the older a man gets. By the time a man reaches the age of 85, he has a 95 percent chance of having to cope with an enlarged prostate, even if he does not have any bothersome symptoms, according to Dr. Whitehead.

At least one man in ten will seek relief in surgery from often debilitating symptoms—frequent, difficult urination; a slow, weak urine stream; or incomplete emptying of the bladder. And the worst part is that these same symptoms can be caused by a simple inflammation or by life-threatening cancer.

All this from a gland that weighs less than an ounce!

There are three basic types of prostate disorders: inflammation of the prostate, or prostatitis; enlargement of the prostate, or benign prostatic hypertrophy (BPH); and cancer of the prostate. Most medical authorities agree that there is very little a man can do to prevent prostate troubles. But treatment for prostate disorders has made great strides, and, as in other health problems, time is of the essence. Getting to the doctor quickly can mean the difference between a long, drawn-out, and possibly life-threatening bout with illness, or a quick path to healing.

PROMPT RELIEF FOR PROSTATITIS

Most prostate problems are usually considered diseases of aging because they tend to get worse as the years add up. But prostatitis usually strikes young men. There are several types of prostatitis, but all share the same basic symptoms: low back pain, fever, pain on urination and under the scrotum, and pelvic pain. Again, the doctor is the person to see, because there are several different types of prostatitis, and the fast track for healing is different in each case.

Take a short course in antibiotics. If your doctor says you have acute bacterial prostatitis, it means that some pesky bacteria have taken up residence in your prostate gland. Temporary residence, that is, because your doctor will prescribe some antibiotics to clear out the neighborhood fast.

Try another round. If your problem is chronic bacterial prostatitis, it means that the bacteria have dug in for the long haul, so a short course of antibiotics may not clear up the problem. A recurrent bladder infection may be the culprit, spilling bacteria over into the prostate and the urinary tract. In this case, the doctor will take a bacterial culture to confirm the diagnosis, and then prescribe an additional course of antibiotics.

BREAKING THE BPH STRANGLEHOLD

For the first two or three decades of a man's pubescent life, his prostate gland remains stable, having grown to the size of a nickel by puberty. But, for reasons unknown to medical science, in middle age the prostate starts to enlarge—sometimes to the size of an orange. This growth, because it's not cancerous, is called benign prostatic hypertrophy, or BPH—although millions of men no doubt wonder how something so disrupting and uncomfortable could be called "benign."

BPH can strangle a man's urethra, which passes through the prostate gland and carries urine from the bladder. He may have extreme difficulty starting the stream, and, once started, it is so weak that the bladder will not completely empty, making it necessary to urinate again in a short time. It's not uncommon for a man with BPH to need to get up in the middle of the night two or three times to urinate. Some men grow impatient and strain so hard to start or increase the flow that they give themselves hernias.

BPH can become even more serious if the urinary tract becomes so constricted that urination is impossible and the bladder becomes full. This can not only be excruciating but life-threatening as well. A thin tube, or catheter, must then be inserted through the urethra to drain the bladder.

"In the old days, either you had the surgery or you learned to live with BPH," says Harold P. McDonald, Jr., M.D., director of the Georgia Prostate Center in Atlanta. Now other treatments are becoming available for BPH, although none is currently believed to be as effective as surgery. So rather than try to live with it, Dr. McDonald advises, "it's better to deal with prostate problems sooner

POTENT WEAPONS IN THE BATTLE AGAINST BPH

Several drugs are currently being tested before being approved for use in treating benign prostatic hypertrophy, or BPH. One of these is Proscar, which blocks the production of dihydrotestosterone, the enzyme that appears to maintain prostatic enlargement. There are other drugs currently available that will block this enzyme and shrink the prostate, but they cause impotence. In about one-third of the men who receive it, according to Seattle urologist Dr. Richard Berger, Proscar shrinks the prostate and improves symptoms but does not cause impotence.

Another drug to ask your doctor about is Terazosin (hytrin), a smooth muscle relaxant. When the prostate is abnormally enlarged, the smooth muscles that line the urinary tract tend to spasm and close off the tube. By relaxing this spasm, Terazosin can relieve symptoms of BPH. Because this drug also lowers blood pressure, it may cause dizziness when you stand up, Dr. Berger advises.

---

rather than later. The nature of the problem is such that it gets better, then three months later it gets worse. Men tend to put off treatment when it's better, but then it gets even worse. And the older you are, the fewer options you have for treatment."

Try TURP. The fastest, most effective treatment for BPH is surgery, specifically the TURP, or transurethral resection of the prostate. In this operation, surgical tools are inserted through the urethra to cut away bits of excess prostate from the gland. The surgery leaves potency intact, although the flow of semen may be redirected backward, leaving the man infertile. You're likely to be in the hospital for four to six days, with recovery lasting as long as eight weeks.

Blow up a balloon. Balloon urethroplasty, or dilation, is definitely a faster road to relief from prostatic enlargement, although the degree and duration of relief are less than that offered by surgery. The procedure, using a local anesthetic, can be done in a doctor's office. A catheter is inserted into the urethra and a special balloon inside the catheter is inflated at the point where the enlarged prostate is strangling the urinary tract. The excess prostatic tissue is pressed outward by the expanding balloon, thus reestablishing room in the urinary tract.

"It doesn't hit the ball over the fence," Dr. McDonald says, "but it gets the man to second base, and that may be enough. About 80 percent of men get 100 percent improvement in their urine flow rate. Now, that may not be all that good if their flow rate is really low to begin with. But it may mean that instead of getting up three or four times in the middle of the night to urinate, they'll get up only once. The improvement lasts about three years."

FASTER FIXES FOR PROSTATE CANCER

Though far less common than BPH and prostatitis, prostate cancer is the most common cancer among men, resulting in about 28,000 deaths every year. Because it causes symptoms only when in the advanced stages, prostate cancer is especially insidious.

Once again, time is of the essence, and a speedy and accurate diagnosis is the essence of saving time.

"Early detection is a man's best hope," Dr. McDonald says. Catching a tumor early "can boost chances of survival and often permits cures with a less radical procedure." Fortunately, medical science has made some time-saving advances in both diagnosis and treatment of prostate cancer.

Get a quick blood test. Fast, accurate diagnosis is the key to speedy healing of a sick prostate. And a new kind of blood test is the first step in diagnosis. Called prostate-specific antigen immunoassay, the test measures concentrations of a protein normally present in the blood only in small amounts. When this protein appears in elevated amounts, prostate disease is definitely present— although not necessarily prostate cancer.

"This is an excellent test for someone over 50 to have yearly," says Carl Killian, Ph.D., of Roswell Park Memorial Institute, Buffalo, New York, where the test was developed. The test can also be used to indicate whether prostate cancer therapy is working, or if the cancer has moved to other parts of the body.

Get a prostate diagnosis at the speed of sound.

HIGH TECH ● THESE SEEDS ARE SOWN TO HEAL

Traditional radical surgery for prostate cancer involves a 3- to 4-hour operation, a week or two in the hospital, and a long convalescence. But there is a new treatment that can be done on an outpatient basis in less than an hour.

"Using ultrasound images as a positioning guide, we inject tiny capsules containing radioactive palladium into the prostate," says Dr. Harold McDonald, Jr., of the Georgia Prostate Center. "For approximately 17 days, the capsules release the major dose of radiation, then gradually become inert. The 17-day period, however, is usually enough to effectively destroy the tumor in most cases. Once killed, the tumor then shrinks, and the dead tissue is gradually absorbed by the body."

Since it is both more powerful and more precise, the therapy even surpasses standard radiation therapy: It delivers 20,000 rads of radiation right to the prostate, versus only 7,000 rads for traditional radiation therapy to the pelvic area where the prostate is located. Because the palladium seeds radiate for only a few centimeters, the higher dose can be delivered to the tumor without damaging nearby tissues.

According to Dr. McDonald, the new treatment offers the same success and survival rate as other therapies—without the side effects of standard radiation or the pain or long hospital stay of surgery. Dr. McDonald's patients "go home right away, play golf the next day, and go back to work the following week."

This procedure is so new that you may have to contact Dr. McDonald to find a clinic near you where it is available. You can contact him at the Georgia Prostate Center, 2550 Windy Hill Road, Suite 215, Marietta, GA 30067.

The ultrasound scan is rapidly becoming an accuracy-boosting part of a basic prostate exam. While the blood test "gives you a hint that there are gremlins at work" and is capable of detecting cancers much earlier than the time-honored digital-rectal exam, according to Dr. McDonald, "the ultrasound scan will pick up twice as much as the other digital exam."

Many urologists use the ultrasound scan, with the blood test and the digital-rectal exam, to make an early diagnosis of cancer or to follow prostate enlargement. Dr. McDonald stores ultrasound images of his patients on

A SPEEDY SELF-EXAM FOR TESTICULAR CANCER

Testicular cancer is the number one cancer killer of men in their twenties and thirties. Yet catching this cancer early makes a complete cure virtually certain. A monthly self-exam is the best way for a man to get a head start on beating the disease.

In this self-exam, you're feeling for a small, hard, painless lump in either testicle. A heavy feeling in the scrotum may also be a sign, along with fluid retention in the scrotum or pain in the groin or lower abdomen. Later signs of testicular cancer are found in the breasts—swelling, tenderness, or discoloration.

- Perform the test in a warm shower or bath when the scrotum is relaxed and the testicles are loose.
- To increase the sensitivity of your fingers, lather your hands with soap.
- Use only gentle pressure. If it hurts, you're squeezing too hard. Pain from squeezing is not a sign of cancer— usually the lumps are painless. And if the cancer is causing pain, you don't have to squeeze to feel it.
- Compare each side of your scrotum for equal heaviness by holding the sac gently in the palms of your hands.
- Inspect each side of the scrotum. Place your index and middle fingers underneath one of the testes with your thumb on top. Use a slow, gentle, rolling motion to feel the egg-shaped glands for lumps.
- Use the same motion to examine the epididymis, the comma-shaped structure (it's actually a long, narrow, convoluted tube) that extends from the top of the testes down along the back side of it. It should be soft and tender.
- Fit your fingers and thumb into the deep groove between the front of the testes and the back of the epididymis. The testes should feel firmer than the epididymis.
- Feel for the vas deferens—the sperm-carrying tube that leads down from the groin into the epididymis. It should be a smooth, firm, movable tube.
- Repeat the above steps for the other side of the scrotum.

Perform this test at least once a month; more often is good practice to learn what you're feeling for and to be able to tell if there's been a change since your last self-exam. If you feel any lump, enlarged area, or change in consistency, see your doctor.

laser disks. Year-to-year comparisons allow him to track the progress of prostatic enlargement.

Get the needle biopsy. If the blood test, digital-rectal exam, and ultrasound test suggest prostate cancer, the next test, according to Dr. McDonald, will be the transrectal needle biopsy, in which a biopsy needle is inserted into the prostate through the rectum. This procedure, which can be done in a physician's office or at a hospital on an outpatient basis, offers an improvement in time and safety over older methods. "It has only a 1 percent complication rate, and it's twice as accurate as previous methods," Dr. McDonald says.

MENTAL PERFORMANCE

You probably think that genes make genius, that smart people are born that way. You probably think this because, as a kid, you got the message: "Whatever you were born with upstairs is what you're stuck with for life."

But consider for a moment a different message, this one from Peter Kline, author of *The Everyday Genius:* "I think the people we've labeled as geniuses have a lot of quick fixes for mental improvement that other people haven't figured out yet." Kline—and many other experts in psychology and education—now believe that the quick fixes geniuses use to improve intellect, creativity, memory, and alertness can work for *anyone.* And, Kline says, "A lot of mental shortcuts not only get the job done faster, they get it done better."

Experts have found methods that can help to:

- Relieve brain-blocking tension in 1 minute.
- Improve your memory in 60 seconds.
- Boost your energy and productivity for long tasks in 10 minutes.

Recent scientific research into human learning has these fast and easy techniques available for you. With the instructions that follow, you can speedily achieve more mindpower in your daily life.

LIVEN UP YOUR INTELLIGENCE

One fast way to improve your intelligence is by forgetting your old IQ score. Intelligence is no longer defined by test results, but by the many abilities you use to learn and progress in life—abilities that you can *always* develop.

"For intelligence to be real you have to be able to do things in the world," says Glenn Doman, chairman of the Institutes for the Achievement of Human Potential in Wyndmoor, Pennsylvania. "Every minute of every hour of every day is an intelligence test."

And the shortest route to a high score on this test is discovering how to make the most of *your* personal intelligence—not somebody else's idea of what your intelligence *should* be.

Discover the seven styles of intelligence. Research in the last ten years has uncovered at least seven different kinds of human intelligence, each of which responds to a different kind of education. The intelligence quotient (IQ) test examines only two of these intelligences (language and logic/mathematical skills). But the remaining five (musical, visual, bodily-kinesthetic, interpersonal, and intrapersonal) offer equally valid ways to learn. (More about what each of those styles means will follow.) And, Kline says, it's easy to figure out which style is yours. Just spend some spare time over the next couple of days making notes about your favorite pursuits and how you learned to do them. Did you start knitting by talking with your mother? Did you take up hiking by first reading about mountain climbers? Seek out patterns in your methods. These are the clues to how you like to learn.

Label your learning style. Now put your learning clues to use by aligning them with a specific intelligence style. Consider how the following types would learn a golf swing:

- Linguistic (language) learners might listen to a tape or buy books describing the best swing.
- Logical learners might analyze the components of a pro's swing before trying it.
- Kinesthetic (body) learners would want to get out there and swing without much study.
- Visual learners would need to see the swing performed and where the ball goes after the shot.
- Musical learners would seek out the rhythm of the swing.
- Interpersonal learners would bond with the instructor and talk about the swing.

- Intrapersonal (self-directed) learners would decide why golf matters to them and invent an individual learning style.

Which learning style best suits your own? Learning will become much easier for you if you adopt the method that is most natural to you, Kline says. Learning is easier—and faster—when it suits your personal style. But that's not the only shortcut.

Do a dynamic decode. Learning something new can be very frustrating—but that's mostly because people think they have to grasp a new subject all at once. "Decode" the secrets of a new subject by dipping into it without expecting to completely understand all the details. Say you're taking a course in computers. Go to the bookstore or the library and browse in the computer section. Look through a few books, skim the introductions, scan the chapter headings. This short intro will give you an overview and ready your mind for more facts.

Tune in to Beethoven's Sixth Symphony or Bach's concertos. This is a particularly good method if you've discovered that you're a "musical" learner. According to Kline, a learning specialist in Bulgaria named Lozanov has found that for some people simply listening to classical or baroque music during study increases retention of new material. (Lozanov's method was particularly successful for learning foreign languages.) Music from the classical and baroque periods has an orderly, logical rhythm that can likewise help order your mental state and speed learning. Excellent (and beautiful) places to start include Bach's, Scarlatti's, and Vivaldi's violin concertos; Beethoven's Fifth, Sixth, and Seventh Symphonies; Brahms's First, Second, and Fourth Symphonies; Handel's Water Music; and Mozart's *Jupiter* Symphony and chamber music.

Spark your surroundings. This is an especially good tip for "visual" learners. The mind can absorb visual cues in the environment even when you don't seem to be paying attention. Take advantage of this time-saver by surrounding yourself with images and symbols related to your goals. If you want to learn Russian, for example, then put the letters of the Russian alphabet up on your walls.

Sketch your thoughts. The visual part of the brain is

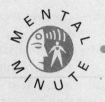

LEARN THE POWER OF VISUAL THINKING

As integrative learning instructor Peter Kline has noted, you can learn all kinds of things much faster—from grocery lists to 3-hour scripts—by turning words into pictures. Just see how easy it is.

Below (upside-down so you can't study it) is a list of ten words. Have someone read them aloud to you, but instead of writing the actual words, quickly draw pictures that symbolize them to you. Spend only a few seconds with each one.

When you've finished, go back and—without using the list—write down the word for each image. Kline says chances are that you'll remember at least nine out of ten.

1. Cat food	6. Light bulb
2. Playful	7. Mind
3. Thoughts	8. Information
4. Confusion	9. Thesaurus
5. Idea	10. God

evolutionarily much older than the logical part. So if you want to access your brain's potent primitive powers, *draw* pictures of new material to learn it faster. Kline recalls a student with a big part to memorize in a 3-hour play. Though that project might ordinarily take a week, she did it in one night because she drew images that reminded her of the words and remembered them instead of just the language. (For more on this technique, see "Learn the Power of Visual Thinking" above.)

Tell yourself that you're smart. Sometimes we don't learn because we tell ourselves that we're not smart. You can create an audio tape to counter that negative self-talk. Fill the tape with positive messages like "I am very creative" or "I enjoy delivering speeches in front of large crowds." You can either record a short message on a tape that repeats (like an answering machine's tape) or record a full tape and use a portion of it each day.

During each session, turn on a piece of classical or baroque music and turn down your affirmation tape to a barely audible hum. Says Kline: "If people consciously hear the words 'I'm very creative,' and they've been told their whole lives that they're not, they will discount the words and the tape won't work." But the combination of music and so-called subliminal persuasion (in which the words are heard by your subconscious—the storehouse of those negative messages) can create "amazingly fast and lasting results," Kline says.

Listen to the tape daily for 15 minutes.

JOLT YOUR CREATIVITY INTO ACTION

"Ask the average individual to name a creative person, and they invariably name the most significant thinkers in the history of the world—people like Einstein, Edison, Leonardo da Vinci, and Michelangelo," says William Shephard, director of programs at the Creative Education Foundation in Buffalo, New York, a nonprofit organization that provides free information and connects people to resources in fields of creativity, innovation, decision making, and problem solving.

Why do we see those people as innovative? Shephard says it's because their ideas were unique, and they were perfectly appropriate to the problem that was being worked on—whether it be a new chapel ceiling, a new theory about the universe to replace an outmoded idea, or a new way to provide a service (like electric lights).

Yet these two criteria can be applied to every situation —not just the problems "geniuses" are working on. "Most of our personal breakthroughs in achievement are not on the same global scale as those of famous individuals, but they are just as important to our day-to-day lives," Shephard says.

And once you start recognizing that you are an innovator, the process can become electrifying. "You can have a 20-volt breakthrough—or a 100,000-volt breakthrough," Shephard says. The point is to learn how to ecognize, respect, and repeat those jolts of creativity into your life.

Grab ideas when you get them. Jotting down an idea only takes a second, but trying to recall a brilliant thought can take hours—if it can be remembered at all. Since great ideas don't occur only when you're sitting at your desk with journal at hand, spend a few minutes readying yourself for the sudden appearance of creativity. Keep a tape recorder in the car. Carry a notebook in your pocket. Put a pad and paper by the bed and one near the shower. Such small preparations may even stir more ideas— creativity thrives if it's acknowledged.

Daydream. "When we were in school, we were told that daydreaming was counterproductive," Shephard says. In fact, daydreaming is an opportunity to let the mind play with new ideas. Kline suggests a technique called image-streaming for quick, constructive daydreaming. Sit quietly, close your eyes, and let ideas float up through your mind for about 15 minutes. Your mind is sure to focus on some of your problems; keep a pad or a tape recorder nearby so you can write down your new ideas immediately.

Defer judgment. A state of mind called flow—receptive and noncritical—is the key to creativity. Rejecting ideas as they come up cuts off flow. "It's like trying to drive a car by putting your foot on the gas and on the brake at the same time," Shephard says. For effective brainstorming, set a short time limit to come up with as many ideas as possible. But don't decide if they're good or bad until you've finished. And even then, he cautions, "apply the brakes judiciously." An idea that seems bad today can seem brilliant tomorrow—or suggest another idea that is the one you've been looking for.

Play games. Kline recommends an "object-combination" game as an easy way to build creativity. Survey the objects in your living room and pick two at random. Think of all the possible relationships between them—wacky or not. Try the game often using different items, or invite your friends to join in and compare answers. Let's see—there's the Elvis lamp, and there's the vase of flowers. How do they relate? Well, both are ceramic, both are blue and white. Elvis is now in the ground covered with flowers. Maybe if he had spent more time smelling the flowers he wouldn't be fertilizing them now. Still, the light from the Elvis lamp illuminates the flowers nicely.

The lamp and vase add balance to the decor: The vase is classy while the lamp is tacky, but the vase is ordinary compared to the lamp's uniqueness. Elvis makes a better lamp than he does a vase. Elvis reminds us of music and rhythm and the vagaries of life, while the flowers remind us of the elemental force and beauty of life.

PRESTO—YOU'RE PROBLEM SOLVING

"Problem solving is a subset of creativity," Shephard says. Creative people use their freedom of mind to come up with quick and original ways to solve puzzling issues at work, at school, and at home. Here's how to begin.

Ask simple questions. "We tend to think we understand our problems," Shephard says. But if we question our assumptions about the problem, we may come up with better solutions. Take a minute or so and ask yourself these questions: Who is involved in this problem? Where did it come from? How much time do we have to solve it? What would happen if we didn't solve it? If I could have a genie solve this problem immediately, what would he do?

Come up with several solutions. A fast way to solve a problem is to think of many solutions—and pick the best one. Stopping at the first solution that comes to mind can keep you from coming up with better ones further down the line.

Promote the positive. The word "problem" has a negative connotation, Shephard says. But if you see only the bad side of a problem, you won't see the opportunities for growth and change it might be offering you. Take a minute and ask yourself "What's good about this problem?" And this isn't just an exercise in hopeless optimism —the positive focus will allow your mind to think clearly and easily.

Use knowledge for quick trips. Take out a pencil and paper and write down on the center of the page one word that summarizes your problem. Then—without judging your thoughts—write or draw pictures of related ideas around that center thought and attach them to the original word like spokes coming out of a wheel. (Work quickly to keep the flow going.) Once you've come up with all the possible connections you may see an aspect of the problem you've never seen before—and a solution you've never thought of.

Take out the garbage while you're figuring out the theory of relativity. Problem solving is much easier if you don't try to force it. If you hit a mental block, stop. That's the advice of psychologist Michael Uhes, Ph.D., of the Human Performance Institute in Lakewood, Colorado. "Do something that's as different from your current task as possible," he says. If you're sitting down, take a walk. If you're balancing your checkbook, clean a drawer. If you're writing a report, do the dishes. The short break will give your mind a chance to *incubate*—a term for what happens when the subconscious takes over the problem-solving task that is baffling your conscious mind. When you return to work, you might find the solution is there waiting for you.

11 FAST WAYS TO IMPROVE YOUR MEMORY

Think of your memory as a high-powered computer. You expect it to keep track of all kinds of information and then pull it out on a second's notice. Well, like a computer, the trick to making your memory function at top level "is getting something into the system efficiently so that it can be retrieved easily," says Forest Scogin, assistant professor of psychology at the University of Alabama. Here are a few ways to do just that.

Do it now. Procrastination is a great enemy of memory, but organization is a great friend, says Danielle Lapp, Stanford University memory researcher and author of *Don't Forget! Easy Exercises for a Better Memory at Any Age.* "Doing something at the time you think of it is much better than expecting yourself to remember it later," she says. This is especially important if you're rushed or feeling emotional. "This is when memory is most fragile," Lapp says.

Get equipped for action. You might, of course, remember to do something when it's either inconvenient or unnecessary to act at that very moment. So you must anticipate the situation and give yourself a visual cue, Lapp says. Have a package of stickers handy and put one where you can't miss seeing it. Say you need to pick up a birthday cake for tomorrow night's dinner party. Put a sticker in a place you can't miss—like on your purse or the dashboard of the car. You'll remember as soon as you see it.

Use this system sparingly, though, Lapp warns: "If you use too many stickers, you might ignore them."

Put the cake on the steering wheel. Another way of remembering errands or appointments coming up is to create visual associations in your head. "Make a mental picture," Lapp suggests. Remember that birthday cake by associating it with your car. "Picture the cake on the steering wheel and comment: not very stable, hmmm . . . ," she says. "Then, when you get into the car and see the steering wheel, you'll remember to go to the bakery."

Put the cat litter box on the kitchen table. In other words, create some chaos to jog your memory. "Pull a chair away from your dining room table if you need to remember something specific and put a note or the item to be remembered on the chair," advises Irene Colsky, Ed.D., adjunct professor of teaching and learning at the University of Miami. Put a pillow next to your bed so you'll step on it when you wake up. Put the packages in the hall so you'll trip on them if you don't take them with you to the post office.

Use your visual brain. Make a visual image out of specific words you have trouble remembering. Danielle Lapp uses the example of her own anthurium plant. Guests were always commenting on it, asking her its name. So she anticipated the situation by making a visual pun of the word. "I imagined an ant (for ant-thurium) crawling on the flower," she says. "Now, I always see the anthurium and the ant together and I always remember right away."

Stop making sense. Another way to use images is to invent strange visual associations between faces and names. Lapp offers the example of her own name and face. "My name is pretty easy because it already means something," she says. "You could just imagine a person's lap."

And the face? "You would look for my most prominent feature," she says. "I have very large blue eyes, so you would pick them out and put them on a lap. So there you have a pair of blue eyeballs on a lap—and that's the visual connection between my face and my name."

Be predictable. Dr. Scogin recommends the Method of Loci (from the Latin for location) as the most basic method of remembering frequently lost items (like keys and glasses). "Always put them in the same place," he says, and take a mental snapshot of it—this is the hook where the keys go, this is the table for the spectacles.

Talk to yourself. Paying attention is important to memory function, Lapp says, so you want to do whatever you can to avoid running your memory on automatic pilot. One easy way is to make a running mental commentary as you do something: "Say to yourself 'I'm putting my glasses on the desk' as you put them there," Lapp suggests.

Make use of all your senses. Memory is jogged most efficiently when you attach more than one sense to it, Lapp explains. She uses the example of parking your car at the mall. "Take a few seconds to consider your surroundings. Listen: You hear a lot of traffic because your parking space is close to a busy highway. Smell: You are near a Chinese restaurant and remember it because you like that gingery smell. Look: You enter near the men's department of the store and notice the clothes by the door."

And the extra minute you spend doing this will pay off later, she says. Chances are very good that when you leave to find your car, at least one of these sensations will lead to it.

Find a motive. "Students have an excellent motivation for learning new material," Lapp says, "but once we've passed that stage we need to come up with an artificial motivation." Tell yourself, for example, that you need to remember this chapter because you want to tell a friend about it: "Joan would be very interested in these tips." Motivation is essential to memory.

Hit the highlights. The tried-and-true method of highlighting important material as you read still works, Dr. Colsky says, but consider these refinements. Use blue to highlight the basic information, and a contrasting color to highlight the most essential sentence from a given paragraph. Then review your material once you've marked it. Memory improves with repetition.

THE SECRETS OF MENTAL ENERGY

A key element of clearer thinking is *mental energy*—being alert throughout the day. There's nothing more frustrating than trying to do mental work when your mind is starting to fade.

Refreshing yourself and maintaining your concentration is little more than a matter of understanding how your body clock functions and using quick and easy techniques for getting yourself back into sync with your own natural energy rhythms. That's the advice of Maria Simonson, Ph.D., director of the Health, Weight, and Stress Clinic at the Johns Hopkins Medical Institutions. Here's how.

Cop those ZZZZs. According to Timothy Roehrs, Ph.D., of the Sleep Center at Henry Ford Hospital in Detroit, "To be more alert, get enough sleep." Sounds simple enough but how much sleep is enough? Dr. Roehrs conducted a study that found that the old idea that 8 hours was good for everyone may not be so—that each person has an individual need and it's often for more than 8. When the participants in Roehrs's research had extra sleep, they were much more alert during the day. To determine your best amount of sleep, go to bed 30 to 60 minutes earlier for several days. When you find yourself awaking naturally (without the alarm) and feeling alert, you have established your optimal sleep time. And once you start really getting enough sleep, you'll have little down time to your waking life.

Rise and shine. "When you first wake up in the morning, stay awake," Dr. Simonson says. Studies of mental alertness show that a good outlook begins at the very start of the day. "Lying in bed can produce negative thoughts and can make you heavy and drowsy if you go back to sleep," she says. So as soon as those eyes open, swing those feet to the floor.

Fuel up on breakfast. Rushing out the door and having a sweet roll at the office may seem like the fastest way to start the day—until you start to slow at 10:00 A.M. The 10 or 15 minutes it takes you to prepare and eat a meal of whole-grain cereal, skim milk, and fruit will be more than returned to you later with increased energy and alertness, Dr. Uhes says. The protein in the milk is vital for your brain to wake up, and since your body metabolizes carbohydrates slowly, the grain and fruit will keep you going until lunch.

Munch a healthy lunch. When midday arrives, Dr. Uhes says, skip the fats. Nothing weighs down mental swiftness faster than a burger, fries, and milkshake at noontime. Jump to the salad side of the menu instead.

Tell yourself how much you like your work. "Those first few minutes of work can be exhausting," Dr. Simonson says. You see the day stretched out before you with piles of work and no certainty as to how to begin. Have stock phrases ready for each morning like "I enjoy my work," "I can't wait to begin," "I'll start with Project A for the next half hour and then decide what to do."

Write to yourself. Your spirits are also less likely to flag if you leave yourself a note each night suggesting where to start in the morning.

Take a 10-minute pep break. Research shows that most people are on a 90-minute cycle of concentration. Pay attention to your work cycles and you're likely to notice that your attention starts to fade at the end of an hour and a half of work, Dr. Simonson says. A 10-minute pep-up period at that point will quickly head you into another productive 90 minutes. Do some easy stretching. Go get a glass of water. Take a short, brisk walk.

March to the beat. Highly rhythmic music can get your body and mind moving, much like soothing music can calm stressed nerves, music therapist Lorna Glassman explains. So if your spirits are flagging, plug in a Sousa march or some other rousing music for a few minutes. Or better yet, pop these spirited sounds into a cassette player and combine them with a 10-minute walk in the fresh air.

Sip an herbal brew. For a pick-me-up in little more than the time it takes the water to boil, keep certain herbal teas nearby. According to herbal expert Nan Koehler, ginger tea is a wonderful natural stimulant.

Brighten your line of sight. Hot colors like orange, yellow, and red can wake you up and make you think. Every time your eye lights on them, the color will help
(continued on page 379)

• PROGRESSIVE RELAXATION

Sinking into the living room recliner after a hard day's work; swinging gently to and fro in the backyard hammock on a drowsy summer Sunday; snoozing in the sun as the trade winds caress your skin and warm sea waters lap at your toes—there's nothing in the world quite like total relaxation. Your mind drifts, your body floats, your cares recede like the tide, you leave stress behind in a matter of minutes.

A comfortable chair, a hammock, or a beach is great for relaxing, but once you learn the technique of progressive relaxation, you'll be able to relax almost anywhere by summoning up a word or an image. And by learning to relax, you can set up the conditions to use visualizations to improve not only your state of mind but also your physical health. It's an excellent way to get the most from several of the Mental Minutes in this book.

Most psychologists and experts in stress relief start their clients on this road to less tension and greater mental power with the Jacobsonian technique of progressive relaxation. The technique follows this basic formula: You control your breathing while relaxing your muscles and focusing on mental cues (which can be scenes, words, or sensations).

Once you've achieved the deep level of calm that this formula promotes, your visualizations will have their greatest benefit. And once you've become highly practiced in this method, you can achieve deep relaxation by just using your cue.

Practice, of course, is vital. You need to do it at least once a day for 20 minutes to become proficient. "If you practice regularly, you're much more likely to develop the skill," says Keith Sedlacek, M.D., medical director of the Stress Regulation Institute in New York City. "Practice is

(continued)

PROGRESSIVE RELAXATION — *Continued*

the key point." And 20 minutes is not that big a piece of your time—about 1.38 percent of your daily allotment of 1,440 minutes.

To begin a relaxation session, find a comfortable place to sit or lie down where you won't be disturbed. Make sure that your head is supported and that your clothes don't bind you.

Now close your eyes and focus on your breathing. You'll want to begin breathing from your diaphragm instead of your chest, explains Dr. Phil Nuernberger of Mind Resource Technologies. "Chest breathing is really used by the body only in emergencies when you need all of the mechanisms of the chest working for you," he says.

Diaphragmatic breathing is much slower and much deeper. You can train yourself to breathe this way by putting your hand on your stomach with the little finger on your navel and the rest of the hand extending up to your chest. "You should feel that hand rise and fall as if a small balloon is filling up your stomach," Nuernberger explains. This system can lower your breaths per minute from 10 to 12 to about 8.

After your breath begins to slow, clear away the cluttered thoughts in your mind by thinking of your favorite place to go to unwind. (Popular spots are the beach, the mountains, and a wooded glade.) Focus on this scene. What does it feel like to be there? Is the sun warming you? Are warm breezes blowing? Are there birds singing? Are the clouds floating by?

Once you feel immersed in these surroundings, you can introduce your cue word or sensation and then begin the progressive relaxation of muscles. (This sylvan setting you've been conjuring can work as your cue if you want, or you can employ something simpler.) Dr. Nuernberger advises that you use a word like "peace" or "love" that has no negative connotations and no ambiguity of meaning. Imagining a bell ringing or a pleasant smell also could work.

(continued)

PROGRESSIVE RELAXATION—*Continued*

Whatever you choose, think of your cue each time you exhale and then begin the muscle relaxation. Start with your left foot. Point it away from you and tense your ankle. Focus on what the muscle feels like tense. Now, relax it, continuing with your diaphragmatic breathing and your cue all the while.

Next, point the toes of the left foot toward you and tense the ankle. After a few seconds, release it and experience what the relaxed state feels like. Tense the calf muscles in your left leg and release them, then tense the left thigh muscles and release them.

Repeat these procedures for your right foot and leg. Work your way up your body, tensing and releasing all the major muscle groups as you go—the buttocks, the abdomen, the chest, and the shoulders, which you can pull back to tense and let go to release. For the neck, try bearing down on the muscles or stiffening them, then relax. And remember—repeat your cue all the while you do this.

Tense and relax all of the muscles in your face. You can even do your lips and tongue by pressing your lips together tightly while holding your tongue on the roof of your mouth.

Squint your eyes closed and wrinkle your nose to tense the muscles in the middle of your face. Raise your eyebrows and wrinkle your forehead to tense your upper face.

A-a-a-a-h. You have just brought thorough relaxation to your body. Now, continue your deep breathing and continue using your cue for a minute or two more. At this point, you can slowly bring yourself back to complete consciousness or you can use your relaxed, receptive mental state to introduce your visualizations.

Obviously, this method has great benefits just as a stress reliever. "I'm amazed at the return in benefits people see by just investing 15 minutes a day in relaxation," Dr. Nuernberger says. But by practicing it regularly, you also can train yourself to induce relaxation and controlled breathing by using only your cue. And then, of course, your visualizations can follow.

your brain stay alert, Dr. Simonson says. Decorate your workspace with touches of these colors—like a bright red mug for your tea, or a photo of the sunrise over your desk. Don't overdue it, though, just use fiery touches on an otherwise neutral space. Too much color can be overstimulating.

HUSTLE YOUR STRESS AWAY

Stress and tension are often self-created, says Gary Grody, Ph.D. "Most people create stress based on their needs and expectations," he says. When reality conflicts with these needs, you feel stressed.

Self-made stress can crop up in every situation—from driving ("I should be at the office now—I'll be in trouble because I'm late."), to the time you spend in front of the mirror in the morning ("The hair dryer broke. I look lousy today.").

But if you create most of the stress in your life, you can *un-create* it as well. Experts have come up with all kinds of fast-action methods to kick stress out the door. Here are a few.

Jot down your thoughts. "I advise my patients to keep a thought journal," Dr. Grody says. Just by writing down the negative thoughts that are flashing through your mind, you see how useless most of them are.

Let Ol' Blue Eyes sing away your stress. Listening to music is a great stress reliever, Lorna Glassman says. And while classical, easy listening, or New Age music are the common choices of many music therapy professionals, it's important to pick your personal favorites. You may find rock or jazz sounds more soothing, if that's your taste. Whatever you pick, however, have some on hand for high-stress times—like airplane trips and dental appointments.

Drink some "tranquil tea." Koehler reports that a cup of chamomile is the best choice for winding down.

Tell yourself to slow down. The times you're faced with a high-stress situation are the ones in which you most need to react carefully, Dr. Uhes says. "I tell patients to repeat to themselves 'Move slowly, think slowly.' " You'll move more carefully in an emergency if you tell yourself to be calm.

Feel yourself breathe for a minute. "This is probably the fastest method of releasing stress," says Phil Nuernberger, Ph.D., president of Mind Resource Technologies in Honesdale, Pennsylvania. Turn your attention from what's going on around you to your own body. Just focus for a minute on the sensation of your breath flowing in and out of your nose. You'll calm down immediately.

Breathe from your belly. Most of us breathe incorrectly. We should be breathing from our diaphragms instead of from our chest. By breathing so deeply that your stomach (instead of your chest) is gently rising and falling (see "Progressive Relaxation" on page 376), you offer yourself a rapid method of stress relief. Diaphragmatic breathing can be used anytime. "No one has to know you're doing it," Dr. Uhes says, "so you can do it under pressure at the office. You can do it when the kids are going cuckoo at the dinner table."

Scan for body tension. Tension can creep into your body—and stay there. Dr. Nuernberger advises a "body scan" for speedy relief. Close your eyes, breathe deeply, and mentally scan your body to find tension. When you hit a tight spot, briefly tense that muscle and then release it while you imagine the area relaxing.

Walk it off. There are few stress relievers better than walking, says adult educator and workplace wellness expert Alan Miller, Ed.D. "It's easy, everyone knows how to do it, and its benefits are almost immediate."

OSTEOPOROSIS

T hroughout life our body deposits minerals into our bones, and just as surely the minerals leave—it's a process of building, tearing down, and rebuilding of bone. During childhood, we deposit more than is removed, resulting in bigger, stronger bones as we grow to adulthood. During early adulthood, deposits balance withdrawals, and we stop growing. In later adulthood, mineral withdrawals exceed deposits—we actually begin to shrink somewhat in size, and our bones become more porous and more easily broken.

If you've lost 30 percent or more of your original bone mass, you have a condition called osteoporosis. Then bones become so weakened that they can be crushed and collapse under the body's weight or break easily in falls. Men and women both lose bone as they age, but women have two extra problems to face: Their bones are smaller to begin with, so any loss is more crucial; and menopause brings about a drop in the hormone estrogen, which allows further bone loss. That's why osteoporosis is primarily a woman's disease.

But osteoporosis is not inevitable. You can take quick, simple steps everyday—starting now—to ensure against this tragic and crippling condition.

- With quick changes in diet, you can replace the calcium that is lost from your bones.
- By swallowing a pill every night at bedtime, you could delay bone loss for up to ten years.
- By taking a 5-minute stroll in the sunshine every other day or so, you can soak up enough vitamin D to toughen your bones.

OSTEOPOROSIS   **381**

- In 30 minutes a day, you can exercise your way to stronger bones.

There is no cure for osteoporosis, although researchers are making strides in finding safe and effective treatments. With osteoporosis, prevention is easier than the cure. Using preventive techniques, you can avoid those lifestyle and diet patterns that can promote bone loss and lay you open to the pain and tragedy of osteoporosis. It's never too late, no matter what your age, sex, or lifestyle.

A QUICK QUIZ FOR RISK

In just 30 seconds you can gauge your risk of developing osteoporosis. Put a quick check mark after every question with a yes answer. The first seven questions have to do with unavoidable risk factors, and the remainder with lifestyle factors.

1. Are you a woman?
2. Are you menopausal?
3. Are you of northern European or Asian descent?
4. Do you have a fair complexion?
5. Do you have a family history of osteoporotic fracture (easily broken bones, especially in older women relatives)
6. Do you have a slender build?
7. Are you allergic to milk and other dairy products?
8. Do you exercise very little?
9. Do you avoid dairy products in your diet?
10. Do you smoke?
11. Do you drink alcohol?
12. Do you consume caffeine?
13. Do you drink carbonated beverages?
14. Do you use a lot of salt in your food?
15. Do you eat a high-protein diet?
16. Do you exercise so much that your period stops?
17. Do you diet so much that you're underweight?

Of course, there's nothing you can do about heredity. But, if you stacked up a lot of yes answers regarding lifestyle, you might be hiking your risk of developing this bone-dissipating condition. Your diet and habits are things you can control. Here's where to start.

A CRASH COURSE ON CALCIUM

Of all the minerals, calcium is the one most often associated with strong bones. Although your bones stop growing in size by the time you're 30 years old, they never outgrow their need for calcium. The rate of building up declines more rapidly than that of tearing down, so the net effect is poorer bone quality and actual loss of bone. Without constant and plentiful calcium supplies, rebuilding falls even further behind. Guaranteeing this supply is a two-step process.

STEMMING THE FLOW

You can immediately take steps to dam that outflowing of the calcium river and create a calcium reservoir. "Be realistic about it, though," says Paul Saltman, Ph.D., nutritionist and professor of biology at the University of California at San Diego. "Don't think you should stop living just to keep the calcium in your body." Just start living better.

Pop the cork back into that bottle. Hold the line after that second drink of alcohol. Booze flushes calcium out of the body. Heavy drinking is a major factor in bone-loss disease, especially among men who suffer from osteoporosis.

Cut your coffee intake in half. Or, even better, switch to decaf. Like alcohol, caffeine flushes calcium out of the body. If you do drink caffeine and don't want to stop, figure that you need an additional 100 milligrams of calcium or ⅓ cup of milk daily to compensate for every two cups of coffee you drink.

Cut your lunchtime burger in half. Excess protein, particularly animal protein, may bind with calcium in the digestive tract, preventing calcium absorption. Many nutrition studies suggest that Americans eat too much protein, anyway. Limit yourself to a couple of small servings daily, preferably lean meats, Dr. Saltman says, and you'll meet your protein requirements with little interference in calcium absorption.

Cut back on tonight's spinach serving. Popeye didn't gulp spinach for his bones. Like other dark green leafy vegetables, spinach is rich in calcium. But unlike its calcium-loaded cousins, its calcium isn't so available for your body to use. That's because spinach is also rich in oxalate and phytate, chemicals that interfere with calcium absorption—not only the calcium in your spinach but in the glass of milk you drink with dinner. But spinach tastes good and is full of other nutrients, so don't eliminate it—just be sure you get your calcium from other sources.

Stop after two soft drinks. Cola and certain other carbonated soft drinks get their sharp taste from phosphorus, which contains phosphate, a component of bone mineral that hooks up to calcium like a horse to a buggy. If you get too much phosphate your body excretes it, and calcium rolls out right along with it. That calcium comes from your bones. Carbonated mineral waters, by the way, do not contain phosphate.

DEPOSITING CALCIUM IN YOUR BONE BANK

The Recommended Dietary Allowance (RDA) for adolescent boys and girls and young adults is 1,200 milligrams of calcium; they need about this much each day to feed their growing bones. The RDA for adult men and women over age 24 is 800 milligrams.

But many experts suggest that the RDA of 800 milligrams is too low. They recommend that adults take 1,000 milligrams. At menopause, things change for women. The National Institutes of Health recommend that a postmenopausal woman on estrogen therapy continue at that 1,000-milligram level. But if you're postmenopausal and *not* taking estrogen, you should be sure to get 1,500 milligrams of calcium daily.

Using the higher recommendation, if you are like many adults, you may be getting only about half of your daily calcium requirement. You can change that quickly.

Kick off the morning with a glass of skim milk. Eight ounces have 300 milligrams of calcium, nearly one-third of your daily allowance before menopause.

Peel open a container of low-fat or nonfat yogurt for lunch. Eight ounces of this creamy dairy nectar contain about 452 milligrams of calcium.

Build a cottage cheese salad for supper. Two cups contain as much calcium as a cup of yogurt.

Learn to love cheddar cheese. It's a great snack food and just 1½ ounces contain a third of your daily calcium need.

Swallow a calcium supplement. Does all that sound like a lot of dairy products? Getting 100 percent of your calcium requirement from food alone means drinking a quart of milk every day, or eating a quart of yogurt or ¼ pound of cheese. Quantities this large may be more than most people are willing to do, Dr. Saltman says. "That's why I'm not afraid to suggest a calcium supplement. It's a quick, easy way to get your recommended daily requirement." Calcium carbonate is one of the best types of supplements; calcium lactate and calcium gluconate are also good. But stay away from bonemeal and dolomite, which may have high levels of lead.

On the road, without a path to proper nutrition or supplements? Dr. Saltman suggests a calcium-based antacid tablet daily—doctors often recommend Tums—as a quick way to meet your calcium needs. Five Tums tablets meets the RDA.

VITAMIN D—CALCIUM'S GOOD BUDDY

Vitamin D is necessary for the absorption of calcium. Figure that most of your vitamin D gets into your body from the sun's ultraviolet radiation acting on your skin. The rest comes through diet, with vitamin D-fortified milk the only major source. Adult men and women need about 200 international units daily. Here's how to be sure you get yours.

Spend 5 minutes out in the sun. Work in the garden. Play with your dog in the park. Sunbathe on your deck. Five to 15 minutes a day ought to do it, according to Michael F. Holick, M.D., Ph.D., of the Boston City Hospital and Boston University School of Medicine. Dr. Holick and his research team studied more than 150 residents at the Hebrew Rehabilitation Center for the Aged and found that nearly 80 percent of them were deficient in vitamin D by the end of winter. So he recommends that elderly people spend 5 to 15 minutes outdoors, two or three times a week, during fair weather.

Drink a glass of milk. Your diet can include nearly all the vitamin D you'll need. Milk is the only dairy product fortified with vitamin D. Contrary to popular belief, yogurt, ice cream, and cheese, as well as all other dairy products are not vitamin D fortified. (But they are still good sources of calcium.) Fish-liver oil and whole fatty fish such as sardines are good natural sources of vitamin D.

Supplement your sunless days. If you're older, or don't get out in the sun much, a vitamin D supplement may be necessary. Many physicians prescribe a daily supplement. But check with your doctor before you decide how much you should be taking, because too much vitamin D can be harmful. (Dr. Holick recommends that people who do not routinely spend time outside take a multivitamin containing 400 international units of vitamin D, especially in the winter.)

TAKE THE ERT TRAIN

Although no one is sure just how sex hormones affect bone, we do know that a woman's risk of osteoporosis depends in large part on how much estrogen her body produces. Back in 1941, researchers theorized that osteoblasts—tiny cells of connective tissue that germinate into bone—depend on estrogen to function. In fact, the hormones of both sexes—estrogen and progesterone in females and testosterone in males—help maintain bone. Thus, loss of these hormones, more sudden in menopausal women and more gradual in aging men, result in bone loss and, in many cases, osteoporosis. For various reasons women are affected twice as severely as men. Quite logically, then, estrogen replacement therapy (ERT) has emerged as the primary way to prevent menopause-induced bone loss.

In fact, when initiated within the first three years of menopause, ERT may actually slow down bone loss. In effect, ERT could delay bone loss for ten years. Once bones become brittle, the damage is done, however, and estrogen replacement is of little use. And ERT is standard for young women who've undergone surgical menopause (removal of the ovaries), which cuts off estrogen production suddenly and completely.

As a result, more and more family physicians and

gynecologists recommend ERT for women who've reached menopause. A few simple steps can help you handle this crucial time of change.

Jot down the date of your last period. Estrogen therapy should begin within your first year of menopause or at least within three years after the last period.

Wake up and take your estrogen. A typical course of treatment might include conjugated estrogens in a dose of 0.625 milligrams a day for 25 days per month and 5 to 10 milligrams of progesterone a day during the last 10 to 14 days of the medication cycle. (Progesterone is another hormone routinely given to balance out the effects of estrogen, and as a side effect, the combination protects against cancer of the uterine lining.) The hormones are available in pills, though sometimes they're administered through creams, skin patches, or vaginal suppositories.

Make calcium part of your daily routine. "Estrogen should be given in addition to, not in place of, calcium," emphasizes David R. Rudy, M.D., a family practice educator in Grosse Pointe, Michigan, and clinical associate professor at Wayne State University School of Medicine in Detroit. He cautions, however, that calcium should not be taken without medical advice.

Toss your cigarettes in the trash bin. "Smoking virtually cancels out the benefits of postmenopausal estrogen replacement therapy," Dr. Rudy says. Doctors theorize that smoking somehow speeds the rate at which your body metabolizes important components of estrogen like estradiol and estrone. Women smokers have lower estrogen levels than women who don't smoke.

ADD MAGNESIUM TO YOUR SUPPLEMENT PROGRAM

Combined with calcium and estrogen replacement therapy, dietary magnesium may help reverse postmenopausal bone loss within a relatively short period of time.

In one study, researchers at Women's Life Care in Anaheim Hills, California, prescribed a daily supplement of vitamins and minerals (including 200 milligrams of magnesium and 500 milligrams of calcium), plus an extra supplement of 400 milligrams of magnesium, to 19 women on estrogen replacement therapy. After as little as six months, tests showed that bone density in the women whose diets were supplemented with magnesium increased 11 percent. In contrast, 7 women who did not take extra magnesium showed no significant improvement.

PUT ON A FEW POUNDS

The old saying "you can never be too rich or too thin" may be good advice for the social climber, but it's bad advice for the bones. Bones get stronger by bearing weight, whether it's plain old body weight or the weight of muscles tugging this way and that. And underweight women typically have lower estrogen levels. No one is advocating obesity, but getting up to normal weight will help.

Go for seconds. If you're underweight, you have permission to go after that second helping at dinner tonight.

And have some ice cream. It's rich in calcium, protein, and calories.

Become a "bodybuilder." You should also begin a muscle-building exercise program. Underweight people can probably afford to put on a little fat, but delicious high-fat foods make this a tricky path. Muscle is denser than fat—it weighs more. A pound of muscle will do more for your bones than a pound of fat, because you can get heavier without ballooning out.

TAKE TIME FOR BONE-TOUGHENING EXERCISE

Nearly all physicians and health experts agree that exercise is good for your bones.

"If you're in your twenties, exercise can help you achieve higher peak bone mass, that is, to develop as much bone as your body can," says Christine Snow-Harter, Ph.D., assistant professor and physiologist at the Exercise and Sport Science Department at Oregon State University. "And the more bone you have, the better off you'll be when you're older. After you pass 30, exercise may help prevent bone loss and maintain bone density."

And not just any exercise, but weight-bearing exercise. No, standing in one place with weight on your shoulders—static loading—won't do. That's the way fat works—it just sits there, kind of like passive exercise for your bones. It's moving about—dynamic loading—that does the trick for the bones. That's because your muscles tug on your bones; that tugging puts stress on the bones, and your bones respond by getting stronger.

You can pick from a wide variety of sports and activities. As long as they involve pitting your bones against pressure, gravity, or weight, you'll reap the benefits—stronger bones. "But we're not preaching marathon running or training for a decathalon," Dr. Snow-Harter says. It's faster and easier than that. "But your activity needs to substantially exceed what it normally takes to get you through your day," she adds. The investment of time pays substantial dividends that are deposited directly into your bones.

Work walking into your schedule. Take a 20-minute walk during your lunch hour. Instead of sitting in traffic to and from work, haul out your walking shoes and trek it: Walking briskly, you can cover 3 miles in an hour. If you toss in brief spurts of jogging, you cover the distance faster and boost the bone-building effect.

Get yourself into the ballgame. Softball keeps you on your feet and moving around, just the kind of exercise you need to toughen bones. Throwing, batting, and catching are weight-bearing exercises for the forearms. The fun, frolic, and camaraderie are side benefits to the bone building.

Go to court. Find a tennis partner and start swinging, rushing the net, pounding a serve. Ninety minutes on the clay a couple of times a week builds muscle and bone, plus gives you your bone-building dose of vitamin D.

Give up the golf cart. Walking the course next time you're playing 18 holes may increase the bone-building effect significantly, and again helps you catch vitamin-D rays.

Add pounds in aerobics. Small hand weights and ankle weights can speed the bone-building effect of all that movement. Get into these weights gradually. Use them within your comfort zone and don't use them for high-impact activities.

Get organized. An hour workout three times a week at a health club gives you a guided, convenient, and concentrated way to strengthen your muscles and bones in an atmosphere where sweating and grunting are socially acceptable, and where training partners at your level can easily be found.

Pump iron. Physiologists are discovering what bodybuilders have known for years: "We have found, particularly in men, that muscle strength independent of body weight is a good predictor of bone mineral density," Dr. Snow-Harter says.

HANDLING OSTEOPOROSIS

So much for preventing weak bones. Now let's face an unpleasant possibility: Your doctor has diagnosed osteoporosis. Like any chronic condition, osteoporosis has both physical and psychological side effects—depression, pain, fear about the future, fear of falls, changes and limitations in employment, social life, and activity. In short, it's bound to put you in the dumps. But there are things you can do—like following the dietary advice for preventing osteoporosis given earlier. And here are some more ideas to get you up and feeling good about life again.

EXERCISE, BUT DO IT RIGHT

Exercise not only can reduce the chance of fracture by increasing bone density, it also works by developing muscle strength, balance, and agility, say Neil M. Resnick, M.D., and Susan L. Greenspan, M.D., of the Division of Aging, Harvard Medical School. But you have to use caution.

"Doing the wrong kind of exercise can make matters worse," says Mary Ellen Riordan, physical therapist and assistant clinical professor in the Department of Physical and Occupational Therapy at Duke University Medical Center. You have to avoid twisting, bending, or lifting too much weight. Riordan offers these guidelines.

Walk around the block—or down the hall and back. "Walking is probably the best kind of aerobic exercise for osteoporosis because it strengthens bones and muscles in the legs and hips without overstressing them," Riordan says. "The idea is to start slow, at a comfortable pace, so you're not huffing and puffing, and build up gradually—as little as an additional minute or two each day." Work up to a mile or two at a stretch.

Climb on a stationary bike. Bicycling can help strengthen your leg bones, but biking on the road poses

WHEN EXERCISE IS OVERDONE

The boom in fitness and sports has brought out the athlete in many women, and doctors are beginning to see the effects of overexercise: Irregular periods or even complete cessation of menses. It usually is seen only in competitive athletes and people whose professions are based on aerobic exercise. But even some ordinary exercisers could be susceptible. A decline or halt in menstruation can mean a drop in estrogen production, and that could lead to increased loss of minerals from bones. The effect may be partially reversible and can be reduced by normal menses, reduced activity, and slight weight gain. "The key word to exercise is—sensible," says Dr. Christine Snow-Harter of the Exercise and Sport Science Department at Oregon State University.

the risks of falls and fractures. For people with osteoporosis, a stationary bike is safer. Begin by setting the resistance so that pedaling takes about the same amount of effort as you'd exert walking on level terrain. And watch your posture! "Don't hunch forward; keep your back straight," Riordan warns. This reduces stress on weakened vertebrae. "A bike with a back support is best," she says.

Call in the coach. In the Duke University Preventive and Therapeutic Program for Osteoporosis (DUPATPO), physical therapists teach people various extension exercises they can perform sitting or standing — arching their trunk backward, or doing modified exercises from a chair. And if you golf, garden, or enjoy other sports and hobbies that involve twisting or bending, you may need to learn new ways to swing a club or wield a hoe in order to avoid fractures. Much depends on your bone density. So to be safe, it's wise to consult a physical therapist who works with people who have osteoporosis. Ask your doctor for a referral.

TAKING CARE WITH CHORES

When it comes to everyday chores, people with osteoporosis can benefit from the same kind of advice given to people with bad backs in general. Riordan offers these tips.

Keep your lifting lightweight. "Don't bend forward," Riordan adds. "Instead, keep your trunk vertical and hold the object close to your body."

Roll up a towel. "A rolled bath towel or inflatable support cushion can help support your neck or lower back (or both) when you're sleeping or sitting," Riordan says. "Spines all curve differently, so experiment with what feels most comfortable to you."

Buy a mechanical reacher—and use it. The next time you're browsing through your local hardware store, medical supply store, or home building center, look for long-handled tools that help you garden and do house-work without reaching or bending.

Rearrange your kitchen. "To further minimize lift-ing and reaching, put things you use most often at chest or waist level," Riordan advises.

A FOUR-DAY COURSE IN COPING WITH WEAK BONES

As with any chronic health condition, osteoporosis can be painful and worrisome. Self-image can suffer. But you don't have to let it get you down. Health care professionals involved in DUPATPO say that people with osteoporosis can help themselves feel better. Here are some highlights from a four-day training session in Duke's ongoing study of middle-aged and elderly people who have either broken a bone or are at high risk for fracture.

Dial a friend. The Duke researchers found that peo-ple felt more comfortable once they realized that it's okay to ask others for help with things like carrying groceries. One man remarked, "I'm not embarrassed to ask my son to do something for me now that I know the doctor says I shouldn't do it." Widows who lived far away from their adult children relied on a strong network of friends in their neighborhoods or churches for practical and emo-tional support.

See every limitation as a challenge and an oppor-tunity. "You may not be able to pick up your favorite grandchild anymore," says Judith Anne Carroll, clinical social worker with the Duke University Osteoporosis program. "But you can play games or interact with them in less strenuous ways."

Follow doctor's orders. More than one person who

ETIDRONATE: TWICE A DAY
KEEPS FRACTURES AWAY

Up to now estrogen and calcitonin have been the only drugs you could take to treat established osteoporosis—that's if you've broken any bones, or if tests show your bones are porous and brittle. But now there may be another drug available—etidronate.

A drug developed primarily as a treatment for Paget's disease, etidronate appears to serve as an inexpensive, safe, and effective treatment for osteoporosis, according to studies in America and Europe.

Like estrogen and calcitonin, etidronate acts by reducing bone resorption. And when compared with estrogen, etidronate seems to have very few side effects and will cost about the same as estrogen treatment.

In a study of 429 women who'd fractured one or more vertebrae, bones grew denser in those who took etidronate twice a day for two years than in women who did not receive the drug. In fact, etidronate was most effective in women whose bones were the weakest at the start of the study. So if your doctor thinks you qualify, etidronate might prevent further bone loss and further fractures.

The Food and Drug Administration hasn't yet approved its use for osteoporosis, but your doctor may prescribe it for you since it has been certified as a safe drug.

participated in the Duke program remarked that doing things for themselves helped their morale tremendously, even though they realized that they sometimes need help. "When I first returned home, I started to feel depressed again. But I went over all the materials, and I made up my mind to follow the doctor's suggestions completely," one woman said. "Now, when I'm feeling even a little low, I start my exercises or create a meal with lots of calcium, and I can make myself feel better emotionally."

FALL-PROOF YOUR LIFE

If you have osteoporosis, another immediate goal is to reduce your chances of breaking a bone. The quickest way to do that is to eliminate hazards. Take 30 minutes or so to make a safety inventory of your home, using the following checklist.

- Remove all loose cords, wires, and throw rugs.
- Make sure other rugs are anchored and smooth.
- Get rid of any clutter you may trip over.
- Make sure stair treads, rails, and runners are secure.
- Install grab bars and nonskid tape in the tub or shower.
- Light up your house: Halls, stairways, and entrances should be well-lit. Put a night light in your bathroom.
- Wear sensible shoes with nonskid soles.
- In the kitchen, place nonskid rubber mats by the stove and sink and clean spills immediately.
- If you're on medication that makes you dizzy, ask your doctor if there's a substitute that doesn't induce dizziness. This is no time to be shy.
- Finally, contact the National Osteoporosis Foundation. It is a national voluntary health agency dedicated to reducing the widespread incidence of osteoporosis. Write to the foundation at 2100 M. Street NW, Suite 602, Washington, DC 20037.

RECOVERY FROM SURGERY

The only way to recover quickly from surgery is to prepare yourself for the physical and mental challenge it presents—you have to *train* for it as though it were an Olympic event. There is mounting medical evidence that preparing yourself mentally and physically can bring you back to health more quickly.

Your preparation doesn't have to be difficult. In fact:

- In just a second, you can press a button that will deliver "coaching" messages to help you face your operation with a positive, relaxed frame of mind.
- In the time it takes you to swallow, you can guard yourself against infections.
- In just a day, you can walk in, have your operation, and go home—with a new kind of surgery.

Here are the particulars.

PREPARE YOURSELF LIKE A CHAMPION

Studies show that patients who prepare in advance lose less blood, experience less pain, and leave the hospital up to two days sooner. Emotional support helps, too. Ask family and friends to keep those visits coming.

If you're getting ready for surgery, now is the prime time to take extra care with your body and your mind. Realize that it is normal to feel anxious as your operation draws close. The more relaxed you can keep yourself, the better off you'll be. Here's how to mentally psych yourself.

Learn as much as you can about your surgery. Studies show that patients who know a lot about what's going to happen have less fear and anxiety both before and after the operation. Even more important, they experience less pain after surgery, recover faster, and return to normal activities much sooner than those who don't prepare. Many hospitals are now providing informational programs for surgery patients, so be sure to inquire about it. Your doctor may also be able to recommend reading materials. Of course, if you're the kind of person who gets squeamish before an operation, or will get *more* frightened learning about it, then skip this step.

Buy a coaching tape. There's a highly effective two-volume tape set you can order. Called "Successful Surgery and Recovery," it's by Emmett E. Miller, M.D., a respected stress-reduction expert.

The tape begins with a progressive relaxation sequence. Then it asks you to remember a good time in the past when you were strong and happy to be alive. From there you move to the present and think beyond your surgery to a time when you'll feel strong and happy again. The tape allows you to let go of negative expectations.

The second half of the tape walks you through the sequence of the surgery so you know what to expect, and it also contains suggestions for how to relax so you'll get a good night's sleep before the operation. The second tape helps people who are recovering from surgery and experiencing pain. Both tapes can be purchased as a set for $15.95 from Emmet E. Miller, M.D., Source Cassette Learning Systems, P.O. Box W, Stanford, CA 94309.

Ask for support. A University of California at San Diego study of 56 men who had coronary bypass operations found that those in the group who were happily married and frequently visited by their wives recovered fastest.

The happily married men needed less pain medication, typically left the intensive care unit earlier, and left the hospital an average of one day earlier than either single men or men who received little emotional support from their wives.

Ask about pre-op antibiotics. Antibiotics have long been given to help prevent infection before major operations. But researchers report in the *New England Journal of Medicine* that antibiotic pretreatment limits infection in simple, clean operations where the drugs previously weren't used. In a study of 1,218 operations (hernia repairs or breast surgery) patients given antibiotics prior to surgery had 48 percent fewer infections during recovery than patients not receiving antibiotic pretreatment. The significance is that fewer infections result in a faster recovery period and less chance of later complications.

EATING FOR A FASTER RECOVERY

There's no doubt. Surgery takes a toll on the body. You need reserves for your body to draw on, so it can meet the extra stress head-on, successfully battle infection, and repair the parts that were cut open. You build those reserves by making sure you are nutritionally fortified.

You can easily get these nutrients in foods or multiple vitamin supplements. Of course, don't take any vitamins without first consulting your doctor.

Here's how to eat for success before surgery.

Take your vitamins. The important nutrients for recuperation are vitamins A, C, B_6 and B_{12}, copper, magnesium, and zinc, says George Blackburn, M.D., Ph.D., associate professor of surgery at Harvard Medical School and chief of the Nutrition/Metabolism Laboratory with the Cancer Research Institute at New England Deaconess Hospital, Boston.

Indulge in dairy foods. If you can tolerate lactose, dairy foods are ideal when you're ill because they're high in nutrients and calories, Dr. Blackburn says. Your pharmacy also sells medical nutrient-rich formulas that are available without a prescription. (Brand names include Resource, Ensure, and Sustacal.) They're easy to digest and contain all the key nutrients, he says.

Ask about vitamin A. A recent research review in the *Journal of American Academy of Dermatology* confirms that vitamin A in the diet stimulates wound healing, especially in people taking steroid drugs. Steroids are often prescribed to control inflammation, but this also makes skin slower to heal. Vitamin A deficiency also slows wound repair. Since vitamin A is the most commonly deficient vitamin in the Western world, eating a
(continued on page 400)

HOW TO CHOOSE THE BEST SURGEON
AND HOSPITAL FOR *YOU*

The surgeon you choose to do your operation and the hospital where it's performed can tilt the balance toward a successful operation and a rapid recovery. Choosing both carefully is one important area where you can assert control.

Here are some tips to help you make the best selection.

Choose experience. Surgeons who perform a specific operation often are more likely to do it successfully. And hospitals where a certain procedure is frequently done also help to ensure a successful outcome.

Of 16 surgical procedures studied by the New York Department of Health, five showed significantly lower mortality rates when performed by doctors and hospitals that do more of the procedures.

Coronary artery bypass, abdominal surgery, partial gastrectomies (removal of part of the stomach), colectomies (removal of part or all of the colon), and gallbladder removal all had significantly lower mortality rates when performed by high-volume providers. For the first four, a surgeon's volume was most important, with hospital volume marginally important. For gallbladder surgery, hospital volume was statistically more important.

It's not surprising that doctors who are more experienced at a particular procedure would lose fewer patients. But hospitals? "Speculation is that hospitals with higher volumes have more experienced backup teams, well-developed protocols for performing particular operations, appropriate equipment, and better monitoring procedures," says Edward L. Hannan, Ph.D., consultant to the Bureau of Health Care Research, New York State Department of Health.

Ask questions. Most people are referred to a surgeon by their family physician, Dr. Hannan says. He recommends that patients ask that referring physician about the surgeon's experience and mortality rate for the particular procedure. Ditto for the hospital. Here are some other pertinent questions.

- If you had to have this operation, who would you choose and why?
- Is your recommendation of this surgeon based on friendship, geographic proximity, reputation, or some independent evaluation of competence?

● How many cases like mine does this surgeon take
  annually?

If you're up to it, you can call the nearest university
hospital, ask to speak to the relevant department chairperson
and ask the same questions.

Steer clear of teaching hospitals in July. July is the
month when newly graduated medical students begin their
postgraduate clinical training, as interns or in first-year resident
positions of specialty programs. These new interns and
residents replace more experienced hospital house staff.
Patients are more likely to experience adverse effects during
this time, according to one study conducted by the Denver
Veteran's Administration Medical Center and the University of
Colorado Health Sciences Center.

The study found that hospital-caused complications such
as adverse drug reactions and surgical and psychiatric complications were highest in July. (In May and June, the complications rate was at its lowest.) Although the quality of hospital
care isn't at its best during July, you're still better off checking
in for necessary surgery than putting it off until springtime,
says Dennis W. Jahnigen, M.D., head of the section of geriatric
medicine in the Department of Internal Medicine at the
Cleveland Clinic. If your surgery is elective, then it's okay to wait
for better circumstances at the hospital.

Ask to see the records. Tell the hospital personnel that
you know they're required by the government to keep mortality
rate records and that the U.S. Health Care Financing Administration (HCFA) publishes the information for everyone to see,
so it isn't privileged information. If they refuse, ask your
primary doctor to get the information for you. If that fails,
contact the Health Standards and Quality Bureau, HCFA, Room
2-D-2 Meadows East, 6325 Security Boulevard, Baltimore, MD
21207, or the regional office of the HCFA nearest you.

The hospital is obligated by the government to provide data
about its mortality rates for 16 specified categories of health
problems. Be aware, however, that the data can be misleading.
Hospitals to whom higher-risk patients are sent may as a
consequence have a less-favorable reported mortality rate. Keep
in mind, too, that the information published by the HCFA deals
only with Medicare cases, not with the total number of cases
diagnosed and treated at that hospital.

vitamin-A-rich diet may also speed healing of cuts or burns in many people who aren't taking steroids.

Severely injured patients, especially burn victims, often develop vitamin A deficiencies. So if you've suffered from a wound or will be undergoing surgery, be sure to get enough vitamin A in your diet. Good sources include beef, chicken, and calf's liver, most cereals, and vegetables like carrots and sweet potatoes.

Be sure not to overdo it with the supplements. Too much vitamin A can cause serious problems, even death. Consult a physician before taking vitamin A.

After surgery, maximum nutrition is also important, but sometimes when you're recuperating, you don't feel like eating. Here's what one doctor recommends.

Listen to your body. If you don't feel like eating, then don't. But limit your fast to about five days, Dr. Blackburn says. (People who are in poor health before their illness should follow a three-day rule, discussed below.) During those five days, let your appetite determine your food intake. Rest and let Mother Nature do her thing. Just make sure to keep yourself well hydrated by drinking plenty of water, juices, and/or broths.

As soon as you start to feel a little hungry, choose

HIGH TECH • THE LASER MAY BE QUICKER THAN THE SCALPEL

Lasers aren't about to eliminate the need for scalpels in surgery, but in certain operations where the laser is the most appropriate instrument, it has resulted in faster and more successful wound healing.

Laser beams offer several advantages. They cut more precisely than the blade of a scalpel, which means less damage to surrounding tissue. The beam cauterizes blood vessels as it cuts, so less blood is lost during surgery. There's also less risk of infection because, typically, nothing enters the incision except the laser's light.

The drawback is that laser surgery can be very expensive. However, many simple procedures can be done on an outpatient basis, sparing you the hassle of checking into a hospital. That's not just quicker healing—it's cheaper healing, too, because you're spared the cost of the hospital stay.

foods that are easily digestible and rich in calories and nutrition.

If you still can't stomach anything after five days, that's when you must think about ignoring what your appetite is telling you. Prolonged fasting can harm your recovery, Dr. Blackburn says. Ask someone to wave your favorite foods under your nose and make yourself take a few bites.

Follow the three-day rule if you've been chronically ill. After three days, start eating, even if it's just milk with a vitamin supplement or medical foods from your pharmacy. And again, if you're unsure and you find you're not hungry, consult your physician, Dr. Blackburn says.

YOUR EARS CAN HELP HEAL

Does the mind shut down temporarily when the anesthesiologist puts you under? New evidence suggests that the contrary is true. What's more exciting is that you can use the consciousness you retain on the operating table to speed and ease your recovery. How? By using positive suggestions.

Henry Bennett, Ph.D., of the University of California at Davis, believes the typical surgical patient is very suggestible and that the central nervous system remains active and responsive, even under anesthesia.

Dr. Bennett designed a study to test this theory. While surgery patients were unconscious from the anesthetic, he played a taped message once into their ears: "I told them that when we interviewed them a few days later about their surgery, the way they would show they had remembered was by touching their left ear."

During an interview with the patients two or more days after the surgery, the patients said they didn't remember hearing any message—yet they sat there tugging on their left ear, Dr. Bennett said. He believes his suggestion automatically activated the ear tugging.

Insist that the operating room be quiet. This is important whether you're completely out or not. Surgery is a serious event, and you deserve better than to have a party atmosphere going on with loud music blaring, jokes being made, and commentary flying back and forth.

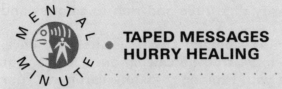

TAPED MESSAGES HURRY HEALING

In a study of 39 women who had undergone a hysterectomy, those who had listened to a positive message tape healed faster than women who'd listened to a blank tape. They spent less time in the hospital, had fewer days of postoperative fever, and were less likely to have problems with gas, diarrhea, or constipation. The women in the first group also were rated as having a better-than-normal recovery by nurses who didn't know which tape the women heard.

The tape reassured the patients that they would not feel sick, would not have pain, and "were doing fine."

The tape isn't very long. In fact, the women listened to just 9 minutes of advice on how to best cope with postoperative procedures, 2 minutes of pointed therapeutic suggestions, and 1 minute's worth of comments about how successfully their surgery was going. The tape was played three times.

Ask if you can bring a Walkman to the operating room. It should have an auto-reverse feature. Don't forget earphones, fresh batteries, and your favorite tapes.

Music played for patients before, during, and after surgery has been shown to reduce anxiety, lessen pain, reduce the need for preoperative and postoperative medication, and speed recovery. In one study, when soothing music was piped into an operating room throughout surgery, the amount of sedative patients required decreased by half.

In another study, the investigator estimated that music had an effect comparable to that of an intravenous dose of 2½ milligrams of Valium. And two studies conducted on surgical patients in Japan indicate that listening to music before and during surgery actually reduces the level of stress hormones in the blood. Since the surgery itself can be loud and the noises strange and disconcerting, the music may just help by blocking out the distressing sounds.

SEASONAL PROBLEMS

A hhh, the great outdoors. In summer there's sunbathing, waterskiing, boating . . . *sunburn, bugs, poison ivy.* And in winter, there's skiing, ice skating, snowmobiling . . . *chapped lips, frostbite, hypothermia.*

We're not trying to rain on your picnic here. It's just that if you're going to work and play safely outdoors, you need to take steps to protect your body from both the burning kiss of summer sun and the icy touch of winter.

STRATEGIES FOR SUMMER'S SIZZLE

It's the camping trip you've dreamed about for the past six months. No telephones. No paperwork. Your only appointment is with a book and a canoe. But if you're not careful, there will be one appointment you'll have to keep when you get back—the one with the doctor.

With a little forethought you can make sure that summer outing is a pleasurable trip rather than a painful jaunt into realms of physical discomfort. You can:

- Rub toothpaste on a bee sting and feel better instantly.
- Gulp down a Gatorade or some other sports drink and stave off muscle cramps in mere seconds.
- Ice down a sunburn and feel better in 10 minutes.

There's a strategy to meet every challenge that summer sends your way. You can stave off sunburn, combat heat cramps, beat heat exhaustion, prevent poison ivy and poison oak, and avoid tick bites and bee stings. Here's how.

OVERCOME OVEREXPOSURE

Last January in the midst of winter's blahs, you promised yourself a glorious, knock-'em-dead summer tan.

Now here it is July and you're trying to live up to that promise. You've been in the sun 1 hour, 2 hours . . . the clock is ticking, ticking. . . .

You *were* aiming for a shade somewhere between golden and goddess brown. But what's going on here?

You're red. Bright red. Watermelon red. Red Cross red.

Now standing in front of the medicine cabinet, you feel like crawling into the freezer. And here's why. A sunburn is a wound. It's your body's response to overexposure to the sun.

Energy from the sun causes biochemical changes within the skin itself, ending with inflammation. The inflammation—a burn—causes damage to the skin, says Rodney Basler, M.D., assistant professor of internal medicine at the University of Nebraska Medical Center.

Repeated sunburn can harm your skin, breaking down its elastic tissues, causing wrinkles, and increasing your risk of skin cancer.

Even getting a tan without burning can damage the immune system by limiting the skin's effectiveness as a barrier to disease, according to a report by the American Medical Association's Council on Scientific Affairs.

"Any suntan is permanent damage. The sun's ultraviolet rays do permanent damage to cells in the skin," says Michael Schreiber, M.D., dermatologist and senior clinical lecturer at the University of Arizona School of Medicine in Tucson. "That damage shows up later in the forties, fifties, and sixties as skin cancers, as wrinkles, as precancers."

However, sunscreens are a simple way to protect yourself while enjoying the outdoors. They take less than 5 minutes to apply all over your body. Look for the sun protection factor, called SPF, on a sunscreen product. The SPF works like this: If your unprotected skin burns in 10 minutes, an SPF of 6 will allow you to stay out in sun for 60 minutes before you burn. The greater the SPF, the higher the protection and the longer you can stay out in the sun.

THE BEST SUNSCREEN FINDER

Skin Characteristics	Recommended SP
Always burns easily, never tans	15 or more
Always burns easily, tans slightly	15 or more
Burns moderately, tans gradually	10 to 15
Burns slightly, always tans well	6 to 10
Rarely burns, tans liberally	4 to 6

An important factor affecting how you'll react to sun is your skin type. People of Celtic backgrounds with fair skin burn easily. If you're not sure about your skin type and the recommended SPF for you, see "The Best Sunscreen Finder" above.

PUT OUT THOSE FLAMES

What should you do when a day in the sun has gone too far, when it's late, when you've fallen asleep in the sun, or just lost track of time?

Hightail it inside. If you're starting to redden while you're outside, you'll be even redder 1 to 4 hours later, Dr. Schreiber says.

Reach for the ice. Place crushed ice in towels and apply to the burned area for 10 minutes. Repeat this treatment three or four times daily for two to three days, Dr. Schreiber recommends.

Pop some antihistamines. Over-the-counter drugs like Benadryl and Chlor-Trimeton will reduce swelling and itching. They should be taken once every 6 hours for the first 48 hours after you've burned, Dr. Schreiber says.

Take some aspirin. To reduce swelling, take two aspirin every 6 hours for two to three days, Dr. Schreiber says.

Go see your doctor. Make an appointment at the first sign of blistering. Bacteria can easily enter the raised skin of a blister, giving you the potential for problems, Dr. Schreiber warns. Dr. Basler says he gives patients with blistering sunburn internal cortisone (to reduce the inflammation) for five days.

Apply Cortaid cream. This product will soothe the area and can be used two or three times daily for the first

48 hours after the burn. Do not use the cream on large blisters because it might cause infections, Dr. Schreiber says.

Spread on a moisturizing cream. Apply a moisturizer like Eucerin to keep the area from drying. Use the cream as needed to keep the area moist.

Jump into a cool tub. This will help reduce swelling. A bath is better than a shower because it's less traumatic to your skin.

Smooth on some aloe vera. Just break off a piece and rub the gel onto your skin as needed for pain. It contains chemicals that help burns heal. And, preparations in the store just don't work like the real thing.

Spray on Solarcaine. This product will numb the painful areas, but be careful using it if you have sensitive skin. It may cause a rash.

Stay inside for a few days. Take one week off from activities in the sun if you get burned.

Cover up. Take special precautions once you've sunburned, because the affected area won't be back to normal for four to six months, Dr. Schreiber says. Keep the area covered with clothing and use sunscreens.

BANISH BURNS FROM YOUR LIFE

The best way to deal with sunburn is to not get one in the first place.

Here are simple things you can do to avoid becoming the lobster of the party.

Slop on the sunscreen. Apply the sunscreen—lots of it—to your skin 30 to 60 minutes before you go outside. Look for a cream or gel with 5 percent para-aminobenzoic acid (PABA) or its esters in ethyl alcohol. (If you're allergic to PABA or its esters, you can use a benzophenone sunscreen.) People in the West and Southwest should use sunscreen liberally year-round, Dr. Basler says.

Dab extra sunscreen on your face and neck. Take a few moments to apply sunscreen with an SPF of at least a 15 on your nose, tops of your ears, cheeks, neck, shoulders, and lips. Or use an opaque cream like zinc oxide on these sensitive areas to maximize protection from the sun.

Reload after getting wet. Be sure to reapply sunscreen after swimming or perspiring heavily. It can wash off, leaving you without protection.

Check the clock. If you must tan, begin slowly. While dermatologists never recommend sunbathing, Dr. Basler offers these guidelines for your first sunbath of the year. You're safe in increasing your time in the sun by 5 minutes per exposure.

- Very fair skin — 5 to 10 minutes
- Moderate pigment — 10 to 15 minutes
- Dark, Latinate — 15 to 20 minutes

Check your pills. Some medications increase your sensitivity to the sun. These include tricyclic antidepressants, antihistamines, diuretics, and oral contraceptives. Make a quick call to your doctor about any medications you may be taking.

Duck inside when the clock strikes twelve. Try to schedule your sunning and other outdoor activities prior to 11:00 A.M. and after 3:00 P.M., daylight saving time. The sun's rays cause the most damage in the hours just before and after high noon.

Get dressed. To keep your cool in the heat while protecting your skin, wear light-colored, loose-fitting clothing.

Grab a cap. Wearing a cap will double the SPF of the sunscreen on your nose and forehead, while a cap alone provides an SPF of 2, Dr. Basler says.

Put on your shades. It takes only a second to put on sunglasses to protect your eyes. Skin cancer can occur on eyelids. Plus, studies have linked sun exposure to cataracts and retina damage. Look for sunglasses that block 75 percent of visible and infrared light and 95 percent of the ultraviolet rays.

TURN DOWN THE HEAT

You're standing at a Main Street curb with a miniature U.S. flag in one hand, a hot dog in the other. It's the Fourth of July parade. You've watched floats, ponies, clowns, and beauty queens march past and there's still no sign of your daughter, who's playing clarinet in the high school band.

Suddenly, you're sweating and feeling queasy. You slowly move through the crowd and sit down on a nearby lawn.

"What's wrong with me?" you wonder.

What's wrong is an overdose of heat. Muscle cramps, heat exhaustion, and heatstroke result from the body trying to maintain a normal temperature during a heat overload, notes James P. Knochel, M.D., chairman of the Department of Internal Medicine at Presbyterian Hospital, Dallas, Texas.

Certain groups of people are more likely to overheat, Dr. Knochel says. If you're a stocky person, you'll generate more heat than someone with a lanky build. Plus, if you have diabetes or cardiovascular disease or are obese, or if you're taking antihistamines, tricyclic antidepressants, alcohol, diuretics, or vasodilators, you're more likely to have heat-related problems.

Yet there are things you can do to treat and prevent these high-temperature upheavals.

BEAT HEAT CRAMPS

Problems from overheating can be as serious as total prostration or as annoying as a leg cramp that puts a crimp in your tennis game. Here's some relief from the pesky problem of heat cramps.

Grab a Gatorade. The quickest way to replace lost water and essential chemicals is to drink Gatorade or other sports drinks. Drink at least one glass every 30 minutes while you're engaging in strenuous activity.

Stretch those balls of fire. You'll feel so much better after you stretch your knotted muscles. While a post-sports massage may sound wonderful, Dr. Knochel says it rarely works and sometimes makes the pain worse.

Walk it out. "You have to cool down just like a racehorse," Dr. Knochel says. "Easy walking for 10 to 15 minutes will prevent cramps from coming on."

DON'T CRAMP YOUR STYLE

You'll enjoy that tennis match, or any other strenuous outdoor activity, if you avoid heat cramps altogether.

Get plenty of sleep. Not enough sack time can cause cramps. Fatigue caused by exercise and lack of sleep will slow your reflexes, impairing blood flow to the muscles and interfering with your ability to lose heat, Dr. Knochel says.

Chow down on the right stuff. Fresh fruits and vegetables, meat, avocadoes, and dried fruits are excellent sources of the potassium you lose during work or exercise. Potassium and other minerals help relax muscles. You lose these minerals when you sweat, so you must replace them or your muscles will cramp. Three ounces of raisins, Dr. Knochel says, will give you half of your daily requirement of potassium.

Take tea. Or select water or some other nonalcoholic beverage. Alcohol is a diuretic—that is, it makes your body excrete water. Drinking alcohol before or during exercise makes you lose even more water.

HEAD OFF HEAT EXHAUSTION

After an afternoon of gardening in the sun, you feel weak, dizzy, nauseated. Though the temperature is in the 90s, your skin is cool. Sounds strange, but it's all part of heat exhaustion. Here's what you can do if the heat gets heavy on you.

Get yourself indoors. Find a room with air conditioning and stay in it until you're thoroughly cooled down, Dr. Knochel advises. If your house isn't air conditioned, go to a mall or see a movie.

Quaff some water or a sports drink. Dehydration is a hallmark of heat exhaustion. You should drink as much water or sports drink as you need to replenish the liquids you lose.

Slap on a moist towel. Drape cool, moist towels over your head, arms, and legs and around your neck. The key is to cool down your body.

Fan down those flames. Fanning air over your body evaporates sweat and helps your own internal air conditioning system work. Sitting in front of a fan will cool you down in no time.

Take a bath. Bathe in cool water, or take sponge baths to really cool off.

SCRATCH OFF POISON IVY

Would you have trouble distinguishing poison ivy from periwinkle, poison oak from a maple leaf cluster, poison sumac from a flourishing fern? Not up on your plant morphology, eh?

You'll know it soon enough if you've walked through any of the terrible threesome. They leave you red, swollen, blistered, and itchy. In fact, about 85 percent of adults are allergic to these plants.

You can curse the little green leaves as you sit and scratch and scratch. Actually, what caused your ire is *urushiol,* an oily substance on the leaves. Wherever the urushiol goes, itching and scratching soon follow.

It's anonymity that makes urushiol a formidable opponent: You can't see it or feel it, says William Epstein, M.D., a professor of dermatology at the University of California at San Francisco.

And the ways you can get urushiol on your skin are limitless! If you take your boot off by grasping the heel and you've stepped in urushiol, then urushiol gets on your hand, Dr. Epstein says. Fido runs by and you reach out and touch his coat. He's rolled in a spot of it, and urushiol gets on your hand again. You go inside, open the refrigerator for a cold drink, shut the door, then rest your hand on the kitchen table as you read the newspaper. Urushiol now is on the refrigerator door, the kitchen table, and the daily news. And because it takes several weeks for urushiol to oxidize, there's plenty of time for all that itching misery to get spread around.

Treatment involves comforting yourself until the itching subsides and the rash runs its course, Dr. Epstein says. Here are a few suggestions about how you can do that.

Apply some calamine. The instructions are easy: "When the skin blisters, dab it on. It's really the simplest thing to do," Dr. Epstein says. He suggests using the lotion as needed to dry up oozing and stop itching.

Stick with plain, pink calamine and avoid buying lotions containing antihistamines because they don't help much, he says.

Take a tablet. Oral antihistamines like Benadryl and Chlor-Trimeton may help relieve itching.

Use a compress. A cool compress applied to the area as needed will ease itching, Dr. Epstein says.

Soak in a cool tub. A cool bath may feel better than a compress and relieve that itch that's driving you crazy.

See your doctor. These are the times you put the calamine down and visit your physician.

- If you are extremely itchy and blistered and can't carry on your normal activities.
- If the rash lasts longer than two weeks.
- If the crust on the rash turns yellow with pus.
- If you've been exposed in a sensitive area such as your face, eyes, hands, or genitals.

BYPASS POISON IVY

If you can prevent an encounter with urushiol, you'll save yourself a lot of grief. But that's easier said than done. If you think you've brushed up against some poison ivy, here are some ways to keep urushiol from bothering you.

Wash with alcohol. Splash the affected area of skin with rubbing alcohol "because it's a good solvent for urushiol," Dr. Epstein says. But don't use alcohol on your skin until you're ready to come home for the day. When you rub alcohol on your skin, you remove protective oils, so any later exposure to urushiol is going to affect your skin even faster.

Douse with water. Follow the alcohol by washing the area with lots of water. If you don't have alcohol and think you've been exposed, wash the area with water as quickly as possible. If you're hiking, pop open your canteen and start pouring, or head for a stream.

Wash your clothes. Throw your clothes in the machine when you get home to rid them of the poisonous agent.

Wash everything else exposed to it. Wash the dog, spray off your boots with water, hose down your tent. You might try adding hydrogen peroxide to water (about 1 part hydrogen peroxide to 20 parts water) for a mix that will neutralize urushiol.

Use solvents. Paint thinner or gasoline can remove urushiol from your golf clubs, a shovel or other hand tools, a baseball bat, your bike tires, or any product you use outdoors. These solvents also work on your skin but are very harsh, Dr. Epstein says, and should not be used often.

Try a cream. At least two barrier creams are available as a defense against poison ivy and poison oak: Ivy

Shield and the industrial cream Stokogard Outdoor Cream. Ask your pharmacist to get them for you, Dr. Epstein suggests. (Another cream, Ivy Block, may also be available.)

GET TICKS OFF

Ticks. They might be called one of God's little jokes on this great big world.

You or your pet is their "host." Some guest—besides giving you a little lump and creepy-crawly feelings when you find one, a tick can give you the potentially serious Lyme disease or Rocky Mountain spotted fever (see "Totally Terrible Ticks: What to Do" below).

Though they can be hard to spot, you can find ticks and remove them. Then simply treat the area. You'll be glad to learn tick encounters can be prevented. But first, let's get the critter off.

Your Uncle Pete in Des Moines probably says a hot pair of tweezers and a jerk of its body will do the trick,

. . . .

TOTALLY TERRIBLE TICKS: WHAT TO DO

Finding a tick on your body gives you the heebie-jeebies, kind of like chewing on a wad of tinfoil. Ordinarily, your problem ends when the critter's life does. But even though he's gone, the tick may have infected you with Lyme disease or Rocky Mountain spotted fever. You can get either from being bitten by an infected tick.

Lyme disease is the bigger problem, with 43 states reporting cases, according to the *New England Journal of Medicine.* If you remove the infected tick within 24 hours after it attaches, your chances of getting Lyme disease are slim, says Jim Gill, Ph.D., a research associate in microbiology at the University of Minnesota at Minneapolis.

Lyme disease doesn't show up right away. It usually takes three days to a few weeks for a red rash to develop where the tick was attached or on other areas of the body. (The rash manifests in only 60 to 80 percent of cases.) Typically, the rash expands, develops a bright red border, and may be hot to the touch. But, this isn't always true.

A person with Lyme disease may experience headaches, fever, fatigue, stiff neck, joint and muscle pain, swollen glands, and dizziness.

Later symptoms, if the disease isn't treated, include abnormal heartbeat, paralysis of facial muscles, arthritis, and severe headaches.

If you experience any of these symptoms and recall that you recently removed a tick or were in an area with Lyme disease cases, call your doctor.

The doctor will give you doxycycline or amoxicillin for up to six weeks to get rid of the rash.

Stronger antibiotics are given for more serious, later-stage symptoms such as paralysis of facial muscles, arthritis, and severe headaches.

Pregnant women who *think* they've been exposed to Lyme disease should see their doctors, because their unborn children may be at risk.

Rocky Mountain spotted fever announces itself with a high fever, says Daniel Fishbein, M.D., a medical epidemiologist at Atlanta's Centers for Disease Control. It can also cause headaches, chills, and aches and pains.

A rash of reddish-purple-black spots shows up on the soles of the feet and on the ankles, hands, or wrists within a week of the tick bite. The rash may spread throughout the body.

A person with this disease may also have problems sleeping and feel agitated.

Aspirin can relieve the aches and pains of Rocky Mountain spotted fever, but if you suspect that you've been infected, see your doctor.

The doctor will prescribe antibiotics such as tetracycline. The fever should subside about two days after treatment begins, but antibiotics must be taken for up to two weeks, Dr. Fishbein says.

Here's an even simpler rule to follow: "If you have *any* suspicious illness within two weeks after removing a tick, see a physician," Dr. Fishbein says.

And save any ticks you remove in a bottle with moist paper, where they can remain for six to eight weeks. Write down the date you found the tick and where you were when you were bitten. If you develop symptoms of either disease, take the tick to your doctor for identification.

while Aunt May scoffs, insisting a drop of nail polish is the only way.

Experts like Roger Drummond, Ph.D., a 30-year research scientist with the U.S. Department of Agriculture, don't like the home remedies. Dr. Drummond writes in *Ticks and What You Can Do about Them* that warming and polishing the little guys doesn't affect them at all, they just keep hanging on, and a quick jerk of the tick's body could leave the head embedded in your skin, increasing your chances of infection. Here are Dr. Drummond's suggestions for getting a tick off.

Do the tick-removal two-step. Grasp the tick as close to the skin as possible with tweezers or your fingers. If you use your fingers, cover the tick with plastic wrap, waxed paper, tissue, or paper toweling to protect yourself from the tick and anything it might be carrying. Then remove the tick with a steady pull. Take your time. Don't crush the tick, pull its body away from its head, or get any of its fluids on your skin—they may cause an infection. (You may want to use The Tick Solution, a new device designed especially for removing ticks.)

Wipe the bite with alcohol. This stings a little, but it disinfects the area.

Wash your hands. This prevents the spread of infection.

KEEP TICKS OFF YOUR TURF

Instead of waiting until the little buggers find you, why not prevent a close encounter with ticks? Here are a few ways to stop ticks from making tracks on you.

Dress in white. So you can more easily see ticks that hitch a ride on you, wear a light-colored, long-sleeved shirt and long pants, Dr. Drummond advises. And tuck your pants into your boots or socks. Keeping your skin covered makes it harder for ticks to attach.

Treat your threads. Use a repellent containing DEET on your clothes, Dr. Drummond recommends. Lay your clothes on the ground, spray one side for 15 seconds, then turn the clothing over and spray again. And, don't forget to treat shoes and socks to protect these critical places.

Permanone Tick Repellent is another choice, though

it's strong and only for clothing. In tests, Permanone provided 100 percent protection against various types of ticks. It's best to spray your clothes and allow Permanone to dry before heading outside.

Dab your skin, too. Look for repellents containing DEET, and apply them directly to your skin. When a tick crawls on you, the repellent makes it drop off.

Take care of pets. It's important to remove ticks from pets so that only Lassie comes home with you. Take a few minutes every day to run a hand carefully through your pet's fur, especially around the collar and the ears. If you find a tick, remove it just as you would from a person. Better yet, keep your pet from getting ticks in the first place by using a tick repellent spray every time your dog romps in the woods or fields.

GET BEES TO BUZZ OFF

Bumblebees. Wasps. Hornets. Yellow jackets. Team names in a high school basketball tournament? No, they're the wrong kind of fliers. These are insects that can sting you. They belong to different families, they have different temperaments, different venoms, and different stingers, but you won't notice much difference in the intense pain and swelling these striped, sharp-tailed buzz bombs create when they make a direct hit on you. It hurts, but unless you're allergic (see "Killer Bee Stings: Don't Be a Victim" on page 417), the pain and swelling will subside. It will take anywhere from a few hours to a few days depending on which pest left you its calling card. Here's what you can do to quickly ease the discomfort in the meantime.

Get the stinger out. Only the honeybee routinely leaves behind a barbed stinger. Using a scraping motion, gently remove the stinger. You can even use your fingernail. It'll only take a second. Don't squeeze the venom sac attached to it, you'll release more venom, says Martin Valentine, M.D., an allergist with the Johns Hopkins Asthma and Allergy Center in Baltimore.

Ice the pain. An ice compress applied to the sting relieves pain and swelling almost immediately. Use ice once every 2 hours during the first day after you've been stung. In addition to cooling, ice "stops the spread of venom," Dr. Valentine says.

Get your leg up. If the sting is on your leg, elevate the leg for about 30 minutes after you've removed the stinger, Dr. Valentine says.

Apply gentle heat. If you're still swollen after the first day on ice, Dr. Valentine advises placing a warm compress or heating pad on the sting as often as possible for one day.

Take aspirin or ibuprofen. Start with two aspirin or one ibuprofen tablet every 4 hours and continue as needed, following directions on the bottle.

Reach for the antihistamines. You may have itching near the sting. Oral antihistamines like Chlor-Trimeton or Benadryl may be taken every 4 to 6 hours to ease the itch, Dr. Valentine says.

Grab the tenderizer. You may soothe the itching by rubbing the area with meat tenderizers made with the enzyme papain.

Take Aim against the pain. Rubbing toothpaste on a sting makes it feel better because the menthol in the paste has a cooling effect, Dr. Valentine says.

Calamine will feel fine. Applied as needed, calamine will help soothe the area.

BEAT THE BEES

The best way to avoid becoming the subject of a stinging tale is to stay away from the airborne critters. Keep these things in mind about preventing stings.

Drop that lipstick. Avoid wearing cosmetics, clothing, or accessories that attract insects: hair spray, cologne, scented soap, perfume, bright colors, print patterns, or shiny jewelry.

Stay calm. If a stinging insect lands on or near you, don't jump. If you stay still, it may buzz off.

Look before you eat. Yellow jackets and hornets, Dr. Valentine reports, have splendiferous palates. "Yellow jackets love steamed crabs and hamburgers," he says. Thus, keep a watchful eye on picnic foods during summer outings.

Cover up. Dress in long pants and long-sleeved shirts when you're outdoors and do keep your shoes on.

KILLER BEE STINGS: DON'T BE A VICTIM

For most people, a bee sting means pain and discomfort. For the unfortunate minority who are allergic, a sting can be life-threatening.

They can experience a total body allergic reaction known as anaphylactic shock. The symptoms include severe swelling in the eyes, lips, or tongue; coughing or wheezing; weakness; itching; stomach cramps; anxiety; nausea and vomiting; trouble breathing; dizziness; bluish skin; and hives. These symptoms can be followed by collapse, unconsciousness, and even death.

If you begin to experience an extreme reaction within 20 minutes of a sting, get medical help immediately, says Marty Aho, R.N., Emergency Medical Service liaison nurse at Yosemite National Park. Many people who know they have allergic reactions carry an emergency kit containing a premeasured dose of epinephrine. These kits are available by prescription, and your doctor can show you how the kit works.

CHAPS AND CHILLS

You don't have to live north of the Arctic Circle to encounter problems related to cold weather. Every year, hikers, campers, skiers, and joggers around the country take winter on the chin—or lips, hands, and ears. In fact, you don't even have to be an outdoor enthusiast to suffer cold-induced health problems. Superheated office buildings can leave your skin as dry as Alaskan tundra. And older people living in underheated apartments are nearly as susceptible to problems like hypothermia as hunters in deer blinds.

Should you find yourself nipped, chapped, or chilled, however, help can be just an instant away. All that is needed is:

- Instant action to relieve hypothermia
- Thirty seconds to apply a cream that protects chapped skin from further damage while it regenerates
- Twenty minutes to rewarm your frost-nipped toes

FAST RELIEF FOR CHAPPED SKIN AND LIPS

Chapped skin is one of the most common consequences of cold, dry weather. And the fact is, you have to be careful both indoors and out to prevent this condition. Indoors, heated air can rob your skin of its moisture, making it susceptible to both drying *and* chapping.

How, exactly, does climate result in chapped skin? "Think of the surface of your skin as a tiled roof," says Leonard Swinyer, M.D., associate clinical professor of medicine in the Division of Dermatology at the University of Utah in Salt Lake City. "Like roofing shingles, overlapping skin cells form a barrier against outside elements. However, when skin cells dry out, they shrink. The cell 'shingles' separate from one another, resulting in a leaky roof easily penetrated by outside elements such as bacteria."

Even without treatment, cells deep within the skin continually generate new moisturizing factors. But this new growth may take 30 days or longer, provided the cells underneath the skin have not been injured. Here's how to help your skin repair itself more quickly.

Take a sponge bath. Bathe only on alternate days, especially if you don't exercise hard or work at a job that leaves you greasy and grungy. You'll cut down on contact with soap and water, which strip away the skin's natural protective oils. Limit hand washing to after using the bathroom and before handling food, to heal chapping.

Use a superfatted soap, like Dove. These have extra lipids for added moisture.

Slip on cotton gloves. For washing dishes and doing other household chores, don't rely on rubber gloves alone to protect chapped skin. They have, in fact, been shown to compound the chapping problem for the allergy prone. For real protection, wear cotton gloves under rubber gloves.

Take a quick bath. Bathe in tepid water using bath oil, and avoid bubble bath. Bath oils will help your skin retain moisture, while bubble baths strip it away. (Just be careful when you climb out of that oil-slick tub.)

Lather up. But spare the soap. Lather only your underarms and groin area, Dr. Swinyer suggests.

Slick on the lotion. Use an oil-free cleansing lotion

such as Cetaphil, available over-the-counter at your pharmacy. Apply it to your face, and pat it dry with a cotton towel. Then reapply the lotion to remoisten your skin, and apply petroleum jelly or an unscented cream right over it. Your skin will begin to regenerate *immediately* after applying moisturizer. Dr. Swinyer suggests making moisturizing part of your everyday regimen.

Cream your sunscreen. Before going outside in the winter, where sun and snow work together against your face, apply a sunscreen rated with an SPF of 15 or higher, and let it dry. Then, to prevent windburn as well as sunburn, put another cream over the sunscreen or use a product that's a sunscreen and moisturizer in one.

Moisturize damp skin. You don't even have to dry yourself completely before you reach for the moisturizer. (In fact, heavy rubbing with a towel only irritates problem skin.) Applying an oil-based lotion or petroleum jelly while you're still damp from the shower or bath helps trap moisture in your damaged skin. Diligent moisturizing can help clear up a case of chapped skin within a week. To avoid recurrence, continue moisturizing four weeks after the problem has cleared.

Plant one on those lips. Like skin, lips dry out fast in winter weather. Heal them fast with a swipe of ChapStick or other lip protectant, says Tom Gossel, Ph.D., professor of pharmacology at Ohio Northern University. And if you suffer from chronically chapped lips, try using a ½ percent hydrocortisone ointment, available over-the-counter, to soothe them. More important, Dr. Gossel notes, keep them protected.

Stick it to your lips. Put a barrier between your lips and the cold air. Lipstick, says Hillard Pearlstein, M.D., assistant clinical professor of dermatology at Mount Sinai School of Medicine in New York City, is a great preventive for chapped lips. And, he adds, the greasier the lipstick, the better for your lips.

Screen out the problem. The sun can dry your lips, even in the winter, causing them to scale and feel rough. Use a lip balm that contains sun protection factor of at least 15, Dr. Pearlstein says.

Moisturize the air. With the flick of a button you can turn dry winter into dewy spring. Humidifiers add moisture to the air, helping to provide immediate relief for dry, chapped skin. You can place a personal-size humidifier on your desk at work, attach a humidifying system to your home heating unit, or plug in a portable humidifier in the most-used room of your house. (One caveat: Unless they're cleaned and serviced regularly according to the manufacturer's directions, humidifiers can breed mold and bacteria, which can cause respiratory infections or allergies to flare up. So be careful to keep your humidifier scrupulously clean and well-maintained.)

After two days, your symptoms may disappear.

Note: If severe chapping persists—talk to your doctor. You may be taking medications that encourage chapping.

TREATING JACK FROST'S BITES

Skiers and lovers of the great outdoors often find that after a couple of hours in the cold, their cheeks, fingers, nose, toes, or the tips of their ears will become somewhat pale. They've got superficial frostbite, a painful or sometimes numbing superficial condition that follows prolonged exposure to the cold.

Deep frostbite is more serious—the extremities, typically the ears, fingers, nose, and toes, actually freeze.

When your skin freezes, you first experience pain, and then, ironically, a warm feeling. When the skin turns white and hard to the touch—like a bar of soap—frostbite has hit. Extreme frostbite is very dangerous—if not handled properly, the affected area may have to be amputated. Anyone who spends time outdoors exposed to the cold runs the risk.

A few simple but smart moves can help you prevent frostbite in the first place. And if you get frostbite despite proper precautions, make sure you see a doctor immediately. Even with immediate treatment, doctors may not be able to tell you for three to eight weeks just how much damage has occurred. A mildly frostbitten area may remain sensitive to the cold for a season or two, but the effects of severe frostbite can last a lifetime.

Prevention is the best treatment, says James Wilkerson, M.D., a veteran of cold-weather climbs on Mount McKinley and coauthor of *Hypothermia, Frostbite, and Other Cold Injures*. But if you do get frostbite despite precautions, there are a number of things you can do to start the healing process.

Double your mittens. Adding an extra pair of mittens can help insulate your hands against cold and wind. It's also a good idea to wear an extra pair of socks, provided your boots aren't so tight that they cut off blood circulation.

Put up your dukes. If you're stuck outdoors, try to shelter your exposed nose and face from the wind by covering your face with your hands, trapping warm air close to your skin.

Head for home. Don't be macho and try to tough out the cold. At the first sign of frostbite, cover the area to warm it up. If it doesn't rewarm and feel normal within a few minutes, get indoors, even if the only available shelter is your car.

G-e-n-t-l-y rewarm your hands and feet. Tempting as it may seem, if you've been frostbitten, *don't* rub your hands and feet vigorously or hold them in front of a heater, fireplace, or woodstove. Rubbing will compound tissue damage, and dry heat will warm it too rapidly. Instead, Dr. Wilkerson recommends submerging the frostbitten area in warm (not hot) water. If you have a thermometer handy, use it—104° to 108°F water is ideal. (If your face gets frostbitten, you can rewarm it by applying a soft cloth that's been soaked in warm water.)

Keep the area submerged for 15 to 30 minutes, or until the tip of the affected area returns to a pinkish color and stays pink when pulled out of the water. The skin should feel warm to the touch. Elevate your feet after they've thawed.

Snap into action at the first signs of danger. Hard, solid, and blanched patches of skin are signs of serious, even deep frostbite. If you haven't done so already, get out of the cold, pronto. Do *not* try to thaw the frostbitten area outdoors, and don't let a thawed area refreeze—it can cause serious tissue damage. With severe frostbite, it's safer to leave it frozen and go to a hospital immediately so the area can be properly thawed.

QUICK THINKING CAN WARD OFF HYPOTHERMIA

Hypothermia is more subtle than frostbite, and it can be more dangerous, possibly even life-threatening. Anytime your body loses heat faster than it's generated, your vital organs—including your brain and nervous system—function more slowly. With mild hypothermia, you shiver, lack coordination, have slurred speech, and start to feel groggy. With moderate hypothermia, shivering subsides, blood pressure and pulse drop, and breathing slows. Severe hypothermia can lead to coma and death. In fact, the person with severe hypothermia will look like a corpse—immobile, cold, and stiff to the touch, with pale, blue-gray skin.

Infants are especially vulnerable to hypothermia—they're so small, any heat loss is significant. Older adults may be more susceptible to the cold because of impaired circulation. And elderly people who are frail and slight of build may have too little body fat to insulate them against the cold.

A short jaunt in the frosty air probably won't bring on hypothermia. But if you plan to spend considerable time outdoors in chilly weather, you should know how to manage the cold, even if you're a seasoned outdoor enthusiast or in good physical shape. Murray Hamlet, D.V.M., director of the Cold Research Division, U.S. Army Research Institute of Environmental Medicine, offers the following advice.

Reach for the fiber-pile. Rule number one: If you're going to spend extended time outdoors—say, building a snow fort with your kids or playing a raucous game of ice hockey with your old college buddies—dress appropriately. Fiber-pile sportswear is the best choice—it contains thousands of tiny air pockets that trap warm air. Once trapped, it stays trapped for a couple of hours or more.

Pull on extra layers. If you're stepping out into the cold, the best warming measure you can take is to dress in layers. This helps trap heat and allows you to peel off clothes as the temperature changes, or as you work up a sweat with exertion. Your inner layer should consist of one of the new synthetic fabrics, like polypropylene, that wick perspiration away from your skin. Silk or wool blends are acceptable as well. The next layers should insulate you by trapping your body heat. A wool shirt, sweater, or pile garment is one of your best options. Your outermost layer should protect you against the elements and allow perspiration to evaporate, so choose a breathable, waterproof jacket or windbreaker.

Donning a few layers of clothes takes from 7 to 12 minutes, but you'll stay warm for hours.

Pack a change of clothes. The great outdoors is a minefield of surprises. You never know when the temperatures will dive or you'll get drenched by a chilling shower. And who can foresee falling into a creek? So as an added precaution, take a few minutes to ransack your drawers and pack up an extra pair of socks, sweater, and trousers. You can carry them with you outdoors in a daypack, or leave them in the car for when you return cold and wet from your hiking, biking, or boating.

Don lightweight togs for exercise. If you're going to be exerting yourself strenuously outdoors, don't bundle up so much that you sweat. Damp clothes lose their insulating properties and combine with cold air to increase heat loss, similar to a super air conditioner when you need it least. Wait until after you've exerted yourself—say, when you reach a rest stop—to pull on your extra clothes, even if you don't feel cold yet.

If you start to shiver, find shelter. And warm yourself with blankets. Stay bundled for at least an hour.

Wolf down some food. Your body needs calories (and lots of them!) to generate heat, raise metabolism, and return your body temperature to normal. So taking 5 minutes to eat a bowl of oatmeal can stoke your furnace for a morning's jaunt.

Drink something hot. Soup, hot cider, or other hot liquids won't warm up the body very much, but they prevent dehydration and make you feel better fast. (Dehydration can aggravate cold injury.)

Hike up the thermostat. Hypothermia can strike even in the "comfort" of your own home, if you have the heat turned way down to conserve fuel. To avoid problems, keep the temperature at 68°F or higher.

Don't just stand there, do something. If you're far from home and begin to shiver, take shelter out of the wind, build a fire, stay hydrated, eat any food you may have brought with you, keep active, and bundle up as much as possible. Doing any one of these things is far better than doing nothing.

Act fast if a friend falters. If not attended to, hypothermia can be a medical emergency. If your companion has been exposed to the cold, lacks coordination, and develops slurred speech, get him indoors at once. If you're stranded or far from shelter, give him warm fluids if possible and get him moving. Walking will help warm your companion and get you closer to shelter. If your companion continues to falter, insulate him as best you can. Anything will do: extra blankets, clothing, even raked up leaves or a snow den (in this case plant a marker so you can find your companion again). Go seek help.

SEXUAL PROBLEMS

S exual problems come in many forms, from impotence and infertility to vaginal dryness and genital herpes. But most have at least one thing in common. Unlike sex itself, which is among the quickest and easiest acts to perform, sexual disorders have a tendency to become long-lasting, burdensome problems that can persist for years—or a lifetime. But that needn't be.

"If you have a problem, such as premature ejaculation or lack of arousal, don't live with it," advises Shirley Zussman, Ed.D., a sex and marital therapist in New York City and codirector of the Association for Male Sexual Dysfunction. "There is help available today for sexual problems."

For example:

- In just 5 seconds, you can practice an exercise that will give stronger orgasms (in women) or firmer erections (in men).
- In just 3 minutes, a man experiencing impotency can activate a device that aids in achieving an erection.
- In just 30 minutes, couples who want to conceive can give semen a better chance to fertilize an egg.

EFFECTIVE SHORTCUTS ON THE ROAD TO FERTILITY

For most couples, fertility is no problem. However, for about one in six couples who want children, getting pregnant can turn into a long struggle—anywhere from 12 months to 12 years, according to Arthur L. Wisot, M.D., a physician on the staff of one of the foremost fertility clinics in the United States. "We've seen patients who have tried for at least that long," Dr. Wisot says. "People will try for years and years and years and not give up. We had a woman in our clinic who had gone through seven in vitro fertilization (IVF) cycles elsewhere and then came here and got pregnant on her first try with us—but her eighth, all told."

At Dr. Wisot's South Bay Hospital IVF Center in Redondo Beach, California, the basic evaluation alone, before any actual treatment begins, can take from three to four months. This evaluation starts out with simple, noninvasive procedures such as a basal body temperature chart for the woman and a series of semen analyses for the man.

But are there any simple, quick "Have I tried everything?" procedures that might also help?

Yes there are, and Dr. Wisot, who is also the coauthor, with David R. Meldrum, M.D., of *New Options for Fertility: A Guide to IVF and Other Assisted Reproduction Methods,* has a complete list of quick checks he discusses with his patients and in his book.

Pick the right time. Timing of intercourse is of the essence when it comes to conception. Keeping a basal body temperature diary is the standard procedure for pinpointing ovulation. But to increase the accuracy of the process, Dr. Wisot recommends an ovulation predictor kit such as Ovu-Quick or Ovu-Kit. These at-home kits allow a woman to test her own urine for signs of ovulation.

Use the missionary position. For the purpose of conception, most people's anatomy works best in the missionary (man above/woman below) position, according to Dr. Wisot.

Women: Maintain the position for 30 minutes or so afterward. Dr. Wisot says the woman should not jump up or turn over immediately after intercourse, but should stay on her back long enough to allow the semen to get a good hold on the cervical mucus.

Avoid the use of lubricants and douches. These can interfere with conception, Dr. Wisot warns.

Get your weight back to normal. Dr. Wisot is particularly concerned about underweight women. "If a woman is severely underweight," he says, "if she has a very low total body fat content, her hormonal regulation could be thrown off. She might ovulate irregularly or not ovulate at all."

Overweight women may jeopardize their fertility, too. A study of 204 infertile women who had never been pregnant found increased problems with ovulation in those who were at least 20 percent over their ideal weight. A woman should reach her ideal weight range six to nine months before trying to get pregnant, says G. William Bates, M.D., former professor of obstetrics and gynecology at the University of South Carolina.

Men: Bypass the hot tub on your way to bed. The hot tub may have become the symbol of the romantic interlude for an entire generation, but men who want to become fathers should skip this step entirely. The testes are hung outside the body for a reason: High temperatures damage or destroy sperm cells. Sinking into a hot tub may relax you into a romantic mood, but the hot water could undo all of nature's efforts to keep your sperm alive and lively. Because one study demonstrated that a single 1-hour bath in a hot tub could impair fertility for six weeks, the hot tub ban is not just a one-nighter. Keep a cool head about bathing for at least six weeks before any planned conception.

Get new underwear. Some physicians even suggest that men who want to become fathers should trade in their briefs for boxer shorts. They suspect that the tighter undies hold the testes too close to the body—and the sperm-damaging body heat.

Quit smoking. This may not be the easiest thing you ever do, but if you're serious and well-motivated, it is sure worth a try if it helps you avoid years of fertility procedures. "There is a very real reduction in sperm count and motility in smokers," Dr. Wisot says.

Ditto drugs and alcohol. Dr. Wisot says that drug and alcohol abuse can also decrease fertility by damaging sperm.

Wake up and smell the decaf. A woman trying to become pregnant could double her chances of success by drinking decaf rather than caffeinated coffee (and other caffeinated beverages). Researchers at the National Insti-

FINDING THE RIGHT FERTILITY CLINIC

A good clinic does make a difference, says Dr. Arthur Wisot of the South Bay Hospital In Vitro Fertilization Center. The right choice can save you time, expense, and frustration. How can you select the right center? Statistics for almost 100 individual clinics were gathered by a congressional survey conducted by U.S. Rep. Ron Wyden (D-Oregon). The results of that survey are available in Dr. Wisot's book *New Options for Fertility: A Guide to IVF and Other Assisted Reproduction Methods* or from the U.S. Government Printing Office ("Consumer Protection Issues Involving IVF Clinics").

A clinic's statistics are not the only way to judge, however. Clinics with higher success rates may not handle tough cases or may handle only a few cases each year, as opposed to larger centers that do take tougher cases. Dr. Wisot gives this advice for finding the center that's right for you.

Ask a friend in the medical community. A doctor or nurse friend may be able to give you the best information about a center's reputation among professionals.

Contact a support group. "Resolve is a support group for people with infertility," Dr. Wisot says. "They know what's going on and can supply a lot of good information."

Ask your own physician. Dr. Wisot rates this as only the third best way to find the right fertility clinic. "Your doctor may send you to a clinic that's not necessarily the best for you, because he or she wants to support his or her hospital or because he or she has an investment in a particular clinic," he says. "This happens quite frequently, so you should go through the first two steps and get some background information."

Dr. Wisot recommends that you not choose your fertility clinic based on advertising, the yellow pages, or the county medical society. The physician's referral service at a prestigious hospital, he says, can be used to find out what clinics serve your area, but that's all.

tute of Environmental Health Sciences, Research Triangle Park, North Carolina, found that women who drank more than the equivalent of one cup of coffee per day were only half as likely to be successful in their attempt to conceive as women who drank less coffee. The more coffee the women drank, the lower their chance of becoming pregnant.

Make love twice in an hour. The sperm count usually decreases with the frequency of ejaculation. However, in men with low sperm count, the second ejaculation within an hour can sometimes actually contain more sperm than the first. In one small study, this was found to be true in 70 percent of men with low sperm count. Having intercourse twice in 1 hour resulted in pregnancy for 25 percent of the couples in the study.

Try taking Robitussin. It may sound like a high-tech old wives' tale, but in this case, the "old wives" happen to be male physicians. Jerome H. Check, M.D., discovered that Robitussin thins the cervical mucus, making it easier for the sperm to swim through to the egg. Marc Cohen, M.D., found that guaifenesin, the active ingredient in Robitussin and some other over-the-counter cold remedies, also makes semen thinner and less viscous. Leaner, looser sperm apparently have a better chance of making their way to the egg and fertilizing it, according to Dr. Cohen. Although he has not yet conducted any controlled studies, Dr. Cohen gives this advice to all his patients, along with the recommendation that men should take 500 milligrams of vitamin C per day to acidify their semen—another fertility-enhancing step.

GET ON THE RIGHT TRACK TO BETTER SEX

Is your sex life everything it could be? Are you basically happy in your relationship but vaguely dissatisfied in the bedroom? Do you sometimes feel that the grass elsewhere is greener, but that there must be a way to make your own grass the greenest in town? Does this mean there's something wrong with you or your relationship, something that will take years of therapy to untangle?

Not at all. There is a fast lane to better sex, and you can use it.

How many times has the following scenario happened to you? You and your partner go out to dinner at your favorite restaurant, then dance the night away at your favorite hot spot . . . and then, despite all your amorous intentions, lapse into a deep sleep the moment your bodies get near the bed. You may have had lovemaking on your minds all night—but by the time you got around to it you were both too tired to even take off your clothes.

Put lovemaking at the top of your list. If you save sex for the last thing you do before sleep, that's the same as putting it at the bottom of your list. If good sex is important, give it the priority it deserves. Would you plan any other important activity at a time when you're likely to be sleepy and physically exhausted? Of course not. "Plan lovemaking for times when you have a little more energy for creativity and imagination. Weekend mornings are a good time. Or afternoons. Or in the early evening," advises Saul H. Rosenthal, M.D., clinical associate professor of psychiatry at the University of Texas Medical School at San Antonio and author of *Sex over 40*.

Make a date for love. As long as intimacy is going to be near the top of your list, why not choose a time in advance? Don't worry about taking the spontaneity out of it. Exciting lovemaking doesn't happen by accident. Besides, what's more tantalizing than looking forward to making love?

Make love in the kitchen. Or in the living room in front of the fireplace, or in the shower, or under the dining room table . . . anywhere but the usual place, the bedroom. "I think people ought to sometimes explore ways of doing things differently," says Wallace Denton, Ed.D., head of child development and family studies at Purdue University. "It may mean driving across town and checking into the local motel."

Change your position on the subject. "Although most people end up with a few favorite positions, it's good to experiment a bit," says Dr. Shirley Zussman. "Some variety in position can make each experience a different kind."

Ask for what you like. Don't expect your partner to be a psychic. You might find yourself waiting years for what you want. Why wait, when you can have it now? "It's important to communicate your needs and wishes and desires," Dr. Zussman says. Easier said than done perhaps? Well, according to Jerome Sherman, Ph.D., president of the national board of directors of the American

Association of Sex Educators, Counselors, and Therapists, "there are two ways to show a partner what you like. One is telling. One is showing. One way of showing your partner what you like is by guiding your partner's hand." Whispering sweet nothings, Dr. Sherman says, "creates a higher level of physical arousal. It helps to share positive feelings during lovemaking. Say things like, 'I'm glad we're here together. That feels good. I feel so close to you now.'"

Read in bed—together. Not just any book. A book about sex. The idea is to quickly loosen up the communication logjam and allow yourselves to talk about sex. By sharing a book or article on the subject, even by reading it out loud at bedtime and discussing your opinions of what you're reading, you can get the ball rolling toward better communication about sex.

Banish the TV from the bedroom. It's your choice: Johnny Carson or good sex. Dr. Zussman says it's a hard habit to break, watching TV at bedtime, but you might be performing the simplest, fastest act to improve your sex life. After all, watching TV not only drains your energy but the 11 o'clock news is not exactly a turn-on.

Switch roles. If one of you is usually the initiator, turn the tables for an instant dose of stimulating change. "It gives each person a chance to have a different role— being the active or passive one," Dr. Zussman says.

Trade your vices for satisfaction. The particular vices we have in mind are smoking and alcohol. The fact that alcohol, a sedative and nervous system depressant, may relax you right out of being able to perform sexually is not news. But did you know that long-term alcohol abuse can also suppress both male and female hormones, putting a further damper on sexual performance?

Chances are, too, that if that post-lovemaking cigarette was one of several smoked during the day, the sex that came before was second-rate. Heavy tobacco use can choke off a happy sex life in two ways. Nicotine constricts the peripheral blood vessels and can make it more difficult to get an erection by decreasing blood flow to the penis. Over the long run, smoking increases the risk of arteriosclerosis, which decreases the blood supply in a much more major way. So, despite the fact that manufacturers use sex in advertising to improve cigarette sales, in reality, cigarettes are a definite drag on your sex life.

Take a walk. Research at Bentley College, in Waltham, Massachusetts, found that vigorous exercise can help older people maintain a high level of sexual interest and activity. The precise reason why exercise seems to help was not pinpointed—most likely because there are several contributing factors. Physically active people do tend to feel younger, have higher self-esteems, and just feel better about their bodies. Exercise also increases testosterone levels, a sure factor in sexual appetite.

Give your sex muscles a mini-workout. Those muscles are the pubococcygeus (PC) muscles, which stretch across the pelvic floor. They are the muscles you squeeze when you want to stop the flow of urine and the passing of bowel movements. And just a few silent, inconspicuous squeezes, called Kegel exercises, a day can help both men and women improve their sexual pleasure. Women have reported Kegel exercises give them stronger orgasms. Men have reported firmer erections, more control over premature ejaculation, and stronger orgasms. And all you have to do is squeeze the muscle, hold the contraction for 3 to 5 seconds, and then release. Your mini-workout can consist of 10 contractions a day at the outset. Then, at your own pace, work up to 50 or 100 silent squeezes a day.

Go ride a bike. Bicycling magazine surveyed its readers and learned that two-thirds of 1,675 respondents believed cycling had made them better lovers. Almost half of them felt cycling had increased their sex drive. And nearly one in seven confessed to having had sex while on the road—at what they called "rest" stops!

But be careful how you sit on the seat! Maybe those cyclists are masochists, after all? Two out of three of the survey respondents also said that cycling can cause numbness, soreness, and infection in the genital area. How you sit on the seat, and the type of seat itself, makes all the difference, apparently. Genital numbness can be caused by sitting on the seat in such a way as to put your weight on the front part of the pubic region. A wider saddle or a saddle pad is the quick remedy.

Seriously, men can even do permanent damage to their sexual apparatus while cycling. If the seat is too narrow, putting your weight on the perineum (the pubic area between the testes and the anus), the arteries that supply blood to the penis can be permanently damaged. Impotence can result, and surgery is the only treatment, once the damage is done. Again, a wider seat, one that supports the body by cradling the two buttock bones, is the best way to prevent this problem.

DEFEATING SEXUAL DYSFUNCTION

It can happen to any man or woman: The man can't get an erection, or the woman isn't interested if he does get one; the man ejaculates prematurely, or the woman has vaginal dryness. Each may be hiding feelings that bear directly on their sexual enjoyment—or lack of it.

But sexual dysfunction doesn't have to be permanent; with the wide range of help available these days, you can defeat dysfunction and begin to enjoy the physical and emotional satisfaction sex can provide.

SPEEDY RELIEF FOR IMPOTENCE

If you're impotent, the quickest way to put yourself on the road to recovery is to put the problem in perspective: You're not alone. Doctors estimate that as many as ten million American men are impotent. The problem appears to be associated with age, with about 1.9 percent of 40-year-olds experiencing it—all the way up to 25 percent of men 65 years old. But once impotence develops, it need not be a lifelong problem. And curing it need not take a lot of time.

For some men who have been unable to achieve or maintain an erection, the solution has been a surgically implanted prosthesis, a device that achieves an erection through mechanical means. But with new and faster methods of treating impotence, mechanical erections are rapidly becoming the treatment of last resort—reserved for only the most severe cases of physiological impotence.

With the availability of medical treatments for impotence increasing all the time, "penile prosthesis is rarely indicated these days," according to Jacques G. Susset, M.D., professor of urology at Brown University. There are several other effective treatments that are not only far less invasive but quicker as well.

First test the system. Normally, a man will have several erections over the course of a night's sleep—unless there is a physical impairment, advise Richard E. Berger, M.D., and Deborah Berger, in their book *Biopotency.* A laboratory can set you up with what is called a Nocturnal Penile Tumescence (NPT) test, which will measure the frequency, rigidity, and duration of your nighttime erections.

NPT tests—even the ones given in labs—are not foolproof. There have been cases of severely depressed men who had abnormal NPT responses but who were helped by psychological therapy. Nevertheless, the information is valuable. But the NPT can involve spending two or three nights sleeping at the laboratory, alone in bed, with tubelike electrodes on your penis.

Cheaper, at-home versions of the NPT test are available, but they still involve learning to operate a suitcase load of high-tech gear, carrying the suitcase home, and connecting yourself to it before you go to bed.

Quicker, easier, and cheaper are the Snap-Gauge and stamp tests. The Snap-Gauge NPT uses a strip of Velcro specially outfitted with little plastic bands, which stretch or break to indicate that a firm erection has taken place. The stamp test, commercially available under the name PotenTest, uses specially designed stamps that, placed around the penis at bedtime, will break along the perforations when you have an erection.

The most equipment-free NPT test is one in which you simply observe your nocturnal erections. It isn't necessary for you to stay awake all night, because these often occur early in the morning. The Bergers say that "finding out that you have just one normal erection is an important piece of information to share with your doctor."

Check out any drugs you may be taking. If the cause of your impotence is a mystery, you might be able to save yourself a lot of the time and expense of a medical investigation by doing some detective work of your own. The first place to check for clues is your medicine cabinet. Many commonly prescribed drugs can cause impotence. Among the classes of such drugs are: blood pressure

TALK IT OVER WITH YOUR PARTNER

The first reaction to sexual dysfunction is often a breakdown of communication between partners, say Dr. Richard E. Berger and Deborah Berger in their book *Biopotency.* That's unfortunate because, the Bergers say, "Understanding and honest communication between partners can be the key to sexual success. Isolation, neglect, and misunderstanding will often only exacerbate the problem. Relationships are sometimes wrecked more by the couple's reaction to the potency problem than by the problem itself."

The Bergers give some ice-breaking suggestions for talking about a potency problem. They advise picking a time when both partners are relaxed—and a place where there will be plenty of privacy. It's always good to begin, they say, by "telling your partner how much you value your relationship." From there, they suggest asking questions and really listening to the answers.

"Don't try to change the way she feels, just try to understand," they advise. To help bring out those feelings, they suggest asking whether the potency problem changes the way your partner feels about you. Ask if the problem has seemed to change her perception of your behavior. Ask what you can do to help the situation. Finally, try to reach an agreement on what course of action to take. Going forward as a couple will save you time, energy, expense, and, as the Bergers say, "Good talkers make great lovers."

---

medications and diuretics, anti-anxiety drugs, antidepressants, tranquilizers, antispasmodics for the bladder and bowel, drugs used to treat irregular heartbeat, drugs used to treat Parkinson's disease, antihistamines, muscle relaxants, anti-ulcer drugs, cholesterol-lowering drugs, female hormones, glucocorticoids, immunosuppressive drugs, anti-arthritis medications, and others.

If you suspect that one of your medications is the cause of your impotence, do not make any changes on your own. Check with your doctor first. Dosages can be adjusted or medications switched. Take heart: The negative effects of drugs on potency are almost always reversible.

Talk to your doctor about an external vacuum device

that produces erections. The device, called the ErecAid System, consists of an acrylic cylinder connected by a short length of flexible tubing to a small hand pump. First, the man slips the cylinder over his penis so that a seal is formed against his body. The pump creates a vacuum in the cylinder, which draws blood into the penis, creating an erection. Before removing the cylinder, the man eases a latex ring from the end of the tube onto the base of the penis to maintain the erection. The entire procedure takes only 2 to 3 minutes—and creates plenty of rigidity for intercourse.

The ErecAid System can help men with psychological and physical causes behind their impotence, including vein leakage, which prevents blood from staying in the penis long enough to maintain a satisfactory erection. As long as the arteries are capable of supplying blood to the penis, the device should work. "What could be a better way to get over a hangup about erections than to actually see one happen with the help of this device?" asks André T. Guay, M.D., head of the Lahey Clinic Medical Center's Endocrinology Section.

A physician can teach a man to use the device, although the ErecAid System comes with a user's manual and an instructional home video. The ErecAid System is available by prescription only from Osbon Medical Systems, Department C, P.O. Drawer 1478, Augusta, GA 30903.

Consider an injectable treatment. The quickest fix for erection problems and impotence (as well as premature ejaculation and performance anxiety) is a 3- to 4-second injection of a drug into the penis. The drug produces a near-instant erection—one that can last anywhere from 10 minutes to 2 hours, regardless of how many times ejaculation takes place.

The injection erection is "good for psychological impotence as well as physical impotence," says to Grant Gwinup, M.D., professor of endocrinology at the University of California at Irvine, who uses the procedure in his practice. The drug overrides the effects of anxiety or lack of confidence because it directly stimulates the vasodilator mechanism that controls blood flow into the penis and, thereby, causes erections.

The dosage of the drug determines the duration of the erection. Physicians usually tailor the dose to the individual.

Dr. Gwinup advises the man suffering from impotence to try to find a urologist who is not going to try to recommend a prosthesis right away. "Use of prostheses should be few and far between now, and only after lengthy trial with medical and injectable treatments," he says. He has no reports of serious side effects with the drug, and the injection produces an erection within 3 to 5 minutes. "It doesn't really hurt—only the slightest discomfort," he reassures.

The drugs used at clinics all over the country are prostaglandin E_1, phentolamine, and papaverine. "Men respond very well to giving themselves the injection," says Sheldon Burman, M.D., director of the Male Sexual Dysfunction Institute in Chicago. "Most men, when they see the results they have, love it."

Get short, intensive therapy for premature ejaculation. Premature ejaculation is now considered a form of impotence, since "impotence is defined as the inability to obtain or maintain an erection at least 25 percent of the time," Dr. Burman says. The good news is that premature ejaculation does not necessarily condemn one to a lifetime of quickies. At Dr. Burman's clinic, the success rate is nearly 100 percent. And the best part is that the therapy seldom takes longer than six weeks.

"Premature ejaculation is usually a psychological problem," Dr. Burman says. "Men suffer from premature ejaculation because of their early, formative experiences with sex—experiences that all share the element of haste.

"What we do in these six sessions is help the patient to replace that old scenario with a different set of elements in a new timetable, " he says. "And that's not very difficult to do. We teach a patient to tune in to his own feelings. Every man has what is called the point of inevitability, the point where nothing in the world is going to keep him from having an ejaculation. Well, before you reach that point, if you know how to listen and how to feel, the body gives you plenty of warning signals that you're going too fast toward that point of inevitability. We teach you how to recognize those signals, then how to lower the excitement rate, at the same time keeping your partner stimulated. With practice you can do this readily and control your ejaculation at will.

"This therapy has nothing to do with conventional, orthodox Freudian analysis or therapy, which can take years and not solve the problem," Dr. Burman says. "It's a completely different process: a results-oriented, behavior-oriented, change-oriented therapy that focuses on the sensations you are presently experiencing. It's quick, intensive, and highly effective. The cure rate is close to 100 percent at our clinic."

This type of therapy, which is done at sex therapy centers all over the country, can also be done over the phone.

Dr. Burman also uses the erection injection method to help premature ejaculators get through the intensive therapy course. "In order to help the patient and his partner have good sex from the moment he walks into the institute," Dr. Burman says, "we teach him how to inject the drug into his own penis. Then it doesn't make any difference whether he ejaculates or not. The treatment alleviates anxiety and is wonderful for performance anxiety.

"Eventually you don't need the drug nearly so often. You start off using it maybe two or three times a week for a couple of weeks and then use it maybe once every four months after that."

QUICK RELIEF FOR WOMEN'S SEXUAL PROBLEMS

Women are not immune to sexual dysfunction. A British study found that 17 percent of women between the ages of 35 and 59 suffered from impaired sexual interest, 17 percent from vaginal dryness, 16 percent from infrequency of orgasm, and 8 percent from painful intercourse. But their problems don't have to take years to fix, anymore than men's.

Dab on a lubricant for vaginal dryness. "In the natural process of aging, those tissues do get dry," advises Dr. Shirley Zussman. And that dryness can make intercourse difficult and painful. But, Dr. Zussman says, the problem can be quickly and easily remedied. A sexual lubricant can quickly and temporarily banish dryness. Or you may want your doctor to examine you first and then

AN ANTIDEPRESSANT THAT GIVES A SEXUAL BOOST

For men and women whose sexual dysfunction is linked with depression, the antidepressant drug Wellbutrin (chemical name: bupropion hydrochloride) may provide a quick route to sexual healing.

Dr. James Goldberg of the Crenshaw Clinic, a sex therapy and research center, says that the drug was originally developed not as an aphrodisiac but as an antidepressant. According to Dr. Goldberg, most antidepressants can have a depressing effect on sexual potency. When Wellbutrin was tested, researchers were surprised to find that the drug actually had *positive* sexual effects—in both men and women.

In one study performed by Dr. Goldberg and Theresa Crenshaw, M.D., Wellbutrin was given to patients who complained of sexual aversion, inhibited desire, inhibited sexual excitement, and inhibited orgasm. Sixty-three percent of the people receiving Wellbutrin reported their sexual functioning much or very much improved. In fact, both the men and women claimed that their sex drive, arousal, and/or orgasms seemed to return to the intensity and frequency more characteristic of their youth.

Does Wellbutrin have a physical or a psychological effect? Dr. Goldberg says that in many cases of sexual dysfunction it is really impossible to separate psychological and physical factors. One bout of impotence, even if caused by a physical ailment, begins to erode confidence and undermines all the psychological supports of sexual functioning.

Wellbutrin helps because, as Dr. Goldberg says, "it is an antidepressant that tunes the system." The drug stimulates the dopamine system in the brain, which controls such functions as attention, movement, alertness, sexual pleasure, and learning.

"In women," Dr. Goldberg says, "their desire increases and they become more assertive. They go beyond becoming more receptive and responsive and begin to take the initiative. One woman who never had orgasms during intercourse was finally able to have them—and she kept on having them, even after the drug was withdrawn."

prescribe a specially formulated vaginal cream containing estrogen. "The cream not only relieves the dryness but restores the health of the tissues," says Dr. Zussman.

Investigate estrogen therapy. Older women suffering from lack of sex drive might ask their doctors about estrogen replacement therapy (ERT). ERT can be helpful in restoring sex drive in women whose decline in libido is brought on by the menopausal or postmenopausal body's decreasing production of hormones. ERT can take the form of vaginal cream, transdermal patch, or oral medications. The transdermal method of administering estrogen therapy is often recommended to women who cannot take the drug orally, because of problems with blood pressure, clotting, or gallbladder or liver disease.

Women whose lowered sex drive does not respond to estrogen therapy might ask their doctors to consider using the drug methyltestosterone, a hormone that often successfully stimulates the libido.

FOR FAST RESULTS, SEEK COUNSELING

It's an interesting fact that a couple's sex life often improves after the first visit to a therapist or counselor, according to James Goldberg, Ph.D., of the Crenshaw Clinic, a sex therapy and research center in San Diego. Dr. Goldberg believes that what happens is the couple is "given permission" to pay attention to their lovemaking in a way that they were unable to do before visiting the therapist.

"Therapy helps you get used to receiving stimulation and even looking for it—and not being discouraged if you don't find it right away," Dr. Goldberg says. "One of the secrets of sex therapy is just to increase the eroticism, increase the attention to sexual stimuli. So even if you have less reaction, you have more to react to. That's why so often in therapy with older people you can get incredible effects, because essentially the people who have not really paid attention to sexual stimuli perhaps all their lives suddenly are paying attention and being stimulated in new ways. Now, this is not a recommendation that you make only that first visit to a therapist and no more. Your problems may require several sessions for lasting improvement. But it's good news that you can expect to find some benefit right away, with the first session."

You can obtain a national directory of certified sex

counselors and therapists from the American Association of Sex Educators, Counselors, and Therapists, 435 North Michigan Avenue, Suite 1717, Chicago, IL 60611.

RAPID RELIEF FOR GENITAL HERPES

Herpes simplex virus (HSV) infects anywhere from 40 percent to 100 percent of the American population. The type that infects the genitals is usually HSV type 2. It's highly contagious and is transmitted by person-to-person contact, *not* necessarily sexual contact: A hand can spread it from the lip to the eye. First signs of infection are usually a genital rash and itching. Lesions soon appear, enlarge, erupt, and ulcerate—they can be very painful. Men get the lesions on the penis, and sometimes the scrotum and inner thighs; women get them on the vulva, vagina, and cervix. The lesions last for one to three weeks. Usually the outbreaks become milder as time goes on, but some people get weekly or monthly outbreaks. Just because there is no lesion doesn't mean the disease can't be spread. There is no cure, but there are effective treatments.

Ask for acyclovir. Acyclovir is still the best medical treatment for herpes, says Carolyn Mabry, coordinator of the Herpes Resource Center hotline in Research Triangle Park, North Carolina. She says that no other treatment seems to speed healing as well as acyclovir. The antiviral drug is available in three different forms: as a topical ointment, a pill, and an intravenous medication that is used mainly for people with very serious cases.

"It's the standard treatment," says Judith M. Hurst, R.N., coordinator and medical adviser to Toledo HELP, a support group for people with herpes, and an obstetric nurse at The Toledo Hospital.

"The only problem with acyclovir," Hurst says, "is that unless it's used early, in the prodromal stage, while the virus is coming to the surface of the skin, it's not as effective. So the sooner it's used the better."

Keep your strength up. "The most important thing is not to impair the immune system," Mabry says. "The body can fight off most infections, but if you're doing things to impair it, like smoking, not getting enough sleep, not getting any exercise—then your body's not

PREVENTING SEXUALLY TRANSMITTED DISEASE

Prevention is the still the best policy when it comes to sexually transmitted diseases (STDs), particularly if you're putting off childbearing until later. STDs such as chlamydia and gonorrhea can cause scarring and closure of the fallopian tubes, thus preventing fertilization.

Short of abstinence or maintaining a faithful relationship with an uninfected partner, condoms are still the most effective means of prevention. Keep in mind, however, that condoms do not afford absolute protection, though they do sharply reduce risk if used properly. One quick way of increasing the protection condoms give is by using a spermicide along with the condom. Spermicides have been shown in laboratory tests to inactivate sexually transmitted agents, including the AIDS virus. Vaginal use of spermicide lowers the risk of gonorrhea, chlamydia, and other STDs.

going to work as well as it could. One of the things we really try to encourage people to do, if for no other reason than to keep their immune system working at its best, is to find some kind of stress management that's helpful for them."

Shore up your emotional supports. Learning that you have herpes is likely to ignite a firestorm of emotions—anger, guilt, sadness. You might consider short-term psychological therapy to help you get over the initial storm. Or you may find a local support group the fastest way to get your mind back on a positive track.

"People share experiences," Hurst says, "they share their thoughts and feelings. It's so important to have someone who knows what they're talking about, since they can't just walk over to their friends' house and talk about their sexual problems. At the support group, you can let yourself go, let your defenses down—and you're not going to have your secrets thrown back in your face.

"And this does help," Hurst says. "In fact, I think this is the only real cure, the only real therapy. The medications are fine, but it really takes the mind to make them work. It takes a positive attitude. It takes the knowledge that you are not the scum of the earth, that you've simply acquired a virus.

"This absolutely shortens the period of suffering for people—and lengthens the intervals between breakouts. When people are in a good emotional relationship, their outbreaks are few and far between. When they're in emotional stress or they lack self-esteem or self-confidence, their episodes are much more frequent. Everyone who is diagnosed with herpes suddenly feels as if they are alone. But the fact is that there are people who will talk about it and help them feel that they are not alone—and that's so vital."

A QUICK TEST FOR CHLAMYDIA

Chlamydia is a bacterial infection transmitted during intercourse. It's called the silent STD because, although it is the most common sexually transmitted disease, it often goes undiagnosed. In half of infected women and one-quarter of infected men, no symptoms occur. When symptoms develop, they usually include genital discharge and pain during urination. If the disease is left untreated, it can result in pelvic inflammatory disease, ectopic pregnancy, and infertility.

One of the reasons chlamydia has gone undiagnosed is that the old test for it was costly and time-consuming. Chlamydia bacteria don't grow well in laboratories and the test often failed.

Today new tests are available that can diagnose chlamydia in the doctor's office within half an hour. One such test, called TestPack Chlamydia, requires the physician to swab a sample from the cervix. The sample is then mixed with certain identifying chemicals that give an answer within minutes. The only drawback is that the physician must be careful to get a sample that contains enough cells for an accurate test.

SKIN AND NAILS

t's time for a little quiz. Which of your organs is bigger than your brain, but not as smart? Grows goose bumps but not feathers? Is more waterproof than a raincoat but not as warm as a fur coat?

Time's up! The correct answer is . . .your skin. Your largest organ, the flexible, expandable, foldable, fragile yet tough, living armor that no high-tech fabric can match. It holds your body together, protects it from the elements and microbes of the world, is nice to touch, and goes well with or without clothes or a tan.

And it can be a problem. It pops up with pimples and boils. It wrinkles with the years. It can get scaly with psoriasis, bumpy with warts, itchy with eczema. And sometimes it even (forgive us, Miss Manners) stinks.

You're the rescue squad for your skin. What do you do when it cries for help?

- A few minutes of icing a potential pimple may nip it in the bud.
- Five minutes of electric heat can cauterize a wart.
- An aspirin paste may relieve shingles pain in 15 to 20 minutes.

To learn more about these safe, fast-working solutions to your skin problem, read on.

NORMALIZE YOUR COMPLEXION IN NOTHING FLAT

You could devote half your life to trying to get the moisture balance in your skin just where it should be—not too dry, not too oily. There are plenty of spas and lots of products out there to play with.

LASER AWAY
PORT-WINE-STAIN BIRTHMARKS

The new "tunable dye" laser is the preferred device to use when removing a type of birthmark known as a port-wine stain. The birthmark, which usually appears as a reddish or purple blotch on the face or neck, is caused by an overabundance of blood vessels near the surface of the skin. The light of the laser can be "tuned" to the precise wavelength that's best for a particular birthmark. As the vessels absorb the light, they heat up and, in a sense, self-destruct. The process leaves little or no scarring.

Before lasers, there were no good surgical options for removing these birthmarks. The argon laser was the first device used, but it left a more noticeable scar. The tunable dye laser procedure may take several office visits before the treatment is complete. Almost all port-wine stains can be altered dramatically, and some can be totally cleared. It's an outpatient procedure each time—no hospital stay is required. For adult patients, it's relatively painless as well. The after-procedure sensation has been compared to a sunburn.

Or you could invest a few minutes wisely and achieve identical results.

Try some "soft soap." When washing very dry and sensitive skin, skip the soap and use a nonirritating cleanser, such as Cetaphil Lotion or Keri Facial Cleanser instead. First splash your skin with lukewarm water, lather for just 1 minute, then rinse thoroughly, says Fredric Haberman, M.D., author of *Your Skin: A Doctor's Guide to a Lifetime of Beauty* and *The Doctor's Beauty Hotline.* Blot gently and follow with moisturizer.

Moisturize when your skin's still wet. It's a little matter of timing, but after your shower, blot yourself gently dry. Then apply moisturizer all over your body, paying special attention to dry, rough areas. It makes a big difference when it comes to getting the most out of this treatment.

Take a quick tepid shower. The longer you stay in the water, and the hotter the water, the more you soak away the skin's natural moisturizing factors.

Dab on a gel-based moisturizer for oily skin. Even

oily skin feels dry from time to time. The smartest way to add moisture to yours without making it feel greasy is to use one of the new gel-based moisturizers, like Nutraderm, Almay Oil-Free, or Prescriptives Oil-Free Skin Renewer, Dr. Haberman says.

Install a humidifier. The winter air in your home is as dry as the Sahara, and in summer, air conditioning pulls moisture from your immediate atmosphere. A humidifier can help keep your skin from drying out.

PIMPLES: READY, SET, CLEAR!

A pimple begins in the hair follicle beneath the surface of the skin. It takes a full 90 days for a hair follicle to become "plugged"—by oil, dead skin, dirt—and develop into a full-scale eruption. If the plug causes the follicle wall to burst, the white blood cells attracted to the break in the follicle lining may begin digesting the collagen around the pore. That's how scars form. To prevent scars, you need to respond immediately to even the mildest cases of acne.

"If you let it go too far, you could have physical and mental scarring for life," warns James E. Fulton, M.D., Ph.D., director of the Acne Research Institute in Newport Beach, California, author of *Dr. Fulton's Step-by-Step Program for Clearing Acne.*

Dermatologists used to prescribe tetracycline pills for their acne patients and kept their fingers crossed. Sometimes they prescribed ultraviolet light treatments, too.

The problem with this antibiotic—besides the side effects—is that it didn't work too well. "It wasn't much more effective than a placebo," Dr. Fulton says.

There have been significant advances since then. Here are faster, more effective ways to control acne and pimples.

Lather on a benzoyl peroxide cleanser. A blackhead doesn't have to last forever. If you've got a crop of them, or whiteheads, you may be surprised at how long it takes your body to get rid of them. This is where benzoyl peroxide can help. Washing with an over-the-counter benzoyl peroxide cleanser morning and evening will help your skin bring the plugs to the surface faster and will also kill the bacteria that cause acne. Benzoyl peroxide cleansers are just the ticket for mild acne, Dr. Fulton says.

Reach for Retin-A. With the discovery of tretinoin, a vitamin A acid derivative (brand name: Retin-A), some acne sufferers are able to see results in as little as six to ten weeks. This topical prescription gel or cream works by causing peeling at the skin's surface and within the follicle itself. This brings plugs to the surface faster, helps prevent new ones from forming, and also helps prevent scarring. Retin-A also makes your skin supersensitive to the sun's rays, so limit your exposure.

Give pimples a 1-2-3 punch. The proper combination of erythromycin, benzoyl peroxide, and Retin-A applied to blackheads, whiteheads, and pimples may bring results much more quickly than any of these medications used alone.

Like Retin-A, benzoyl peroxide promotes peeling. Additionally, it sinks right into the pores and kills acne-causing bacteria. The topical antibiotic erythromycin also kills acne bacteria.

By combining these prescription medications, you may see results in two weeks and complete clearing within two months, Dr. Fulton says. His patients use erythromycin lotion in the morning and then apply benzoyl peroxide gel in the evening, washing it off after an hour or two. At bedtime, they apply a conditioning lotion that contains a 0.25 percent solution of vitamin A acid to help peel out impactions.

Ask your dermatologist if this regimen is right for you.

Use ice to defuse flare-ups. You have an important meeting tomorrow, and that familiar funny feeling on your chin that tells you a pimple is on its way. Fight back fast by applying ice to the danger zone for 3 to 5 minutes. Then be sure to get a good night's sleep, Dr. Fulton says. The ice will halt the inflammation, and this may help the lining of the follicle wall to heal itself.

Keep your fingers off it. The worst thing you can do now is fiddle with the potential pimple. If you accidentally push the acne plug deeper into the skin, you may cause the follicle wall to rupture and guarantee yourself a nasty-looking pimple. If the rupture occurs close to the skin's surface, it will take your body at least a week to clear the resulting pustule. If the rupture occurs deeper in the skin, you could develop a nodule, a deep, undefined red bump that takes several weeks to clear.

Try a new antibiotic gel for adult acne. It's a prescription drug (brand name: MetroGel) containing metronidazole, a powerful antibiotic that's difficult to tolerate in oral doses. When rubbed directly on the skin, it's virtually free of side effects. In clinical tests, metronidazole gel reduced adult acne—rosacea—inflammation rapidly during the first three weeks of therapy, achieving maximum results by the ninth week.

Metronidazole gel won't give everyone with rosacea a completely clear face in three weeks. Right now, nothing is 100 percent effective for everybody. But it does provide a significant reduction in the disease faster and better than anything else. Ask your dermatologist about it.

Try prednisone for post-30, menstrual-cycle flare-ups. If you're one of an increasing number of women who are having their first acne flare-ups in their thirties, forties, and fifties, you may find better results with prednisone, a drug that alters your body's hormone balance. Prednisone therapy typically lasts a couple of months, Dr. Fulton says. You may have to wait several weeks before you start seeing results.

Typically, acne develops at age 12 and resolves by age 23, Dr. Fulton says. Acne in adult women may be related to the use or discontinuation of oral contraceptives, or to the effect of stress on the normal hormonal fluctuations that occur each menstrual cycle.

Zap zits with zinc. Zinc is a mild anti-inflammatory, Dr. Fulton says. For people who suffer from acne cysts, pustules, and nodules, it can decrease the white blood cells that fatten acne lesions.

Dr. Fulton recommends limiting your zinc intake to 100 milligrams a day because the body can't absorb any more than that. Check with your doctor, of course, before you add any vitamin or mineral supplement to your diet.

Shrink a cyst with steroids. For nodules and cysts, your doctor can inject an anti-inflammatory corticosteroid, which shrinks them dramatically in 48 hours.

The problem with these injections is that they don't remove the initial impaction, or plug. So the area may flare up again, Dr. Fulton says.

BANISH THAT BOIL

An immune system in good working order takes about two weeks to dispatch the typical boil. But some boils linger longer. The toughest ones to get rid of are the boils that pop up on your bottom or other areas of your body where clothing can rub against them and aggravate them.

Boils are the result of a bacterial infection that begins in a hair follicle. White blood cells rush to the area to fight the infection. Pus accumulates, formed from the mounting numbers of dead blood cells, skin cells, and bacteria. Once the boil bursts and the pus drains, the skin can begin to heal.

Here's how you can make that happen faster.

Give it a shot. Injecting a boil with a steroid solution helps it to heal fast, according to Stephen Schleicher, M.D., codirector of The Dermatology Center, based in Philadelphia. The treatment can be performed in the doctor's office.

Apply moist heat. If you're really intent on getting rid of that boil fast, apply a hot, wet compress to the area for 20 to 30 minutes four times a day. The moist heat helps draw blood to the site, which can make the boil come to a head faster, Dr. Schleicher says.

Ask your doctor about taking antibiotics. Prescription antibiotics can tackle that boil in three to four days, Dr. Schleicher says. In fact, oral antibiotics are your *best* course of action for a boil that has lingered or for battling a persistent crop of boils.

Give it the needle. You can safely lance a small boil if you carefully follow these instructions from dermatologist Rodney Basler, M.D., assistant professor of medicine at the University of Nebraska Medical Center.

Wait until the boil has come to a head—you'll be able to see the white pus beneath a thin layer of skin. Hold a needle in a flame to sterilize it, let it cool, and then give the head a small prick. Gently squeeze the boil to help the contents out. Dr. Basler says it's rare that squeezing pushes the infection deeper, and it's likely that a doctor would also squeeze it.

Apply an antibiotic ointment. After the boil is opened — whether naturally or with your help — you may want to smear on over-the-counter antibiotic ointments Neosporin or Bacitracin Sterile.

Keep it draining. Continue to apply the warm compresses after the boil is opened, Dr. Basler says. This helps the boil heal faster.

Bandage it if you want. After the boil is open and draining, a bandage can help to keep it clean and keep the exudate off your clothes.

RUB OUT CHAFING

You've set out to do something wonderful for your body — exercise — and your skin's chafing to pay you back. An angry red welt rises between your thighs after you walk. Raw, red areas cover your fanny where you've been sitting on your bicycle. Is there any hope of continuing your exercise program and getting rid of this chafing?

Lubricate your body. If walking or running is rubbing you raw between the legs, under the arms, or where your shirt or pants rub against your skin, the easiest solution is a 60-second rubdown with a lubricant gel or cream, such as petroleum jelly. Many come in tiny tubes that you can carry in your hand or stash in your pocket.

Aerosol the problem. Or give yourself a 10-second spray with an aerosol wound covering over your tender area.

Take a powder. Talcum powder will act to reduce friction just the way petroleum jelly does, by helping the skin to slip around without catching and rubbing.

Vent yourself. Take a little sweat, add a little skin-to-skin contact, and you'll get a problem with chafing, Dr. Fredric Haberman says. Wear lightweight, vented clothing to cool your body as you move.

Make your protection stick. It takes only a couple of seconds to stick an adhesive bandage over rubbed nipples, if that's where your chafing is worst. Or, you can try small patches of moleskin to protect your nipples from friction with your clothing.

Cotton up to underwear. Be sure to wear cotton underwear under your nylon clothing, separating the abrasive fabric from your delicate skin.

Do away with the woolies. Wool is an unkind cloth that may be a source of your problem. Wear all-cotton clothing instead, says Hillard Pearlstein, M.D., an assistant clinical professor of dermatology at Mount Sinai School of Medicine in New York City.

Elasticize your thighs. If your thighs are chafed, try wrapping each with an elastic bandage. Instead of skin against skin, the friction will be bandage against bandage.

Pad your seat. If your chafing is more like a saddle sore—from riding a bicycle or a horse—you can prevent that problem by padding your fanny before you sit down. Avoid wearing jeans, for instance, because the heavy seams will rub and irritate. Instead, try a pair of jodhpurs —lightweight pants with tiny seams—or bicycling pants lined with chamois. Get a well-padded bike seat, too.

ECZEMA: BREAK THE CYCLE OF ITCHING

Call it eczema or dermatitis, but it still comes down to the same thing: itchy, red, swollen, or crusting skin. This affliction comes in four basic varieties, and while each is controllable, none is presently curable.

In adults, *atopic dermatitis* produces intense itching and thickened, discolored skin. You'll recognize *nummular dermatitis* by its red patches of weepy or crusting skin. Flaking skin (including dandruff) is a red flag for *seborrheic dermatitis. Contact dermatitis* is what you get when your skin meets up with an allergen, like poison ivy.

Hydrocortisone creams and oral antihistamines are often employed in the battle against eczema. Other typical treatments include coal tar creams and ultraviolet light radiation therapy.

Here's how to get relief in the meantime.

Use antiscratching therapy to speed the healing of eczema. Eczema is a problem not only because it causes dry, flaking skin but also because it itches. That promotes scratching, which makes the condition worse. Eczema patients in a Swedish study were instructed in how to resist the scratching urge and saw significantly greater improvements from hydrocortisone cream application than patients who were given the cream only.

Antiscratching therapy was given in two sessions. The first taught patients to press firmly on the affected area for 1 minute whenever they felt the urge to scratch, and then to move their hands to their thighs or to another object. The second session instructed the patients to avoid the affected area entirely; they were told to move their hands to their thighs or to grasp an object directly. Results: After four weeks, patients given the antiscratch therapy plus cream had nearly twice the improvement of the patients given the cream only.

Pull on a pair of glove liners. The few seconds it takes to don clean, white, cotton glove liners underneath your heavy-duty rubber gloves can spare your hands days of irritation. If you have dishes or gardening to do, or if your hobby requires that you work with acids and solvents, make sure your hands are protected. Nelson Lee Novick, M.D., associate clinical professor of dermatology at Mount Sinai School of Medicine and author of *Super Skin: A Leading Dermatologist's Guide to the Latest Breakthroughs in Skin Care,* suggests you buy a few pairs of glove liners so you can launder them often. Perspiration and grease buildup can trigger irritation, he says.

Switch to a soap substitute. Even the few minutes you spend washing your face and hands can be used profitably if you switch to a soap substitute like Cetaphil or Neutrogena—they won't aggravate your eczema by drying out your skin. Purpose soap is another good choice, says Nicholas Lowe, M.D., director of the Southern California Dermatology and Psoriasis Treatment Center and clinical professor of dermatology at the University of Southern California at Los Angeles.

Take a quick dip into a moisturizing bath. A nightly soak in a tub filled with lukewarm water and colloidal oatmeal can help make you more comfortable.

Spread on the cream. As soon as you get out of the tub, apply your prescription cream or a fragrance-free emollient. Vaseline petroleum jelly works fine, too, Dr. Lowe says.

● SCRATCH THAT SCRATCH

What would you rather do—scratch or talk? During a study conducted by Swedish scientists, 16 people with eczema were split into two groups. Half were given a corticosteroid cream to prevent itching and the other half received the same cream and two antiscratching training sessions. The results: After 28 days, scratching dropped markedly for both, but the trainees scratched about half as much.

You can try the training with a friend or neighbor. First describe and demonstrate to them how you scratch. This step helps you recognize the early signs of scratching. Describe the situations that seem to set off your scratching. Discuss the unpleasant aspects of scratching—it's bad for your skin, it's embarrassing, whatever.

Concentrate on putting your hands on the itchy area for a full minute without scratching. At the end of the minute, move your hands to your thighs or grab something.

Imagine the situation that makes you want to scratch the most. Pretend you're in that situation and hold the itchy area for a full minute without scratching. Then grasp your thighs again.

Sit down with your helper for a final discussion and test. Have your helper remind you to use your mental exercises when you have the urge to scratch.

AGING SKIN: PROMISING NEW WAYS TO TURN BACK THE CLOCK

Maybe someday the truth will catch up with all those cosmetic company advertisements and there really will be a miracle lotion you can rub on your wrinkles tonight, assured that tomorrow you'll awaken with the dewy skin of youth.

For now, you'd better give yourself several months if

you're bent on dramatic improvement before that class reunion. Techniques exist that diminish fine lines, fade out age spots, and renew that youthful glow. They do require some persistence, however. Your reward? Results that just weren't possible before.

Here's how.

Iron out wrinkles with Retin-A. If you're serious about minimizing your wrinkles, forget the cosmetics counter. Ask your dermatologist about a prescription for Retin-A, a gel or cream derived from vitamin A acid. Within three to six months of daily use, this product can visibly eradicate many of the fine superficial wrinkles around the eyes, mouth, and upper cheekbones, Dr. Haberman says.

"Retin-A seems to turn back the clock," Dr. Haberman says. "Along with restoring some support and resiliency to aging or sun-damaged skin, it actually promotes a faster turnover of cells and increased production of tiny blood vessels that supply oxygen and nourishment to the skin. This gives the skin a healthy, rosy, younger look.

Studies also indicate that it can help prevent new wrinkles from forming.

Most doctors recommend cutting back to weekly or twice-weekly applications once you've been using Retin-A for a year. "Once you stop, the antiaging benefits stop as well," Dr. Haberman says.

In a double-blind study at the University of Michigan, 30 people used Retin-A daily on one forearm with sun damage and a placebo cream on the other. The arms treated with Retin-A showed significant improvement compared with the placebo-treated arms. The only side effect the Retin-A users experienced was skin irritation.

You can help prevent the irritating effects of Retin-A if you eliminate from your skin care program all harsh soaps, exfoliation lotions, and any products that contain alcohol. Instead, use mild soap substitutes, like Purpose or SFC Lotion. Rinse your soap substitute off with warm water, then wait half an hour before you apply the Retin-A, Dr. Haberman advises. Also, be sure to use a sunscreen with an SPF of 15 or higher, all day, every day, Dr. Haberman cautions.

Alternate Retin-A and Lac-Hydrin Lotion to improve

skin coloration. Lac-Hydrin Lotion is a new moisturizing drug, available by prescription only, that contains 12 percent lactic acid. Its effects on the skin continue from 3 to 14 days after its last application, according to Dr. Novick.

"The combination seems to even out mottled, discolored skin, diminish fine wrinkles, and eliminate age spots and sun spots. It can help smooth out the skin postoperatively, too," Dr. Novick says.

Even though it's a moisturizer, Lac-Hydrin Lotion is available by prescription only. Ask your dermatologist about it.

Consider a chemical peel to help nature along. "Exfoliation clears away the debris of dead flakes and allows better-looking skin to show through," Dr. Haberman says. It also encourages skin to renew itself. This new skin is more supple, has more of a light-reflecting glow, and appears to have fewer tiny lines.

Trichloroacetic acid is often used by dermatologists to "peel" a specific area of skin or the entire face, speeding up and evening out exfoliation. If you opt for a full face peel, the chemical treatment takes only a minute, but your skin will probably need about two weeks to recover. During that time, scabs will form, then fall off. Your skin will hurt and appear red for six weeks to six months before it returns to its normal color. During this time, it's important to stay out of the sun.

Take Retin-A beforehand to help a chemical peel heal fast. "I've found that using Retin-A as few as three weeks prior to a chemical peel seems to improve the rate of healing afterward," Dr. Novick says. "It makes the skin healthier and younger looking than the chemical peel alone."

NAIL CARE IN (NEARLY) NO TIME AT ALL

You've probably never stopped to think about the effect of aging on your nails, but the truth is that your nails do change with age. After age 25, their rate of growth begins to taper off steadily. After 35, you might find that brittleness and splitting are more troublesome than they've ever been.

With a minimal amount of care, you can keep your

nails healthy and attractive through the years. Here's what our experts suggest for the most common nail problems.

Give your nails a lube job. Your brittle nails will benefit most from a nightly soak in plain warm water. Fifteen to 20 minutes of soaking is best, says Richard K. Scher, M.D., head of the nail disease section at Columbia Presbyterian Medical Center in New York City. If you have a favorite before-bed television program, you can soak your nails and watch at the same time. Once 20 minutes have elapsed, dry your nails and apply a moisturizer.

Clip your nails. A good set of nail clippers can help you trim back your nails in nothing flat. If yours are brittle, this is a good investment of time. Shorter nails are much less prone to injury than longer nails, Dr. Scher says.

Soak 'em before you clip 'em. Before you cut them, soak your nails for 15 minutes in a solution made from 1 part bath oil and 4 parts water. Then apply a moisturizer like Complex 15, an over-the-counter product that contains phospholipids, the component that makes nails flexible.

Opt for a nail-polish touchup. Covering over the chipped color will take you less time than removing your nail polish and applying new polish. You'll be doing your nails a favor, too, Dr. Scher says, since nail polish remover can really dehydrate nails. Dr. Scher's advice is to limit its use as much as you can.

Carefully snip hangnails with a clean pair of scissors. If you don't, your hangnail is likely to hang around for another week or two, the time it takes your body to get rid of it. Hangnails are easy to avoid: Just keep your hands and nails well-moisturized, Dr. Scher says. (Hangnails, of course, don't refer to your nails but to the skin around the nails.)

PSORIASIS: GET LONGER-LASTING RELIEF

If you have psoriasis, certain production centers in your skin are stuck in overdrive. A normal skin cell takes 28 to 30 days to mature. In psoriasis, cells move to the surface in a mere 3 days. Instead of being shed, they clump together to create that silvery, scaling look. The redness you see is from blood vessels just beneath the surface that are feeding all that growth.

Psoriasis can range in seriousness from mild to severely disabling. It tends to be chronic. You may find that yours follows a cycle of remissions and flare-ups.

While there is no cure at present, there are ways to help clear psoriasis plaques and prevent new flare-ups. Current therapies include topical treatments like coal tars, anthralin, and hydrocortisone creams; drugs like Tegison that are taken orally; and a combination therapy called PUVA that teams ultraviolet light with psoralen, a drug that increases your sensitivity to light. These treatments have side effects, so all cases of psoriasis require a doctor's care.

What else can you do? This is what our experts advise.

Layer on that moisturizer. Psoriasis sufferers tend to overlook the importance of proper moisturizing, says John H. Hanifin, M.D., professor of dermatology at Oregon Health Sciences University. You have to apply the moisturizer within 3 minutes after you finish bathing, while your skin is still damp. Which moisturizers are best? Those that come in cream or ointment form, Dr. Hanifin says. A lotion is not potent enough for your needs.

Slip into a sauna suit. If your psoriasis covers large areas of your body, you may want to ask your doctor about the benefits of a specially made nylon "sauna suit" that can help keep your skin moist. Some people sleep in them, but you'll need specific instructions from your doctor about how you can best use it, Dr. Hanifin says. If your doctor approves, a suit can be ordered through Sleep Sauna, 211 Nevin Lane, Lower Gwynedd, PA 19002.

Learn to relax. A number of independent studies suggest that emotional stress can precipitate episodes of psoriasis. If you observe yourself closely, you're likely to find a relationship between psoriasis flare-ups and major episodes of stress in your life, says Eugene Farber, M.D., president of the Psoriasis Research Institute in Palo Alto, California. "From what I've seen in my practice, if you use the best ointments and medicine alone, you don't get nearly as good a result as when you emphasize stress reduction along with it." A good way to reduce stress is to practice the progressive relaxation technique outlined on page 376.

Ask your doctor about fish oil. Several studies suggest that fish-oil supplements may prove useful for psoriasis sufferers.

In a British study, 28 people who were given ten capsules daily of fish oil showed significant improvement in itching and scaling after eight weeks. There was no such change in the placebo group.

In a Danish study, 58 percent of the people put on a low-fat diet and given daily fish-oil supplements showed "moderate to excellent" improvement after four months.

Of course, these results are very preliminary. If you are interested in trying fish oil, be sure to consult your doctor. Increased consumption of fish oil may lead to toxic levels of vitamins A and D and produce other undesirable side effects.

Take the spa approach. If your psoriasis responds to ultraviolet light therapy and psoralen pills (PUVA), but you find that psoralen pills make you queasy, ask your dermatologist whether psoralen baths are for you. Certain psoriasis treatment centers are now experimenting with this therapy.

Therapy consists of three baths each week for five to seven weeks. You're likely to need maintenance treatments to keep the psoriasis in remission. This is not a home therapy. Psoralen makes your skin extremely sensitive to light and you could really harm your skin if this therapy is not given under medical supervision, Dr. Lowe says.

CLEAR OUT COLD SORES

You've been out skiing all day, enjoying the sun and the snow and the great feeling of being outdoors. And now you're getting ready to sit by the fire in the lodge, spin a few daring ski tales, and flirt a little. Your hair is great. Your body is great. Your face . . . ooops. Is that a cold sore lurking on your lip?

Could be, says David Burt, D.D.S., a Bethlehem, Pennsylvania, dentist. People often assume that weather is a cause of cold sores or fever blisters (they're the same thing), but the truth is, they're caused by a herpes virus that's triggered by intense exposure to ultraviolet light, like that reflected off the snow while you ski. It can happen if you go to the beach and bake in the sun awhile. Fever, a cold, and stress can trigger an attack of these irritating ulcers, too.

When you don't have the sores on your lips, the virus is hiding in the ganglia, the nerve cells in front of your ears, in such a low level of activity that your body can't detect and kill them. But give them a nice, sunny day and these bugs decide to take a road trip, right down to your lips. They call ahead to wherever they plan to camp, sending a tingling, itchy sensation up to 12 hours before arrival. Then boom, they pop up a crusty, oozing tent and stay put 7 to 14 days.

You may be able to evict these little pests before their vacation is over if you act swiftly.

Break the connection. If you get cold sores, ask your doctor or dentist about a prescription for acyclovir ointment. This is one of the half-dozen antiviral drugs that can be used against the herpes virus. If you dab it on the minute you feel your skin tingling in that old, familiar way, you may prevent a sore from appearing.

"If you get it in place soon enough, the cold sore may go away without even showing up," Dr. Burt says. "Forty percent of my patients do not ever get the lesion. They carry a tube of the stuff with them because they never know when they'll get that tingling feeling."

Block the sun. Always wear a sun block, especially over those areas where you get the cold sores, Dr. Burt advises. Use a lip balm with a sun protection factor of at least 15.

Chill out. Applying ice directly to the sore for 10 minutes four to five times a day may send the virus scuttling right back to the ganglia, cutting the time you have to suffer.

Wash and dry. Keep your sore clean and dry, Dr. Burt says. Washing with soap and water, then patting it dry, will keep it from getting worse.

Swap brushes. Switching to a new toothbrush at the right time may stop the spread of herpes in your mouth, say researchers at the University of Oklahoma. A moist toothbrush can harbor the herpes virus for up to seven days, spreading the virus to the lips and throughout the mouth each time you use it to brush. Drying the brush and rinsing it with mouthwash won't kill the germs.

Researchers say you should use three new toothbrushes during each outbreak. The first new brush should be opened in the prodrome, or tingly, phase just before the blister appears. Get another new brush when the blister breaks. Get the third brush when the blister disappears.

Dry it up. Soothe the sore by applying a wet, warm face cloth over the area. Then, set your hair dryer on low, and blow-dry the cloth. This will ease some of the pain.

B-eat your sores to the punch. It wouldn't hurt to try adding a vitamin B supplement to your diet, says Fred Magaziner, D.D.S., spokesman for the Academy of General Dentistry. Studies show that some of these vitamins, such as riboflavin and folate, are especially good at preventing sores around the edges and in the corners of the mouth.

Touch it with a tenacious gel. One over-the-counter drug, a gel called Zilactin, forms a healing, flexible film over sore spots, according to the *Oral Surgery, Oral Medicine, and Oral Pathology Journal*. Studies at the University of Alabama School of Dentistry and Comprehensive Cancer Center found this ointment will ease the pain and stick to the wet membranes in your mouth for 8 hours.

Limit your arginine. If you avoid some of the arginine-rich foods in your diet, such as chocolate, peas, nuts, and gelatin, you'll be depriving your body of the amino acid that feeds the metabolism of the herpes virus and helps your cold sores thrive.

Sniff it out. Camphor, which gives the over-the-counter medicine Campho-Phenique its trademark smell, will dry your sore and help it go away, Dr. Burt says. Be cautious, though, this medication could dry your blister out so much that your lesion will crack and bleed.

Think zinc. To help speed healing, apply a water-based zinc solution the minute you feel the tingling. Zinc may inhibit the herpes virus from duplicating.

In a six-year study in Boston, 200 people were treated with a 0.025 percent solution of zinc sulfate in camphorated water. The solution was applied every 30 to 60 minutes during the onset of the sore. Sores healed in an average 5.3 days.

Kiss carefully. If you have a herpes sore in any form, from first stage tingling to last stage dry scab, don't kiss anyone. Especially don't kiss anyone with cracked lips or sores on their mouth. You're contagious.

Don't touch. Wash your hands carefully any time you touch your sore. You can spread the herpes virus to your eyes or your genitals if you aren't cautious.

Clean cups. Clean cups. Everyone had to keep moving at the Mad Hatter's tea party. He'd yell "Clean cups. Clean cups. Move down. Clean cups," and Alice and all the other partygoers in this classic tale would shift seats.

Think of using this philosophy in your own home. Be sure everyone has his own clean cup in the bathroom, for instance. Family members shouldn't share washcloths, towels, or toothbrushes either, because this virus thrives for days on the dampness and can spread.

SNUFF OUT SHINGLES PAIN

Shingles (herpes zoster) is a viral infection of the central nervous system that can lead to blistering, weeping skin along the route of the affected nerve. You might feel itching, burning, excruciating pain—or general numbness.

When you first get shingles, you're best off leaving your skin to heal on its own and seeking a pain reliever that works internally (unless your doctor advises you differently.) Topical pain relievers are best used for the discomfort that can linger after your skin heals.

Time is the only sure cure for shingles. Here's what our experts advise for easing discomfort fast.

Ask for Zovirax. This prescription medication is taken orally at the first sign of shingles. It heals lesions quickly and keeps new eruptions from forming.

Reach for the aspirin. When shingles pain strikes, desensitize yourself quickly with aspirin. A regular or extra-strength dose could deliver all the pain relief you need to get by while your body recovers.

If you find aspirin isn't strong enough, tell your doctor.

You may need another type of anti-inflammatory drug, available by prescription only, to calm the affected nerve endings.

Try an aspirin paste. Post-herpetic neuralgia is the nerve pain that can linger after your herpes zoster blisters have healed. A very small Boston University School of Medicine study conducted by neurologist Marilyn Kassiner, M.D., found that four out of six patients suffering from post-herpetic neuralgia experienced significant relief 15 to 20 minutes after applying an aspirin paste directly to the affected area. A fifth patient experienced some relief. All other treatments had failed for these people, who were in great pain.

This technique may work for you. To make the paste, crush an aspirin tablet and add it to 2 tablespoons of Vaseline Intensive Care lotion. Apply the paste where you need it three or four times a day.

Don't try this remedy if you are allergic to aspirin. And if the treatment doesn't work within 15 to 20 minutes, it's not going to work at all for you.

Squeeze on Zostrix. If you still have pain after your herpes zoster blisters have healed, try a tube of Zostrix for some convenient rub-on relief. You can purchase this ointment without a prescription.

Zostrix works as a counterirritant. Its active ingredient is capsaicin, the "hot" ingredient in red pepper that gives Zostrix its sting. Scientists believe that the capsaicin, by causing pain itself, depletes the chemical needed to transmit pain impulses between the nerve cells and prevents the body from making more of this chemical.

Be aware that it may take you two weeks or more of rubbing Zostrix on five times a day to see if it is going to work for you. See your doctor. Of course, if you have shingles, you should be under a doctor's care. But if your pain is resistant to Zostrix, or if it lasts more than a month, be sure to tell your doctor, Dr. Schleicher says. If you ignore your discomfort you could end up with persistent pain.

WHISK AWAY WARTS

If that wart of yours absolutely, positively has to disappear overnight, you have treatment options available to you that your grandpa would envy.

Of course, you may be one of those people who decide that the most time-saving treatment of all is to let nature take its course. Most warts disappear naturally, often within a few months. But it may take your immune system two years or more to triumph over the wart-causing human papilloma virus and remove that growth from your skin.

If two years is too long to wait, size up your priorities so you can determine your best treatment option. Are you willing to use an over-the-counter product once a day for up to 12 weeks? If you're in a rush, you can spend the money and endure some discomfort to have your doctor whisk the wart away in minutes.

Realize from the outset that no wart treatment comes with a guarantee that the wart won't recur. The papilloma virus is contagious and may have already spread to an area of your skin where resistance is weak.

If you have a bump that you think is a wart, but you're not sure, see your doctor.

Here are the fastest ways to handle a wart.

Nip it in the bud. The earlier you catch the wart, the greater your chances of banishing it quickly, Dr. Schleicher says. In its early stages, a wart resembles a tiny, flesh-colored, solid pimple. You can combat it with an over-the-counter preparation for warts. "These are usually made of some sort of acid solution, like salicylic acid, and may work on the smaller varieties of warts," Dr. Schleicher says.

You'll probably get the most benefit from these over-the-counter products if you first soak the wart for 15 to 20 minutes, allow it to dry, then rub it with a pumice stone. Apply the medication and give it time to dry before you cover it with a waterproof bandage.

Patch it over. Dermal patches deliver a solution of salicylic acid that is absorbed by the skin. You apply them at night and remove them in the morning. It may take up to 12 weeks to completely remove the wart.

The patches are not safe for people with diabetes or impaired circulation. They are available by prescription only, Dr. Schleicher says.

Juice it with a few volts. Electrocautery is quick and relatively painless. Dr. Novick is enthusiastic about the use of this procedure, which is performed under local anesthesia and uses a heat-producing electric current. He says the procedure takes about 5 minutes and causes little pain. This technique can cause scarring, however.

Freeze it off. No, we're not suggesting that you pack your wart in ice. But you could ask your doctor about cryosurgery, a technique in which the wart is sprayed or swabbed with liquid nitrogen.

The procedure takes only a few minutes, although it may need to be repeated on several occasions for deep warts. It often causes a blister to develop, and the wart is usually removed with the blister roof. You'll feel moderate to severe throbbing pain afterward. The pain can last a few minutes to a few hours, depending upon where the wart was located.

This technique can cause scarring and may make the treated area different in color than the area around it.

Alpha-interferon can combat recurrence. Alpha-interferon injections have been approved by the Food and Drug Administration as a new treatment for genital warts. A protein that fights virus infections, interferon is injected directly into the warts. In studies, this treatment has been found to work better than freezing, burning, or chemical peel at preventing recurrences of warts. But it's more costly and time-consuming, researchers say.

BANISH BODY ODOR

Body odor is such a social embarrassment that you can't rid yourself of it fast enough. Who wants to clear out a room when they take off their shoes or raise their arms?

Not you.

Keeping your special fragrance within the bounds of olfactory etiquette is a simple matter of making use of these quick methods. Along with using a deodorant or antiperspirant, here are some other effective measures.

Scrub with a prescription soap. Most body odor is caused by bacteria that thrive on apocrine sweat, which is what your underarm and crotch areas secrete. The best way to neutralize this bacteria is to wash thoroughly, at least once a day, with a prescription antibacterial soap— such as pHisoHex and Hibiclens—says dermatologist John F. Romano, M.D.

Can the curry. Unfortunately, the very seasonings that impart so much flavor to your foods can make your body smell rather dicey. If body odor is a problem for you, try eliminating garlic and spices such as curry or cumin, Dr. Romano suggests. If you love each of these flavorings, try eliminating one at a time. If you can find that only one is really causing you a problem, you won't have so much to give up.

Stay cool. There's a link between stress and body odor. Anything you can do to keep yourself cool and calm can help you thwart the problem. Try practicing the progressive relaxation technique described on page 376.

Zero in on zinc. As a last resort, try taking zinc supplements. Their effectiveness in beating body odor hasn't been medically proven, but there is some anecdotal evidence that they work. One doctor says that 25 to 50 milligrams of zinc daily has helped eliminate body odor for six of his patients. Of course, don't use any mineral supplement without first getting your doctor's okay.

SLEEP

n apartment 3B, Karen's tossing and turning is tying her bedsheets in knots. Just one floor above, Jeff's snoring is a cross between a cough and a shout. Across town, drifting into the curb at the corner of Elm and Poplar, Roberta is dozing gently at the wheel.

Karen, not surprisingly, will be scratchy-eyed and grouchy tomorrow from lack of sleep. But so will Jeff, who mistakenly thought he actually got a good night's sleep. And Roberta? She'll be yawning at her customers and counting the hours until her lunchtime nap.

Each of these bleary-eyed blunderers has a specific sleeping problem. Karen's problem is insomnia: She wakes up in the middle of the night and can't get back to sleep. Jeff's is sleep apnea, and this breathing pattern leads to shallow, unrefreshing sleep patterns. Roberta's is excessive fatigue resulting from sleep deprivation: Her husband's a heavy-duty snorer.

How are these people to get their needed rest, and how much sleep do they really need?

The so-called good night's sleep changes with age. As newborns, we start out requiring 16 hours a day. By the time we're 65 or so, we can make do with just 6. The turning point in our sleep requirement comes at about age 50, when sleep cycles change. That's when we seem to have more middle-of-the-night awakenings, shorter dreams, and less overall sleep.

Whatever the specific need, it's often not filled. About a third of all adults have a sleep problem at one time or another, says Peter Hauri, Ph.D., codirector of the sleep disorder clinic at the Mayo Clinic in Rochester, Minnesota, where he treats common problems like insomnia and daytime sleepiness, but also helps people who miss sleep because of snoring and restless leg syndrome.

Although some causes of insomnia need medical care, most people can be helped with a few simple adjustments in their sleep styles, says Dennis Hill, M.D., a neurologist who is medical director of the Sleep Disorders Clinic at University Hospital in Charlotte, North Carolina. It generally takes only four to six weeks for these adjustments to turn into habits that trigger the sleep response.

But there are fast-action tactics you can begin with right now.

- Eating the right foods before bedtime
- Moving a single item in your bedroom
- Inducing restful slumber simply by breathing right
- Eliminating daytime drowsiness by sitting in front of a special light box for 2 hours

Nighty-night, don't let the bedbugs bite, see you in the morning light!

HINTS THAT HURRY THE SANDMAN

You're lying there, staring at the clock's luminous dial. You want to sleep, but you can't. Chances are, you took a late afternoon nap, or maybe you're stressed out or excited. This kind of insomnia is usually temporary and lasts from several days to a few weeks. Here's how to cure it fast.

Have a full day. Researchers at Loughborough University in England found that people who have an active day are more likely to have restful sleep at night. They studied volunteers, who spent periods of four days in the sleep lab. On one of the four days, the volunteers went to a distant city where they shopped, went to a museum, visited an amusement park and zoo, and then watched a movie. That night the volunteers conked out earlier and had longer-than-usual periods of restful sleep. They awoke feeling refreshed.

Paint your bedroom. Light colors are best. Look for peach, pink, pale green, and aqua to be the best for soothing you into slumber.

Set aside some quiet time. Before bedtime, begin a ritual you will follow each night. Take about 10 minutes to reflect on your day's activities. Plan tomorrow's. Try to work out solutions to problems, then put your cares aside.

Keep strict mealtimes. Regular meals tell your body that its internal clock is working properly, Dr. Hill says. Also, avoid eating heavy meals at bedtime, when they can cause reflux or heartburn.

Turn your evening snack into a sleeping pill. One of the amino acids in food, called L-tryptophan, can help you get to sleep faster. Here's how it works: You eat a late-evening carbohydrate-rich snack such as rice cakes, dry cereal, air-popped popcorn, potatoes, corn, bagels, or a muffin. As your body digests the carbohydrates, the pancreas releases insulin, decreasing the bloodstream concentration of all amino acids but tryptophan. The now-strong tryptophan levels reach the brain, where they are used to manufacture a chemical called serotonin. Serotonin is the body's own prescription for sleep, and as your brain uses it, feelings of stress and tension slip away. Most people need only an ounce or so of carbohydrates to get the tranquilizing effect within 20 to 30 minutes.

Try milk. You may be tempted to reach for that old standby, a glass of warm milk. The carbohydrates may help you sleep, but some studies show that milk can be an eye-opener, because it has enough protein in it to block the sleep-inducing effects of the carbohydrates. Try it to see how it works for you.

Go to a clambake. You should not only eat the clams, but ask for a helping of oysters, too. Copper and iron, minerals found in these seafoods, are vital to a good night's sleep, according to research by James G. Penland, Ph.D., of the U.S. Department of Agriculture Human Nutrition Research Center at Grand Forks, North Dakota.

Dr. Penland found that women who got only a third of the recommended amounts of these minerals took longer to fall asleep, woke more often in the night, and felt worse upon awakening.

Just ¼ cup of oysters supplies the Recommended Dietary Allowance (RDA) of copper. A serving of clams has 80 to 100 percent of the RDA of iron.

Other foods to consider are nuts, liver, tofu, and refried beans for copper, and red meat, dried fruit, spinach, and garbanzo beans for iron.

Can the coffee. Coffee, cola, chocolate, and your insom-

NINE NEW WAYS TO "COUNT SHEEP"

Counting sheep is just fine, but any boring repetitive thought pattern will push activity from your mind, according to Donald R. Sweeney, M.D., Ph.D., author of *Overcoming Insomnia.* He advises his patients to do one of the following.

Count the ceiling tiles. And when you're finished, count them again.

Subtract, working backward from 768 by 17. This taxing exercise should soon make you drowsy.

Write from 1 to 100 on an imaginary blackboard. After you write each number, pick up your imaginary eraser and erase. Then go on to the next number. If you make it all the way to 100, do the exercise backward.

Recite Hiawatha. Or some other poem. When you're finished, recite it again, spelling each word.

Make it a contest. Think of a category and fill it: American states or four-legged animals.

Tell yourself a story. Focus not on events but on details. Are there strings hanging from the hero's shirt? How many bricks are there in the building?

Take an imaginary trip. Find a setting: a beach, the middle of a forest, a mountaintop. Concentrate on the sounds around you: the crash of the waves, the birds in the trees, the whistling of the wind. Smell the salt spray of the ocean. Feel the heat of the sun.

Attend to the small stuff. Feel the way the sheets touch your toes. Listen to the sound of the furnace turning on and off. Hear the creaking of the house as wind rushes around the corners. Feel your stomach juices settle. Spend time with every creak and squeak of your body.

Bore yourself to sleep. Find a technical manual or instructions for building a swing set. Or, when all else fails, read this paragraph over and over. Don't reward your sleepless self with a pleasant activity. Make your reading bore you to sleep.

If you haven't fallen asleep in 15 to 30 minutes, give up. You'll have missed the sleep window in your body's circadian cycle, and lying in bed awake isn't going to help. Dr. Sweeney recommends moving to a different room to perform a repetitious activity, such as needlepoint, pasting stamps into an album, or solving an easy crossword puzzle. After 45 minutes, return to bed.

nia have something in common—caffeine. Caffeine is a long-acting drug, Dr. Hill says.

Avoid caffeine after noon and you'll fall asleep faster at night. Also, skip sugary snacks at night, according to Dr. Hauri.

Bag the booze. A glass of wine or a shot of whiskey at bedtime may help you fall asleep, but in 3 or 4 hours, when the effect wears off, you'll be up again, irritated and agitated.

"It's very important to have alcohol out of your system when you sleep," Dr. Hill says. "It is a sedative, but it fragments sleep and takes away the deep sleep, the dreaming sleep. A cocktail at dinner is fine, but nothing after 7:00 P.M."

Be a creature of habit. That bedtime ritual you followed as a child—wash your face, brush your teeth, use the toilet—can be just as relaxing today. Make the last hour or so before bedtime a routine. Check the locks, turn out the lights, do your personal grooming in a certain order each night before climbing between the sheets. The preparations will give you the necessary sense of security to fall asleep, and your body will learn that those actions are a prelude to bedtime.

Draw a hot bath. A bedtime soak in the tub is a traditional—and effective—tranquilizer, thought to work by relaxing the muscles, Dr. Hill says.

Another theory holds that hot water raises the temperature in the brain, too, by about 1°F, according to a study at Loughborough University. To be effective, run a bath 100° to 102°F and soak for no more than 15 minutes. The small change in your brain temperature, the scientists reported, can cause an increase in deeper stages of sleep. Now some researchers suggest that using a hair dryer hood can send you to sleepytown, too.

Try a lullaby. In just two weeks, you can teach yourself to fall asleep on cue. The cue? The same music each night at bedtime. Here's what you need to do: Listen to various compositions to find one that seems restful. Turn out the light, then flip on the music you selected. Listen to it over and over until you fall asleep. Use this particular tune only when you're ready to sleep. Eventually hearing that lullaby will alert your snooze response and you'll drift off with the first few notes.

• READ THIS AND SLEEP

Many experts recommend imagery or visualizations to relax the body and fall asleep. Keith Sedlacek, M.D., author of *The Sedlacek Technique: Finding the Calm within You,* recommends a warming exercise combined with mental imagery to bring on drowsiness. Today this exercise will take 10 minutes. If you practice it daily, in four to six weeks you'll be able to do it within seconds.

Close your eyes and picture yourself lying in a hammock strung between two giant oak trees. It's warm enough that you need only a T-shirt and shorts. A soft breeze ruffles the leaves overhead, showing you tiny patches of blue sky and white clouds. The hammock gently sways back and forth as the trees bend back and forth.

Feel the relaxing warmth on the top of your head as the sun touches your hair. Your head feels warm and relaxed. The warmth flows down your head onto your shoulders. They feel warm and heavy.

The warmth flows down toward your hands and gently into your hands. They feel warm and heavy.

You breathe, slowly and regularly.

The breeze flutters the leaves in a sigh. The sun is like a yellow blanket against your exposed skin. The hammock moves like a cradle with you in it.

Warmth flows down to your heart. Your breathing is slow, regular. You may feel your heart beating calmly.

The relaxing warmth flows into your thighs, and they become warm and heavy. Your legs become warm. Your feet are washed with warmth.

The warmth wells up in your abdomen and stomach. Your heart feels warm and easy.

Your body is quiet and calm. Your mind is calm and quiet. Your body feels heavy with the warmth of the sun.

Enjoy the calm, warm, relaxed feeling. End the exercise by counting to three. The feelings may be subtle at first but will grow as your experience grows.

THREE O'CLOCK AND ALL ISN'T WELL

It's 3:00 A.M. You know that. Five minutes ago it was 2:55 A.M. And when you look at the clock again, it's going to be 3:05. Then 3:10, 3:15, and 3:20.

So what can you do to keep from watching the clock?

Drop it in a drawer. That's what Dr. Hauri recommends everyone do as part of their bedtime ritual. Set the clock, he says, then shove it under the bed, turn its face to the wall, or stick it in with your underwear.

"It's the time pressure that's disturbing," Dr. Hauri says. "You can't possibly relax if you watch the seconds ticking away and you're calculating how many hours of sleep you have left before you have to get up."

Get rid of the clock, "and until the alarm rings, don't know what time it is. Be time-free. Trying to sleep is the pits. You must never try to sleep. Sleep comes when you don't worry about it," Dr. Hauri explains.

Get up and relax. If you can't sleep at any time during the night, don't just toss and turn. Get up and do something relaxing. Watch the late, late movie. Read something boring. Just be sure whatever you do is on the boring side. Experts warn that you'll never get sleepy working on a report you need to complete, doing your income taxes, or even reading that wonderful spy novel. Sex may or may not help you sleep—if it works for you, do it.

TV or not TV? There are two kinds of insomniacs, Dr. Hauri says. One type benefits from a television or book in the bedroom to help ease them back to dreamland in the middle of the night. If you nod off during the nightly news or never quite finish the end of a chapter before you have to put a book down, then you're that type of insomniac.

However, if you're a person who says you can fall asleep anywhere except the bedroom, then banish all activities except sleeping from the bedroom.

Block it all out. Your spouse is sawing logs loudly enough to wake the neighbors. A street light shines in your eyes like the midsummer sun. Or maybe you are tossing and turning because you're cold. Get yourself a pair of earplugs to block the noise. Add some eyeshades to extinguish the light. Plug in the electric blanket and slumber in constant warmth.

SLEEPINESS: THE SUN IS UP, BUT YOU'RE NOT

Think of your body's sleeping and waking demands as operating in a time zone all their own. Scientists call this your circadian rhythm. And what that means is, your body has a 24-hour internal clock that regulates hormones, hunger, mood, alertness, sexual desire, and sleep. And, like any good clock, it functions best when it's not fiddled with, Dr. Hill says. That's why scheduling is so important to preventing insomnia.

"Most people are chronically sleep deprived," Dr. Hill says. "But it's not how long you sleep, it's how well you perform during the day that counts. If a person is sleeping 3 or 4 hours a night but has no problem, then that's all right. If they're feeling sleepy all day, then it's time to do something."

Lighten up. Chronically poor sleepers who just can't get started in the morning may benefit from resetting their circadian rhythms. Researchers at the National Institute of Mental Health are using bright lights in the morning to put body clocks back in time.

People sit in front of high-intensity, full-spectrum fluorescent lights for 2 hours each morning for several weeks. The lights signal the body that it's morning and time to get going. In the evening, these people wear dark glasses so the body knows it's time to slow down.

You can get these special lights (which are about the size of a suitcase and cost several hundred dollars) by writing to The Sun Net, P.O. Box 10606, Rockville, MD 20850.

You can also accomplish the same thing by getting out in the sunshine as soon as you get up.

Push the clock. Shift work plays havoc with getting the needed 40 winks. Research shows that if your schedule rotates clockwise—day to evening to night—rather than counterclockwise, you'll handle the changes more easily. Also, shift changes are easier to handle in a 10-day cycle than in a 7-day cycle.

Take a walk. When your I-need-a-nap feeling hits, don't nap, warns Donald R. Sweeney, M.D., Ph.D., author of *Overcoming Insomnia: A Medical Program for Problem Sleepers*. Arrange your daily schedule so that your usual sleepy time of day is filled with a stimulating task.

Return phone calls or take a brisk walk. Minimize the urge to nap. It will go away. (If it doesn't, see "Now, a Note about Napping" on the opposite page.)

WHAT TO DO WHEN YOU'RE MESMERIZED TO SLEEP

Repetitive work, and especially driving, can lull the senses into sleep. Dr. Hauri recommends his patients try a few sense-jangling tricks to stay awake.

Take a jog around the parked car. If you're driving, park the car in a safe spot and jog around it a couple of times.

Sing. Turn on the radio and sing something bright and lively.

Say 10-4, good buddy. "Truck drivers have CB radios for the companionship they provide, and to help them stay awake," Dr. Hauri says.

Quaff a cup of caffeine. Coffee, iced tea, cola—choose your favorite and hoist it. But be prepared to pay the price later—you may have a hard time falling asleep when you've finished your drive.

HOW TO GIVE RESTLESS LEGS A REST

One frequent sleeping problem brought on by age, Dr. Hill says, is slow movements of the feet or legs during sleep, called restless leg syndrome. These movements, often described as crawling sensations in the legs, are more than just a chronic annoyance that severely disrupts sleep and causes insomnia, especially in the elderly. No one knows the cause of the sensations, although some researchers think it could be an imbalance in the brain's chemistry.

However slow the movements, they can be disturbing to both the sleep "dancer" and the partner slumbering nearby.

Walk it off. Getting up and walking around seems to be the fastest way to stop that drowsy dance.

Stroll a while before bedtime. Sometimes this light exercise will reduce the sleepytime shuffle. Exercise releases chemicals in the brain, called endorphins, that may promote restful snoozing.

Change temperatures. Some people say soaking their feet in cool (not cold) water stops the movements. Others say the warmth of a heating pad stops the "limb-o."

Pop a multivitamin. Iron deficiency may be a cause of restless legs, several studies show. Folate deficiency has also been considered a culprit. A multivitamin will fill those deficiencies, according to Lawrence Z. Stern, M.D., professor of neurology and director of the Mucio F. Delgado Clinic for Neuromuscular Disorders at the University of Arizona Health Sciences Center in Tucson.

Ask your doctor about medication. The prescription drugs Sinemet and Klonopin offer good results, Dr. Hill says.

NOW, A NOTE ABOUT NAPPING

Some experts say you should get your sleep at night and minimize the need for napping during the day. But an after-lunch catnap is a time-honored tradition. Approximately half the world's population takes an afternoon siesta. Winston Churchill and John F. Kennedy were famous nappers. And 55 percent of college students nap, often in the afternoon, according to David Dinges, Ph.D., a psychologist at the Institute of the Pennsylvania Hospital in Philadelphia.

One survey showed that naps are good for us, too. Among hospital patients who reported taking a 30-minute nap, there was a 30 percent lower incidence of heart disease than among those who don't stretch out for stolen slumber.

Still, sleep experts say that some types of siestas can cause our circadian rhythm to miss a beat. So if you're going to nap, do it right. And fast.

Keep it short. If you must retire, keep it no longer than the length of a sleep cycle. That is, rest from 60 to 90 minutes.

Make sleep positively preventive. If you know you're going to be up late or even all night, take your nap *before* you lose sleep, not afterward. A study at the Institute of the Pennsylvania Hospital tested 40 young men. The men stayed up for 56 hours, with only a 2-hour nap allowed. After that marathon, the men were tested for alertness and feelings of sleepiness. Those who took their naps early in the ordeal were more alert after it was over than those who slept at the very end. Preventive sleeping, the team concluded, is better than makeup work.

Lie down between 2:00 and 3:00 P.M. That's the ideal time to fit sleeping into your body's natural rhythm. Morning naps are usually light and evening snoozes are too deep. Afternoon provides just the right amount of refreshing sleep.

Give a little, get a little. If you get 90 minutes of sleep during a daytime nap, expect to have 90 minutes less sleep that night to keep your body in sync with its natural rhythm.

SNORE WARS: CALLING A TRUCE

While men are more likely to snore than women, a study of 2,000 people in Toronto, Canada, showed that more than half of the women snored, too.

At least two people suffer when there's a snorer in the family. There's the person who endures the noise and loses sleep. The other person is the snorer, whose uvula and soft palate—tissue at the back of the throat—relax and vibrate during sleep. For some, these floppy throat muscles collapse around the tongue, blocking the airway for 10 to 60 seconds or more and creating a condition called sleep apnea. For some people, this blockage can cause them to awaken 50 to 100 times an hour, Dr. Hill says, causing fragmented sleep and drowsy days.

"These people will fall asleep during a conversation, in church, or at work. They have difficulty concentrating, their memory is poor, and some are depressed," Dr. Hill says.

Doctors take sleep apnea seriously. Some 2,000 to 3,000 people die yearly, they suspect, because of suffocation caused by this disorder.

People with apnea spend very little of their night in the deep sleep stages that are necessary for rest. Sleepiness can be just one of the side effects. Apnea also may contribute to high blood pressure, heart attack, and stroke.

Your doctor can prescribe medications to help prevent snoring. However, some of these drugs also may keep you awake or inhibit the dreaming stage of sleep.

SHORT-CIRCUITING SNORING WITH A THROAT-LIFT

Sometimes surgery to enlarge part of the throat, called uvulopalato-pharyngoplasty, or UPPP, is required to end snoring. The surgeon removes excess tissue, including the uvula (the little punching bag over your tongue), the tonsils, and part of the soft palate (the back upper portion of your mouth and throat). This expands the airway, lessening vibration during sleep. Doctors sometimes call this operation a face-lift on the back of the throat.

Doctors recommend this surgery for severe snorers who have been unsuccessful with other methods of treatment and who also have sleep apnea. It is also recommended if there is an obstruction in the throat that causes apnea.

After the operation, which has a success rate of about 95 percent, the patient's throat is sore for a week or ten days.

For the person listening to the snorts and snores, earplugs or a change of venue (another bedroom) may be the only choices. However, there are some things the snorers themselves can do to diminish the din.

Spray your nose with a little salt water. An over-the-counter saline spray will moisten mucous membranes, making it a little easier to breathe. The spray, which contains salt and water in the same proportion as in the body's blood plasma, won't have the rebound effect that another nasal spray might. You can try making your own saline nose spray by dissolving ½ teaspoon of salt (⅓ teaspoon if you have high blood pressure) in 8 ounces of warm water. Collect the solution in a nasal aspirator. Hold your nose straight back and snort the water into your nostril. Then spit out the water and blow your nose. Be careful if you're making your own spray, however. If you use too much salt you might burn your nose.

Start a diet today. Just by losing some weight, you may get over your snoring and apnea. Increased tissue in the neck and throat, along with poor muscle tone, constricts the air passageway. Further, a large abdomen pressing against your diaphragm when you lie on your back decreases the size of your lungs and the amount of air you breathe with each breath.

At least one study shows that a weight loss of 10 to 25 percent can eliminate apnea or reduce its frequency. Another study of men who were more than twice their ideal body weight and whose apnea caused them to stop breathing 70 times each hour showed that the incidence of apnea was cut to 10 awakenings per hour when they lost 30 to 60 percent of their weight.

Sleep on a firm mattress. Use a low pillow to keep the neck straight and reduce obstruction in the throat that might be causing the snoring, advises Derek S. Lipman, M.D., author of *Stop Your Husband from Snoring*.

Snooze on your stomach. You may not snore if you lie on your stomach. Put your arm under the pillow to steady your head.

Slumber on your side. Mold pillows to fit your stomach and back to make sleeping on your side more comfortable.

Find a new use for old tennis balls. Sew a pocket between the shoulders of your pajama top or onto the back of a T-shirt. Insert a ball. When you roll onto your back while asleep, your body will gently shift to another position without you waking.

Toss your pillow. If you *must* sleep on your back, remove the pillows from your bed. Lying flat allows your throat to become one smooth pipe, with no snore-causing "kinks." Tuck a small pad under your chin to keep your mouth closed.

Elevate your bed. Raising your upper torso, not just your head, can help minimize the noise. Put a couple of bricks under the legs at the head of your bed.

Stub out the butt. Smoking causes changes in the tissues of your respiratory system that contribute to snoring, Dr. Lipman says. The irritation, for instance, increases mucus production in your throat and nose and makes those membranes swell, leaving less room for the air to get through.

Nix the nightcap. A drink at bedtime increases muscle relaxation (including those in your throat) and aggravates snoring and sleep apnea, Dr. Lipman says.

In one study of middle-aged men who seldom snored, drinking substantial amounts of alcohol triggered snoring. In another study of a group of people with mild sleep apnea, alcohol increased the frequency and severity of the apnea. In fact, warns Dr. Lipman, alcohol can be the factor that turns heavy snorers into apnea victims.

As for drinking in general, people who snore mildly should drink in moderation. Heavy snorers and people with apnea should abstain or drastically reduce alcohol consumption.

Read the label on your medication. Some over-the-counter medications affect the body in the same way alcohol does. Some cold cures, for instance, contain muscle relaxants that can affect breathing. People with apnea should always check with their doctors before using nasal sprays, decongestants, or other over-the-counter medications.

Slip by the sedatives. Sleeping pills may help you sleep temporarily, but because they relax the head and neck muscles, they may make snoring worse.

Prop open your airway. Your doctor may prescribe a soft plastic mouthpiece that fits firmly over the teeth and expands the airway by pulling the jawbone forward. One type pulls the tongue forward and widens your airway at the same time. Another appliance lifts the soft palate and keeps the jaw in a forward position.

HIGH TECH • A SPECIAL DEVICE FOR PROBLEM SLEEPERS

Snorers with sleep apnea (a condition in which the throat relaxes and closes during sleep) can try a special device that may restore normal breathing during slumber.

The method is called nasal continuous positive airway pressure, or Nasal CPAP. The sleeper wears a special mask that feeds pressurized air into the nose. The pressure holds the throat open, ending both the noise of snoring and the obstruction causing the apnea. The machine that delivers the air is the size of a small computer terminal and weighs between 9 and 18 pounds.

If a doctor at a sleep clinic prescribes this device, you'll spend the night at the clinic and a technician will determine your proper air pressure while you sleep. If you wake refreshed, the pressure is correct. With your doctor's prescription, you can rent or buy one of these devices from a medical supply company that specializes in home respiratory equipment. Studies show the Nasal CPAP is effective for about 85 percent of all apnea patients.

THROAT PROBLEMS

magine your throat as a highway, a two-way street between you and a dry, dusty world. Traffic never stops, does it? You breathe exhaust, call for a taxi, cough. You chair meetings, talk long-distance, scold the kids. It's a mighty busy place, your throat. Too busy to put to bed for a week.

Don't let sore throats and pesky coughs slow you down. And don't let laryngitis leave you speechless.

- In just a few seconds, you can coat your throat so every swallow slides right down.
- In just several minutes, you can thin cough-producing phlegm.
- In just a few months, you can change your speech patterns and leave hoarseness behind.

Sometimes a sore throat can be the result of a serious infection, like streptococcus bacteria. In this case you should see a doctor. But usually it's something you can handle easily at home.

SOOTHE THAT SORE THROAT

A sore throat is nature's way of reminding us how much we take for granted. Eating and drinking, for instance. A sore throat makes water feel like a handful of tacks. It makes Jell-O feel like sandpaper. As for going out to dinner, forget it — why waste a good meal on a bad throat? What to do?

Give it a rest. Colds and flu, which often bring sore throats, tend to stick around. That means your sore throat sticks around, too.

• SOOTHING SORENESS
WITH IMAGERY

Simple remedies play their part in soothing a sore throat. But don't forget your mind—it's powerful medicine, says Dr. Martin Rossman, author of *Healing Yourself: A Step-by-Step Program for Better Health through Imagery.*

"For many people, visually imagining healing brings about symptomatic relief and sometimes helps bring about a cure," he says. Indeed, Dr. Rossman says, studies indicate you can improve your circulation just by concentrating on your blood flow. Endorphins, the body's natural painkillers, also respond to mind commands. Both are important in relieving all kinds of throat problems.

If you put your mind to work, you can ease a sore throat in as little as 15 minutes, Dr. Rossman says. Before your mind can go to work, it needs some peace and quiet. So first practice the technique outlined in "Progressive Relaxation" on page 376.

Now, Dr. Rossman says, "Choose your image. Focus your attention directly on where you have the pain. Imagine it in as much detail as you can."

Everyone imagines things differently, so let your mind go. And be thorough: Make your throat a real place. Give it textures, shapes, and colors. Hang some drapes if you want, or add a potted plant. Imagine it any way you want.

"I imagine a janitor with a bucket filled with a very smooth antiseptic solution," Dr. Rossman says. "He's wiping down the sides of my throat, every nook and cranny."

It's important that you find an image you like: You may prefer a more anatomical version, where your body fights the inflammation, or a more spiritual version, full of healing rays of white or golden light.

Imaging gets easier, and more effective, with practice, Dr. Rossman says. For a sore throat, repeat the exercise several times a day. If you don't notice improvement right away, don't get discouraged, he says. Keep practicing. "It's inexpensive, it's entirely nontoxic, and it can't hurt."

"Someone once said that to recover from a common flu takes the energy of a 40-mile hike with a 40-pound backpack," says Martin L. Rossman, M.D., clinical associate in medicine at the University of California at San Francisco. So give you *and* your throat the day off. Better a day in bed than a week in misery.

Keep it moist. A dry, sore throat, like a hot engine, needs lots of lubrication. Slippery-elm lozenges coat your throat and reduce painful friction, Dr. Rossman says.

Think zinc. Zinc lozenges can help the kind of sore throat that's associated with a cold. The zinc heads straight for the sore spot in your throat, says Eleonore Blaurock-Busch, Ph.D., director of Trace Minerals International and a nutrition counselor at Alpine Chiropractic Center in Boulder, Colorado. If you zap your sore throat with zinc every 2 to 3 hours, "You will feel soothing effects within a day," she says.

Take a gargle. A warm saltwater gargle reduces painful swelling in minutes, Dr. Blaurock-Busch says. It also kills germs. Just add a teaspoon of salt to a cup of warm water, tip your head back, and gargle away. You can gargle as often as you want relief, she says. ·

Fight inflammation with ibuprofen. This nonprescription drug is as effective a pain reliever and inflammation fighter as its cousin, aspirin, but it may be easier on your stomach. Follow the directions and precautions on the bottle.

TAKING CARE OF COUGHS

There's nothing like a nagging, tickling, wracking cough to distract you and attract an unwilling audience. Coughers have broken ribs during severe attacks, and listeners may be forgiven for wishing themselves elsewhere. Even worse, coughs, like unruly children, act up at the most inconvenient times—such as during the opening movement of the symphony.

"Your body doesn't cough because it thinks it's fun," Dr. Blaurock-Busch says. "It's a mechanism to bring up mucus." Here are ways to send that pesky cough packing as soon as it's outlived its usefulness.

Take a swig of cough syrup. Thick, gummy phlegm isn't leaving without some help. You can make it easier for your cough to expel phlegm by diluting it with over-the-counter expectorants containing guaifenesin, an ingredient in many cold remedies and cough syrups.

Go south of the border. For dinner, at least. Fiery foods like chili, Tabasco, and garlic put mucus on the run in minutes, Dr. Rossman says, helping your lungs cough the stuff out of the way. Garlic even doubles as a mild antibiotic.

Don't have a taste for tacos? "You can take four to six drops of Tabasco in half a glass of water and it will stimulate secretions in your lungs," he says. Naturally, people with a sensitive stomach should be cautious with hot-sauce remedies. But when you want to get the juices flowing, a "hot" drink several times a day hits the spot.

Savor some soup. Grandma always said chicken soup is the best cough buster. The heat of a steaming bowl of broth helps clear your chest before your spoon scrapes bottom, Dr. Blaurock-Busch says. Best of all, you don't need a prescription.

Lace your tea with honey and lemon. Besides tasting good, this traditional combination really seems helpful for relieving coughs and congestion, says Hueston King, M.D., an otolaryngologist and clinical associate professor of otolaryngology at the University of Texas Southwest Medical Center.

Add some oil. Aromatic oils often ease coughs in minutes, Dr. King says. Incidentally, you don't *have* to rub oil on your chest; a dab under your nose works just fine. "It promotes mucus secretion," Dr. King says. "It works almost immediately" to get mucus on the move, enabling you to cough productively.

Moisturize the air. Switch on the vaporizer and leave it on until your cough is gone. The warmth and moisture help dilute and loosen phlegm. Add shots of spearmint or peppermint oil to fire things up. Like chili, they produce a chemical heat that liquefies phlegm. And clean the vaporizer daily: The moisture that soothes your cough also is friendly to molds and bacteria.

Get steamed. You need a lot of hot, wet air when your lungs are trying to cough out phlegm. So run a hot bath or take a steaming shower, says Elliot Dick, Ph.D., professor of preventive medicine and director of the Respiratory Virus Research Lab at the University of Wisconsin.

He also recommends vaporizing your head. "It helps to put your head over a steaming pot, particularly one that has a little menthol in it," Dr. Dick says. "It makes a momentary but vast difference." Drape a towel over your head to trap the steam.

HANDLING A TICKLISH SITUATION

Despite the cute-sounding name, there's nothing funny about a tickle. Your throat feels dry, scratchy. Maybe something's stuck? You cough, try to clear your throat, cough again . . . and again . . . and again. Nothing comes up and the tickle's still there. Now your throat is sore, too. So is anyone around you. What can you do to swiftly stifle the tickle?

Drink lots of water. Make that *lots* of water. "If it's just a tickle and no soreness, it's probably just dryness," Dr. King says. Older people are especially prone to dryness, he says, but everyone can use extra fluids. Besides, the more you lubricate your throat, the less irritation you'll have in the first place.

Cool your uvula. Look in the mirror and say, "Ahh." See that bit of tissue hanging down at the back of your throat like a punching bag? That's your uvula, and if it's swollen, it may create a tickle. A tall drink of cold water, by reducing the swelling, may take out the tickle, says Dr. King.

Reach for the salt. A saltwater gargle can give quick relief, Dr. King says.

Stop the urge to scratch that itch. A throat tickle, like an itch, gets worse the more you scratch it. How do you scratch a throat tickle? With just one good cough, one loud throat clearing. But if you give in to the urge to scratch this itch, the tickle gets worse because you just irritate it more. One way to calm the urge to scratch is with a cough syrup containing dextromethorphan, an ingredient that calms coughs within an hour.

SAVING YOUR VOICE

It's opening night. After months of rehearsals, late nights, and soliloquies, you're ready to play Hamlet—except that last-minute laryngitis made your voice quite, quite hoarse.

(Actually, there's more of a donkeylike quality to it.) You stay home and someone else gets the glory. Good night, sweet prince!

What can you do to stop laryngitis—an inflammation of the vocal cords—from stealing the show? If it's acute laryngitis, not much. Acute laryngitis often accompanies colds or other viral infections and can turn the most melodious voice hoarse and gravelly—or in some cases, turn it off entirely. In this case, your voice will return when the virus leaves.

Chronic laryngitis, on the other hand, is persistent. It often comes from overusing (or misusing) your voice, and it responds well to voice management. Rescue your voice from the croaks and whispers with these fast, easy methods.

Don't let "chronic" start. Acute laryngitis and hoarseness typically last a few days—*if* you rest your voice, says Robert J. Feder, M.D., an otolaryngologist at UCLA. If you don't rest your voice, it can last for weeks. Rest means talk softly, and smile rather than laugh. And don't whisper: It's tough on your vocal cords, he says.

Stop talking. At least until you absolutely *must* talk. If you feel your voice going, give it a break for a few hours, Dr. Feder advises. "If you have to talk for an hour, be quiet another hour," he says.

Shut your mouth. "The best thing is to close your mouth and breathe through your nose," Dr. Feder says. Mouth breathing dries your vocal cords, which increases hoarseness.

Take a long drink of water. Keeping your body—and vocal cords—hydrated will help you get your voice up and talking in a few days. How much water? "About ten glasses every day," Dr. Feder says. "It's an awful lot, but push yourself."

Keep your throat warm and moist. "The best thing is steam," Dr. Feder says. "Use it 5 minutes, four times a day."

Avoid harsh fumes. If you're breathing paint by day and cleaning solutions by night, your voice (not to mention your lungs) will suffer. If you can't avoid the fumes, at least breathe through your nose. Wear a respirator or mask. Ventilate your work area.

Ask your doctor for steroids. Sometimes the play—or the after-dinner speech or courtroom trial—must go on.

NEWS FOR NODES

In *The Godfather*, Vito Corleone's hoarse, gravelly voice has just the right sound for a New York boss of organized mayhem. However, most people don't want to talk like they have a mouthful of cotton. Had the Godfather been so inclined, he might have visited his neighborhood doctor for an offer he couldn't refuse.

Chronic hoarseness often is caused by nodules on the vocal cords, says New Jersey otolaryngologist Jason Surow, M.D. Although the nodules (also called singer's nodes and screamer's nodes) may be quite a bit smaller than the tip of a sharpened pencil, they can wreak havoc on your voice. "I like to refer to them as calluses on the vocal cords," Dr. Surow says. "They're caused by a thickening of the membrane at the point at which the vocal cords vibrate most exuberantly."

Fortunately, they respond well to treatment. Surgery to remove the nodules—performed in minutes with microscopic instruments or laser—is safe and effective. And to keep them from coming back, Dr. Surow would prescribe speech therapy. He calls it speech hygiene. No, speech hygiene isn't cleaning up your language. It's cleaning up the way you *use* your voice. If you give your voice regular, intensive workouts, you also have to give it regular rest, Dr. Surow advises. Keep the volume down. Avoid excessive coughing or throat clearing—both needlessly stress the vocal cords.

And avoid using "harsh glottal attacks" to frame your sentences, he says. "That means making the sounds with so forceful an attempt that it causes an injury to the voice box." In other words, say "Hello" even when you mean "HELLO!" You'll get your point across, and your voice will thank you for taking it easy.

Steroids quickly reduce the swelling that causes hoarseness, Dr. Feder says. Because they can have severe side effects, steroids aren't routinely prescribed. Ask your doctor about them only as a last resort.

See a speech therapist. People who are constantly hoarse with chronic laryngitis, or people who have scream-er's nodes or singer's nodes (small "calluses" on the vocal cords), may improve with two to three months of speech therapy, Dr. Feder says. That beats a lifetime of sounding like the Godfather.

GAGGING YOUR GAGS

Oh-oh, you say. Here it comes. Sure enough, when your dentist goes to work with her probe — gag! She tries again. You gag again. Darn it, you just can't help yourself. *You* know she's not going to drop the probe down your throat, but your throat isn't too sure.

Gagging may be an embarrassing problem, but it isn't rare, dentists say. Far from it. As much as 20 percent of people older than 50 — and perhaps 2 to 3 percent of younger folks — are gaggers, says Irwin Smigel, D.D.S., president of the American Society for Dental Aesthetics.

Why? No one knows, Dr. Smigel says. Gaggers may be unusually sensitive to oral manipulations. They may be extremely frightened of dental work. Whatever the cause, gagging is uncomfortable for patients and time-consuming for dentists. What can you do?

Numb your mouth. Some dentists apply a topical anesthetic to the soft palate, the back part of the roof of your mouth, which is most likely to be sensitive to gagging, Dr. Smigel says. If you're a gagger, ask your dentist to do both of you a favor and anesthetize your soft palate.

Brush it off. Some people gag even when they brush their teeth. Try firmly pushing the head of your toothbrush against the inside of your cheek when a gag starts, Dr. Smigel suggests.

Pass the salt. Try eliminating a gag reflex by putting salt on your tongue. No one knows why this works, says Kenneth Burrell, D.D.S., director of the Council on Dental Therapeutics. There may be a chemical explanation, or perhaps the salt simply is a useful distraction, he says.

Look for distractions. "In some cases, the gaggers have a feeling that they have lost control," Dr. Burrell says. "If there is some way you can get them to participate in the process, that diminishes the gag reflex." He says he asks gaggers to help out by holding the saliva ejector — that little pipe that gurgles away under your tongue and keeps your mouth dry. They concentrate on their task and "forget" to gag.

Instead of just sitting in the dentist's chair and waiting for the worst, look around. Any distraction will help. Is there a poster of Garfield on the ceiling? Count his whiskers. Count ceiling dots. Count the pores and wrinkles on your dentist's face. Concentrate on anything that isn't your mouth.

Change your breathing. Try taking rapid, shallow breaths—or slow, deep breaths. People who experiment with breathing patterns often finish entire sessions without gagging, Dr. Burrell says.

Listen to music. The whine of dental drills isn't especially restful. Bring some tapes. Crank up the rock and roll. Imagine yourself far away—maybe on a distant island where no one says, "Open wide."

Naturally, you can't whip every throat problem into shape in 5 minutes. Some coughs won't be tamed. Some sore throats stay sore until they get bored and leave. Maybe 5 minutes with the dentist is all you can stand—today.

That's okay. You're not looking for miracles, but to feel better as soon as you possibly can. So get started. It just takes a little time.

TRAVEL

D id your tropical cruise turn you more green than tan? Did your tour of Greece include you as one of the ruins? And did that fast jet to Africa leave you lagging in Lagos?

If so, let this tour guide of quick travel treatments make all your *voyages* truly *bon*. For example, learn how you can:

- Unpop your ears on a plane in 10 seconds.
- Relieve motion sickness in 1 minute.
- Cut your chances of getting *turista* by 65 percent.
- Recover from altitude sickness in 30 minutes.
- Reduce jet lag from a week to one day.

FAST WAYS TO SLOW MOTION SICKNESS

If you've named your sloop the Mal-de-Mer, and your idea of Chinese torture is flying to Beijing, you've probably experienced the dreadful symptoms of motion sickness. Whether you're carsick, seasick, or airsick, the symptoms are all the same: light-headedness, pallor, sweating, queasiness, then nausea and vomiting.

The cause of all this misery is a conflict of sensory input. Your inner ear (which registers information about movement) tells your brain you're moving. But your eyes say you're not. Your brain doesn't know how to deal with this confusing input, and the result is motion sickness.

This illness, like the flight itself, has a point of no return. Once you start vomiting, there's little hope of returning to good health until you get off the moving conveyance. So at the first twinge of queasiness, try these simple strategies to put a quick end to motion sickness.

Sit still, with your head tilted back. Stabilizing your head minimizes the disorientation that seems to cause motion sickness.

Stare at a fixed object, or fix your gaze 45 degrees above the horizon. On an airplane, close your eyes if that doesn't work.

Avoid food odors and smoke. If you are bothered by odors, tie a bandanna over your nose and mouth to help filter the air.

If you dread travel because you've suffered motion sickness in the past, try these preventive measures.

Skip the bon voyage party. Fatigue, alcohol consumption, and/or a hangover worsen the symptoms of motion sickness.

Ask for a seat where motion is minimal. The most stable areas are amidships in a boat or in the front seat of a car. (Drive whenever possible. Drivers almost never get motion sickness.) On a train, face forward and sit near a window. On a bus, sit up front, so you can see the road and anticipate and adapt to curves and bumps.

On a plane, ask for a seat over the wing, on the right side of the plane, suggests aviation medical expert Howard Rodenberg, M.D., of the Truman Medical Center in Kansas City, Missouri. Since most flight patterns turn left, he points out, you won't swing around as much.

Try ginger. Sold in health food stores, powdered ginger capsules may be more effective in preventing motion sickness than Dramamine (a commonly used over-the-counter anti-motion-sickness drug containing dimenhydrinate), according to a study reported in *Lancet.* Researchers gave the testers one of three treatments: two capsules of powdered ginger (940 milligrams total); a standard, 100-milligram dose of Dramamine; or two capsules of an inactive herb, then strapped them into a revolving chair. The six people who took ginger were able to spin 50 percent longer before getting queasy than the six taking the drug. People who took neither ginger nor Dramamine fared worst of all: Three out of six threw up.

Ginger is considered safe. You can take two 450-milligram capsules about 10 minutes before your flight or cruise, and two more later if you start to feel queasy. (Dimenhydrinate is taken 30 to 60 minutes before travel begins, and may cause drowsiness.)

Scope out the patch. If nothing else works and it's imperative that you avoid motion sickness, you may want to consider wearing a "scop patch," or transdermal scopalamine. A potent prescription medicine, scopalamine is slowly absorbed through the skin from a patch worn behind your ear. Scop patches prevent motion-induced nausea but don't make you sleepy like Dramamine and other over-the-counter motion sickness drugs. Keep in mind, though, that scop patches should be worn for no longer than three days. Scopalamine is related to belladonna, and even at recommended doses, it can trigger a number of disturbing side effects, from minor annoyances like parchment-dry mouth to severe disorientation and, more seriously, high blood pressure and cardiac arrhythmias.

DODGING DISTRESS FROM MICROORGANISMS

Each year, *turista,* or traveler's diarrhea, strikes more than a million visitors to Mexico. Attacks of "urgent diarrhea" also affect up to half of all travelers to other areas of Latin America, as well as to Africa, Asia, and the Middle East. Part of the cause is inadequate sanitation, making traveler's diarrhea more common in developing tropical areas. But travelers anywhere, even in first-world nations, can come down with the tourist two-step. In one recent year, 25,000 cases of *turista*-like gastrointestinal distress occurred in London. And although it's rare, Mexican citizens have been known to suffer problems resembling *turista* on visits to Tucson!

In most instances, traveler's diarrhea in a developing country results from swallowing food or drink contaminated with *E. coli* or other kinds of bacteria (although viruses and parasites can cause diarrhea, too). Yet one of the pleasures of traveling is sampling the local cuisine. And whether you're at home or away, you need to drink water—about 3½ to 9 pints a day.

So what's a poor traveler to do?

GIVING TURISTA *THE OLD HEAVE-HO*

Turista is quirky. Some people can eat or drink just about anything and not get diarrhea, while others take great pains to avoid bowel-wrenching bugs and get *turista* anyway.

So if you get *turista* despite fastidious eating habits and hygiene, here's what to do.

Drink up. "Primary treatment for traveler's diarrhea is fluid replacement to prevent dehydration," says Charles D. Ericsson, M.D., professor of medicine at the University of Texas Health Sciences Center in Houston. For mild diarrhea, doctors recommend carbonated beverages, juice, clear broth, mineral water, and purified water, plus salted crackers.

For moderate to severe cases, they suggest the following rehydration formula: In one glass, combine 8 ounces of purified water with ¼ teaspoon baking soda. In another, combine 8 ounces of fruit juice (orange or apple, for instance) with ½ teaspoon corn syrup or honey and a pinch of salt. Drink a few sips from one, then a few sips from the other, continuing to alternate sips until you finish both glasses or your thirst is quenched, whichever comes first (about 10 minutes). Then continue to drink safe liquids until diarrhea subsides. (Avoid alcoholic beverages, coffee and, of course, contaminated water.)

Open a can of soup. With your plumbing in turmoil, you're better off sticking with a bland diet of clear soup, crackers, and toast for a day or so. As diarrhea subsides, add bulkier foods like rice, baked potatoes, and chicken soup with rice or noodles, Dr. Ericsson says. After a day or so, as your stools resume their proper consistency, add baked fish or poultry, applesauce, and bananas.

Try Imodium. The urge to "take something" for diarrhea is almost as powerful as the urge to hit the bathroom during an attack. Most bouts of mild diarrhea last two to three days and subside on their own. But that's a long time to be severely inconvenienced if you need to run to a bathroom at unpredictable moments. It can ruin a business meeting or overland bus tour. Taking Imodium or other similarly acting over-the-counter antimotility medicines can bring diarrhea to an abrupt halt. They work even better than your old pink friend, Pepto-Bismol.

Say gracias to Pepto-Bismol, adios to turista. Pepto-Bismol can help settle mild to moderate cases of diarrhea, although it's not as effective as Imodium. The recommended dose is 1 ounce every half hour after diarrhea begins for a total of 8 ounces, two days in a row. Remember,

THE MILKSHAKE THAT COWED *TURISTA*

Someday soon, travelers may be inoculated against *turista*. Scientists from the University of Maryland may have come up with a concoction that can give traveler's diarrhea a run for its money. Since a type of bacteria called *E. coli* is the most common cause of *turista,* the researchers decided to test the effects of a concentrate made from the milk of cows that had been immunized against that very bacteria.

The results are encouraging: Ten volunteers given the concentrate proved immune to a drink contaminated with *E. coli.* Of another ten volunteers who drank a formula made of milk from cows not immunized against the bug, nine developed diarrhea, cramps, and other symptoms.

Carol O. Tacket, M.D., head of the study, is continuing her research and hopes it will someday lead to a remedy for traveler's diarrhea.

though—Pepto-Bismol is *medicine.* It contains salicylates —aspirin is a salicylate. So if you're already taking aspirin for other health conditions, like arthritis, be careful. You could overdose.

Attack with antibiotics. Before you leave home, it's a good idea to ask your physician for advice and a prescription for antibiotics, Dr. Ericsson suggests. In a recent study, he found that diarrhea was cut down to 1 hour or less in moderate to severe cases with two doses of antibiotics in combination with Imodium. "You can take Imodium as often as you need to," Dr. Ericsson says. If you continue to have cramping, fever, or bloody stools after a day or so of treatment, seek medical help.

HEADING TURISTA *OFF AT THE PASS*

Even experienced globetrotters will tell you that getting the trots is almost inevitable at one time or place or another. But there are several time-saving tips that can help you avoid *turista* in the first place.

Learn this simple phrase. A quick way to remember the rules for avoiding *turista* is to memorize this dictum: "Boil it, cook it, peel it, or forget it." (Details follow.)

Boil water for 1 minute. To sterilize tap water for drinking, cooking, or brushing your teeth, the U.S. Public Health Service advises travelers to bring water to a vigorous boil for 1 minute and let it cool to room temperature before using. William B. Strum, M.D., a gastroenterologist at the Scripps Clinic in La Jolla, California, suggests hotel guests should use an electric-coil heater in a cup of water. (To avoid a fire, read the directions and heed the voltage.)

Disinfect with iodine. If boiling water isn't practical, you can disinfect it. Use 2 percent tincture of iodine (available in pharmacies and sporting goods stores.) Add ten drops or one tablet to a quart of clear water. Let stand for 30 minutes before using. Longer stand times may be necessary for very cold or cloudy water. (*Never* drink untreated water from mountain streams or wash food in it.)

Say aqua puraficada, por favor. This means "purified water, please" in areas of Latin America. Otherwise, any kind of bottled or carbonated beverage is generally safe, provided it's served in the original container. Be sure to wipe off the mouth of the bottle before drinking the beverage.

Order drinks with no ice. Freezing doesn't kill germs, so ice made from contaminated water is still contaminated. (And regardless of what anyone may tell you, alcohol does *not* decontaminate water or ice.)

Sidestep street vendors. Limited or nonexistent sanitation facilities or refrigeration makes eating food purchased from street vendors riskier than restaurant dining.

Eat well-cooked food only, served steaming hot. The U.S. Public Health Service tells people not to eat raw (or undercooked) meat or seafood, and most raw fruits and vegetables. (Fruit is okay if you can peel it first.) Also verboten are milk, butter, ice cream, custard, and uncooked cheese.

Wash and dry your hands thoroughly before handling food. Not all traveler's diarrhea can be blamed on other people's bad habits. Be sure you wash your hands before eating or preparing food, especially after using the toilet. Taking an extra 2 minutes to practice good hygiene is prudent at home or abroad. If you can't wash your hands, at least hold your sandwich, fruit, or other "finger food" with a paper napkin.

Rinse your mouth with your toothbrush. A few drops of water won't hurt you as you brush your teeth, but risking swallowing a mouthful of water might. After brushing your teeth, rinse your toothbrush with hot tap water and use the rinsed toothbrush to clean away excess paste.

Reach for Pepto-Bismol. Did you know bismuth subsalicylate actually kills germs? Commercially sold as Pepto-Bismol, it can cut your chances of getting traveler's diarrhea by 65 percent. You can start taking it the day you leave home and continue for two days after your return. But even if you take Pepto-Bismol, it's still a good idea to watch what you eat and drink. And don't be concerned if the Pepto turns your tongue and stools black—it's a harmless side effect of Big Pink.

The recommended dosage to prevent diarrhea is two chewable tablets four times a day, for up to 21 days. Again, if you're already taking aspirin (a salicylate), keep in mind that Pepto-Bismol contains salicylates. Be careful not to overdose.

Think twice before taking preventive antibiotics. Taken ahead of time, antibiotics like doxycycline, co-trimoxazole, and norfloxacin can cut your chances of coming down with diarrhea by 90 percent. Antibiotics stymie troublemaking bacteria before they can take hold in your stomach and intestines.

But the problem is that antibiotics taken over a long period of time have potentially serious side effects—notably skin disorders or a rare but fatal rash called Stevens-Johnson syndrome. And taken indiscriminately, or not taken for the full course, antibiotics promote the growth of antibiotic-resistant organisms.

So it's best to reserve antibiotic use for treatment of infection rather than trying to prevent infection. And closely follow your doctor's instructions on its uses.

A SOLUTION FOR JET LAG

If you skip lunch, you might feel tired and irritable. Skip a few time zones, however, and you'll feel a whole lot worse. Like lights and appliances you can set to turn on and off when you're away from home, your brain, digestive tract, bowels, and other organs work on preset timers, too. In fact, every cell in your body functions in day/night cycles, roughly based on so many hours of light and activity followed by an equally predictable period of dark and rest. Now that air travel makes it possible to pass through many different time zones, east or west, in just a few hours, you can stretch or shrink periods of light and dark, throwing off your internal timers. You may land in London at noon, but your brain and other organs think it's 7:00 A.M. The resulting discomfort and disorientation is "transmeridianal fatigue," commonly called jet lag.

Common jet lag symptoms include irritability, diminished alertness, fatigue, insomnia, constipation, and depression. Normally, it takes your body one day to adjust for each time zone crossed. But a special anti-jet-lag program devised by Charles F. Ehret, Ph.D., an expert in chronobiology (the study of biological cycles) can help you reset your body clock in just a day or day and a half, even if you've traveled across five or six time zones. The program is fairly elaborate and uses various internal and external cues called zeitgebers—light, food, caffeine, exercise, and social interaction (like conversation or paperwork). But here, in abbreviated form, are some simple steps to ease the transition to a new time zone.

Get some extra sleep before you depart. "Sleep deprivation is a big part of jet lag," Dr. Ehret explains. "So if you can, pad your sleep time by 15 minutes or half an hour. If you normally get 7½ hours of sleep a night, get 8. Don't do a lot of last-minute shopping or partying. Start out well-rested."

Wake up with isometric exercises. If you're landing in London or Zurich at 3:00 A.M. (home time), you can help wake up your body in time for breakfast at destination time by squeezing a ball in the palms of your hands for 5 minutes, pressing your hands together in front of your chest, doing deep-knee bends in the back of the plane, and otherwise stretching your body into wakefulness, Dr. Ehret says.

Talk to your neighbor. Another way to cue your brain that a new day is beginning after as much in-flight rest or sleep as you can manage to enjoy (even if your watch says it's the middle of the night) is to engage in lively conversation for 15 or 20 minutes. If that's not practical, do some paperwork or other intense intellectual activity, Dr. Ehret says.

A COMPUTERIZED REMEDY FOR JET LAG

Calculating what you should eat, when you should sleep, and each of the essential other factors for overcoming jet lag can be time-consuming and confusing. Now a computer can do it for you, in seconds. Dr. Charles F. Ehret developed the program, called Jet Ready, and it's available from Kinetic Software, 12672 Skyline Boulevard, Woodside, CA 94062 (415-851-4484; Fax 415-851-2457). Your travel agent just punches in your itinerary and the computer tells you how to manipulate your intake of food, sleep, light, exercise, caffeine, and other zeitgebers to prevent jet lag.

Eat a high-protein breakfast. Food is another useful tool for cueing your body that a new day has begun. So if it's morning at your destination, eat breakfast on time! Last night's in-flight supper menu heated and served especially for you at this time works well. Concentrated sources of protein — cottage cheese or other dairy products, skim milk and bran flakes cereal, lean meat — sustains blood sugar energy throughout the morning, according to Dr. Ehret.

If you arrive at night, hit the sheets. Even though it's still happy hour at home in Houston, it's already bedtime in London. So go to sleep strictly on time if you can or even half an hour earlier than usual. Again, the idea is to slip into the local time frame as soon as possible.

Set your alarm, and arise at sunup. You may be tempted to skip breakfast and sleep late the first morning after you arrive. Don't.

Step out into the light. If you're eastbound, an early-morning walk or jog outdoors in bright light on the first and second days after arrival is an excellent way to quickly get into sync with your new time and destination, Dr. Ehret says. If you're westbound, get out in the late afternoon or early evening. "Anchoring" your day with 15 or 30 minutes of exposure to bright light, morning and evening on the following days, with lunches *al fresco* whenever the weather permits, is especially important if you're cooped up in business meetings or a convention hall most of the day.

Eat lunch precisely on time. "Eating meals on time is a key anchor for phase shifting," Dr. Ehret says. "If possible, eat outdoors, with others, to combine social cues—like conversation and activity—with light and with exercise before and after the meals, to maximize the effect."

HOW TO UNCLOG YOUR EARS

Some people can tell when an aircraft is descending without looking at the scenery: Their ears feel "full" and start to hurt in response to small increases in air pressure against one or both eardrums as the aircraft descends. Sometimes your ears can equalize the pressure on their own, and sometimes they can't. Here are some simple steps you can take to quickly stop the pain.

Pinch your nose and blow gently. Any blockage in the eustachian tube (connecting the back of your nose to your ears) can prevent equalization. Pinching your nose shut and exhaling through the blocked airway for a second or two usually relieves discomfort.

Gulp and chew gum. Repeated swallowing, drinking, or gum chewing may also help equalize pressure in your ear passages.

Open wide and say Ahhh. Yawning or moving your lower jaw from side to side every minute or so can also open the eustachian tubes and clear the ears.

ANTIDOTES FOR ALTITUDE SICKNESS

The world's highest places—like the Himalaya mountains of Tibet or the city of Machu Picchu in the Andes of Peru—are sources of wonder and exhilaration. But ascend too high, too fast, and you're likely to experience a type of physical distress aptly called altitude or mountain sickness. Symptoms of mild altitude sickness include loss of appetite, throbbing headache, nausea, vomiting, sleeplessness, a feeling of fullness in the chest, or some combination of symptoms triggered as your body struggles to adjust to the change in atmosphere at higher elevations. Even physically fit people are susceptible.

The cause of the problem is a lack of available oxygen. Because there is less oxygen in the air at high elevations, your heart and lungs have to work harder to provide the amount of oxygen needed by your body. As a result you feel tired, sick, and not surprisingly, out of sorts.

You don't have to trek across the mountains of Nepal to suffer altitude sickness, though. In the United States, skiers have been known to experience the effects at as low as 8,000 feet. And according to the *Western Journal of Medicine*, more than 60 percent of climbers on Mount Rainier, Washington, suffer at least mild altitude sickness.

Still, more than 40 million people around the world live at elevations of 8,000 feet or higher, so obviously a body can and will adjust, given time. Here are some ways to enjoy your own peak experiences.

Be a slowpoke. The greatest risk seems to be the speed of ascent, not the altitude reached. So, eager as you may be to plant your flag at the summit, don't start your trek by bolting uphill like a billy goat. As you ascend, you'll gradually breathe faster to compensate for the air's thinness. Other changes will occur, too, as your body adapts to the higher elevation. Remember the story of the race between the tortoise and the hare? Be a tortoise.

Take 1,000 steps, then make camp. Doctors say climbers should allow one day to ascend 1,000 feet at elevations of 10,000 to 14,000 feet and two days to ascend 1,000 feet at elevations above 14,000 feet.

"Staging" your climb in this way will delay reaching the summit, but it's the best way to prevent altitude-induced illness. Gradual ascent, by the way, is safer than relying on drugs, which may mask early, important warning signs of altitude sickness, a condition that can be fatal if it's not managed correctly.

Declare a one-day R and R. If possible, plan to stay at one altitude for a day or two, allowing time for your body to recover and adjust before you climb higher. Richard Dawood, author of *How to Stay Healthy Abroad*, recommends a "rest day" for every 3,000 feet of ascent above 9,000 feet.

Top off your canteen with H_2O, not C_2H_6O. Alcohol will only add to the problem of dehydration, which is common at higher altitudes and may contribute to altitude sickness. Instead, drink lots of water—1½ quarts a day.

Snack all day. In addition to rest and fluids, you need steady nourishment. Eat small, frequent, carbohydrate-rich meals and snacks.

Take a breather. In fact, take several. Ten to 12 deep breaths every 4 to 6 minutes can help increase oxygen levels in your blood, according to James A. Wilkerson, M.D., a climber-physician and specialist in environmental and high-altitude medicine.

Go downhill fast. With rest, most people will recover from mild altitude sickness in time to continue their ascent. But if you don't feel any better after three or four days, descend *promptly,* while you're still able to walk under your own power. If mild altitude sickness pro-

A PSYCHOLOGIST'S TIPS FOR FEARLESS FLYING

"Airplane apprehension" isn't a newscast euphemism for a plane hijacking. It's just another name for plain old fear of flying—the nervous feeling that once you board a plane, just about *anything* can happen.

All the statistics saying that you're 70 times safer in a plane than a car mean nothing to the fearful flyer. "Fearful flyers do not even know how to think like normal, relaxed flyers," says Albert G. Forgione, Ph.D., who's helped more than 4,000 people overcome the worry of air travel. "All they know how to do is worry, which isn't thinking at all, but the rehearsing and rerehearsing of negative expectations based on feelings, not knowledge. So the first step in overcoming fear of flying is a technique called thought stopping, to control what's going through your mind, followed by some relaxation training."

A few minutes of active relaxation can prevent many hours of worry. Here's Dr. Forgione's program, in a nutshell.

Put the brakes on fear. "The moment you sense you're starting to worry, tell yourself 'stop,' " Dr. Forgione says. "Then take a slow deep breath. Next, s-l-o-w-l-y

(continued)

A PSYCHOLOGIST'S TIPS
FOR FEARLESS FLYING—*Continued*

exhale, while thinking 'relax.' Finally, smile and imagine a pleasant setting, like sitting on a sunny beach under a palm tree." This exercise, practiced every time you feel a wave of anxiety coming on, can break the chain of worry before it escalates into a full-blown anxiety attack.

Breathe with your belly, not your chest. "Abdominal breathing slows your heart rate, in addition to being more efficient than upper-chest breathing, which speeds up your heart rate and increases anxiety," Dr. Forgione says. "It helps to put a small pillow at the small of your back, to compensate for the typical airline seat, which is designed to pitch you forward in a semicrash position."

Relax one muscle at a time. Anxious people usually scream at themselves to relax when they're tense, but in fact, it causes even greater anxiety, and fearful flyers are no exception. So Dr. Forgione teaches them, "Gradually tense and relax each muscle group. Start with your feet, thighs, buttocks, stomach muscles, hands, shoulders, face, and forehead. At the same time, take slow, deep breaths, and exhale slowly, like a deflating balloon. As you do, repeat to yourself,' relax.' That way, the next time you tell yourself to relax, you'll know how!"

Start practicing the day your airline tickets arrive. "Anxious moments are no time for analysis," Dr. Forgione says. "And in truth, most of the agony occurs on the ground, before you board." So practice breathing and relaxation training before the day of the flight, be it the next day, the next week, or next Christmas."

Place your hands in your lap, not on the armrests. "The typical white-knuckle flyer spends the whole flight grabbing the seat arms. They feel every vibration in the aircraft, heightening anxiety," Dr. Forgione explains.

Order juice or decaf. Consuming too much sugar, caffeine, booze, or carbonated beverages before or during a flight will leave you wired, bloated, and dehydrated, exacerbating anxiety. "Instead, eat a low-sodium snack every 3 hours, like crackers and peanut butter or dried fruit, and drink fruit juice, even if you have to pack your own food," Dr. Forgione says.

gresses to pulmonary edema (fluid accumulation in the lungs) or other severe disorders, the chance of recovery grows dim. On the other hand, descending as little as 500 or 1,000 feet may bring dramatic improvement.

Dr. Wilkerson recalls an instance where a woman hiking in Nepal got altitude sickness at 12,000 feet. She didn't even know her name. She was carried downhill about 500 feet by a Sherpa, and within just 30 minutes, she was coherent again. "The improvement can be that dramatic," Dr. Wilkerson says.

WEIGHT LOSS

s today the first day of your new, slimmer life? Are you ready to lose weight and get fit for the very last time — because you're going to stay that way? If your answer is yes, then you're ready to use these fast-action strategies dieters have found for unloading extra weight and building a better body.

- Take 10 seconds to add a calorie-burning taste-booster to your food.
- Do 30 seconds of simple arithmetic to help drop your diet below 30 percent fat.
- Do 2 minutes of planning that can keep you from a snack-attack binge.
- Learn a 10-minute trick that can put an end to overeating.

GET READY TO LOSE

Successful dieters share a few common traits. The first and probably most important is that their motivation to lose weight comes from within. To have the perseverance you need for success, *you* must want to become thinner. A second trait is the willingness of successful dieters to involve their minds as well as their tummies in the dieting process. You have to think up a plan, again one that works for *you,* and follow it.

Start by being selfish. "If someone tries to lose weight because their doctor or spouse told them to, that's the kiss of death for their diet," says John P. Foreyt, Ph.D., of the Nutrition Research Clinic and Baylor College of Medicine, Houston, Texas. "People tend to drop out quickly if they're trying to lose weight for someone else. You're much more likely to stick with it if you're doing it out of self-motivation.

Write it out. "Write down your reasons for losing weight and refer back to them when you're tempted to stray," Dr. Foreyt says. "Pick something that's personally compelling —what turns me on might not motivate you."

Take a look back. Check for the breakdown point in your last weight-loss attempt, see what caused it, and leave that technique out of your new game plan.

Do a little homework. To lose a pound of fat, you need to burn up 3,500 calories over and above what you take in. People who don't realize this tend to become disappointed when they aren't losing a pound a day, even though that kind of fat loss is next to impossible. Find out what your physician thinks is a reasonable weight-loss schedule for you. Believe it or not, it might be a little more lenient than the one you cook up on your own.

Make small changes. Change little behavior patterns, things that you can accomplish with a fair chance of success. For example, start off the first week by no longer snacking in the car. Then, boycott food in front of the TV. As you get one small section of your life under control, go on to the next.

Give yourself a gentle reminder. Don't go out and buy a bikini or dress four sizes too slim. What ends up happening is you keep trying the clothes on, and when they don't fit, you're reminded that things aren't moving along as fast as you'd like. Then the whole project starts to look impossible. Cut out a picture of that swimsuit or dress and put it on the refrigerator as a gentle reminder.

Make a flexible plan. "Know how many calories or how many foods from each food group you're going to eat each day," recommends Dr. Foreyt. "If you overeat at one meal, plan to eat less at the other meals."

Grade success fairly. Everyone deviates from their weight-loss plan at some point. Keep in mind that if you blow your diet as much as one-fifth of the time, that's still an 80 percent success rate, which on a grading scale of A to F would give you a B—no reason to drop out!

Get a hobby. This could mean going to the movies a little more than usual, taking up hang gliding, or collecting coins. But make it something you can truly get lost in, something that, for a time, lets you forget the world—and food—around you.

Set small goals. Plan on rewarding yourself after every 2, 3, or 5 pounds and make those rewards progressively more grand as you go along.

Gear up. Get yourself some bright, exciting exercise clothes. Make your mind say, 'I'm going to put them on, I'm going to get ready, and I'm going to feel good about doing this.

Accept yourself. Most weight-loss programs put the cart before the horse and imply you can accept yourself after you lose weight. If you see yourself as a crumb for being overweight, you can't possibly succeed, because your assessment will be a self-fulfilling promise.

Do it now. Don't tell yourself that weight loss is always easy, therefore you can conveniently lose, if and when you get around to it. After all, if something is such a snap to accomplish, it's hardly worth putting forth the effort.

Stock up on humor. When chocolate-eclair deprivation leaves you a little blue, administer a dose of the Marx brothers. A couple of laughs will put everything, including your diet, in a better light.

ADOPT A WEIGHT-LOSS MINDSET

Thinking like a thin person can help you to become one. When you review a menu, plan your evening, put together a grocery shopping list—imagine the way a slender person would do it. Then imitate that model.

Fast every day. But only from 9:00 P.M. until you go to bed. These are the hours when self-control tends to fall asleep while our eyes are still watching TV.

Keep farmers' hours. Tuck yourself in an hour earlier than usual. That will make it a lot easier to maintain your post-9:00 P.M. fast. It'll also get you out of bed earlier, so you can find time for exercise.

Phrase it light. When you look at a menu or buffet table heavy and congested with food, say to yourself, "I'm a person who doesn't eat very much." Does it work? About half the time—good for a couple of pounds not gained each year. Try it. Remember, you're not saying you don't like to eat, just that you're satisfied with a reasonable amount.

Save the best for last. Contract with yourself to do

something that's difficult yet beneficial, before allowing yourself a more pleasurable activity. For example, exercise before you allow yourself to read a book or watch TV.

Use a cuff. If your blood pressure's on the high side, buy a home blood pressure monitor and take your reading every morning. As you lose weight, you should see a gradual decrease in pressure. That in turn can be an important motivator for continued weight loss.

Know your cholesterol. For the same reason you want to know your blood pressure, you should know your cholesterol reading. Losing excess poundage can often bring cholesterol down, too. Seeing that work, over time, tells you your weight loss is doing great things for your health.

DEVELOP A STRATEGY

Every successful plan involves some up-front work. If you are going to overcome years of impulsive eating, or develop a taste for foods you never ate in the past, you're going to need some solid strategy.

Write it down. Keep a food diary, which includes not only what you eat but when and where. You'll be able to identify patterns and "food cues" that stimulate you to overeat.

Identify your habits. The following food habits seem to make you store more fat, regardless of how many calories you eat, said Japanese researchers at the International Symposium on the Dietary and Metabolic Basis of Obesity and Its Prevention.

- Gorging just before resting. Example: Eating a large meal before hitting the sack.
- Eating refined, processed grains, not whole grains. Example: White bread instead of whole wheat bread.
- Consumption of soft, digestible foods rather than hard, more difficult-to-digest foods. Example: Eating applesauce instead of apples.

Learn to read labels. Fat in prepared foods shouldn't exceed 30 percent of the total calories. Figure the percent of fat per serving with this formula: Grams of fat per serving times 9 divided by total calories per serving.

If the answer exceeds 30 percent, leave the package on the shelf or eat the food only in small portions.

Get the cold facts. Convenience-minded dieters have made low-calorie frozen dinners a multi-billion-dollar business. They're microwaveable, they're easy, and they automatically limit portion size. But so-called lean or light frozen foods aren't always low in fat. Some have more than half their calories from fat.

Learn the label lingo. Supermarket labels can be misleading. Here's what some mean.

Lean: No more than 10 percent fat by weight—not by calories.

Extra lean: No more than 5 percent fat by weight—not calories. (When applied to raw meat, Lean and Extra lean mean it has no more than 30 percent of its calories from fat.)

Leaner: At least 25 percent less fat (by weight) than the original product.

Dietetic: One or more ingredient—usually sodium or sugar—has been changed, restricted, or substituted. Dietetic items are not necessarily lower in calories.

Sugarless/sugar-free: Contains no table sugar (sucrose), but might contain corn syrup, fructose, honey, sorbitol, or other sweeteners. Not necessarily lower in calories.

Low in calories: No more than 40 calories per serving, or no more than 0.4 calories per gram.

Reduced calories: One-third fewer calories than the product it most closely resembles; meat and poultry items must contain 25 percent fewer calories than similar products.

No cholesterol: There is no legal definition. Items carrying this label may still contain saturated fats, which raise blood cholesterol. Be aware that "No Cholesterol" labels do not mean "No Fat."

Eat your breakfast. Breakfast serves as a "metabolic kicker." The body needs fluids and a range of nutrients in the morning to get started. And breakfast will ward off the afternoon munchies.

Shop with a list. It can help you resist flashy displays of high-fat foods, fragrant bakery counters, and other lures that encourage impulse buying.

Research psychologists from Lincoln University in Jefferson City, Missouri, found that women who prepare menus for the entire week and convert these menus to shopping lists that are organized by store aisle not only purchase fewer calories but avoid wandering and impulse buying.

Make a ten-most-wanted list. Write down ten foods that are low in calories, low in fat, and that you actually like to eat. (If you have never liked carrots, it won't do you any good to put them on your list.) Then make sure that all ten of them are in your refrigerator or pantry.

Learn ten new recipes. Most people have about ten recipes that they enjoy and use again and again. If you can learn ten alternative, low-fat recipes that you enjoy cooking and eating—maybe even low-fat versions of the same dishes—you'll go a long way toward ensuring a healthy diet.

Know thyself. A strong urge for sweets is an urge only made worse by total denial. Nutritionists offer this solution: If you know it's going to lead to bingeing, don't try to deprive yourself of sweets totally. Instead, incorporate controlled portions of sweets into your daily diet.

Plan a snack. Four o'clock in the afternoon seems to be the witching hour for many would-be dieters. Instead of trying to stick it out and failing, plan a snack for this or any other particularly tempting time, says Christine Beebe, R.N., who specializes in diabetes management. Take the calories from somewhere else in your day. The trick is planning: It protects you from impulsively eating something you'd rather not.

FOOD SECRETS THAT SLIM WHILE YOU EAT

The rice diet, the grapefruit diet, the put-nothing-in-your-mouth-but-cottage-cheese diet all are bound to be unsuccessful. Human beings crave variety, not only for taste satisfaction but for nutrition as well. Any one-food plan will last only so long before the person following it goes absolutely bonkers. Here are some tips that will help you keep to your regimen.

Eat a variety of foods. A good meal should include three types of food—three different colors—at several different temperatures. This kind of eating is best for your body and triggers feelings of satisfaction.

Slow down. When you do eat, take your time. A meal should last at least 20 or, ideally, 30 minutes. You need time to chew thoroughly, to concentrate on enjoying the sensations of eating: taste and smell. You'll feel more satisfied.

Try the carb trick. Start your meal with a high-carbohydrate food, like a pasta appetizer, bread without butter, or a bean or noodle soup. That should lessen your fat craving as the meal wears on, and then you won't be as likely to want a high-fat dessert.

Spice up your food. Spiking rat food with capsaicin (the "red hot" in red pepper) makes rats eat more food but store less fat, says a Japanese study. The researchers conclude that capsaicin might help prevent obesity. This confirms other studies that have shown that hot, spicy foods, like chili and mustard sauce, have the potential for increasing metabolic rate. Burning calories simply by eating hot, spicy food is good news for lovers of tongue-tingling ethnic cuisine.

Take up a collection. Refrigerate canned meats, soups, gravies, and other canned foods containing fat. The fat will collect and rise to the top so you can scrape it off.

Ease into skim. Switching from whole to skim milk can spare you a lot of fat. Help your taste buds make the switch. Start out by mixing whole milk with 2 percent milk. After a month or so, try 2 percent mixed with 1 percent, and so on.

Be fruitful and subtract. Don't butter your toast. Use fruit preserves or fruit butters.

Grab the margarine. Do you feel you need butter or margarine on your bread? When you begin thinking about your next meal, cut off a wedge of your favorite spread and let it warm outside the refrigerator. You can cover your bread with only one-quarter of the calories you'd use if your spread were cold.

Choose the kindest cut. Trimming the fat can make a tremendous difference in the fat and calorie content of beef: A 6-ounce sirloin steak, for example, contains 480 calories and lots of fat. Trim away all the visible fat and you've got a 360-calorie steak with almost half the fat eliminated. In addition, a study done at Texas A&M University says trimming all the visible fat *before* you broil meat can cut the fat by nearly 20 percent compared with trimming fat after the meat is cooked. The invisible fat inside will keep the meat tender and juicy.

Shake it, don't bake with it. Sprinkle-on butter substitute doesn't taste just like butter, but it also doesn't contain cholesterol or fat. You can't cook with these products, but they will flavor eggs, vegetables, and popcorn.

Spritz a salad. Look for salad sprays, low-calorie salad dressings in pump-type bottles. You'll use less if you spray it on.

Brown bag your popcorn. Regular popcorn cooked in a microwave oven has about a third of the calories and fat of microwaveable brands. Place regular popcorn in a brown paper bag and fold over the top. Put it in the center of your microwave and cook 3 to 4 minutes on high. Don't add oil or other ingredients until after the popcorn is cooked.

Be a smart cookie. When you have to have a cookie, reach for a "hard" variety. Soft store-bought cookies generally have a higher fat content, getting as much as half of their calories from fat.

INCREASING FAT-FREE FLAVOR

Foods with a high fat content are often deeply satisfying. And when you don't pat on the butter, dry toast or baked potatoes can be mighty unappealing. So don't eat them! By switching to completely different foods, and by using spices and herbs, you can create meals and snacks that are truly gratifying.

Add spice to your life. You've already heard one reason to spice your food, now here's another. Spices are the most concentrated forms of flavor—exactly what your taste buds need when your stomach is growling. Research from the Monell Chemical Senses Center in Philadelphia shows that good taste, not monotony, is the key to losing weight.

Be food fickle. Eating more kinds of food may help you eat less of each. Why? By the third bite of any one food, you can barely taste it anymore. So switch from food to food, never eating two bites of the same food in a row. This strategy increases the impact of taste, odor, and texture sensations.

Heat it and eat it. Cold food is not always a hot idea. Hot food wafts more odor into the nose, just as it releases aroma into your kitchen, and satisfies your hunger. So eat popcorn fresh out of the popper. Or sip some soup.

Gnaw more. For years, behavioral psychologists have been urging us to chew food longer. Why? The longer you chew, the more time your stomach has to register that it's full. Also, chewing creates currents of air, which force odors into the nose, telling your body that you're satisfied.

Choose ethnic eating. Do your diet a favor, and make it Mexican, Indian, or Middle Eastern, advises registered dietitian Barbara Cerio, assistant professor at the Rochester Institute of Technology. That's because these foods usually feature rice and beans (either in the main course or as side dishes), which are low in fat, are healthy sources of protein and fiber, and contain essential amino acids. As an added bonus, these meals are usually cheaper than other ethnic specialties.

Add crunch to your salad. Instead of croutons on your salad, add melba toast to provide crunch without lots of calories. Most commercial croutons are loaded with oil. In contrast, melba toast is almost fat free. Two slices of melba toast broken onto your salad will add only about 35 calories, and you can choose a different flavor every day.

Zap that fat. Whenever a recipe calls for sautéed onions, garlic, or other veggies, microwave them. You'll soften them and bring out their full flavor without a bit of fat. If you need chopped, sautéed onions, for instance, place the onions in a custard cup, cover with vented plastic wrap, and microwave on full power until tender. One-third cup takes 2 minutes.

WEIGHT WATCHING WHILE EATING

Here you are, face to face with a dinner plate. And the aroma of food is making your mouth water. How can you remain vigilant, firm, committed to your program? Here's how.

Eat alone. The more people with you at a meal, the more you're likely to eat. That's what Georgia State University researchers found when they paid 63 adults to maintain diaries noting everything they ate, how hungry they were, and how many people were around. Compared with solitary meals, the average social meal contained more calories (591 versus 410 calories) and more fat (230 versus 157 calories). Researchers considered several reasons: Maybe you're encouraged to eat more; maybe diners eat like everyone else ("If everyone has dessert, so will I."); maybe you don't want to insult the cook.

Water down your appetite. Drink two cups of water before each meal. This may fill you up and it guarantees exercise (back and forth from the restroom.)

Learn 1-minute meal management. To control the amount of food you eat at mealtime, establish a time-out halfway through your meals. One trick: Put a large pot of cold water on the stove when you sit down to eat. When it boils (in about 10 minutes), get up and make a pot of herb tea. When you go back to the table, you probably won't feel like eating much anymore.

Get food out of sight, out of mind. It's Friday morning, and you know your receptionist has set out doughnuts on her desk. Do you try to convince yourself that you really don't want some cream-filled extravagance, or do you skulk in the back door and avoid the whole situation? If you're a skulker, you're more likely to lose weight, according to a new study conducted by Gerald A. Bennett, Ph.D., at Birch Hill Hospital in Rochdale, England. Food-avoidance strategies (such as tossing out leftovers, storing food in opaque containers, etc.) work better than just resisting temptation.

Cut your portions in half. This is an easy way to cut calories while still enjoying all your favorite foods.

Watch out for vacations. A study from Kent State University confirms it—people eat more fat and less nutritious foods when they eat snacks and meals away from home. But if you watch what you eat, you can stick with your resolve and still eat well.

Carry a low-fat snack survival kit. Avoid those high-fat snack stands. Pack your kit with goodies such as rice cakes, fruit, diet soda, air-popped popcorn, bagels, whole-grain crackers, bran muffins, and graham crackers.

In restaurants, treat yourself—but not too much. "A good rule is to choose no more than one special-occasion food per meal," suggests registered dietitian Sonja O'Conner, author of *The New American Diet*. In other words, don't choose a steak, plus sour cream and butter for your potato, plus Roquefort dressing for your salad, plus butter for your bread, plus cheesecake for dessert."

Don't make food the focal point of a trip. So says Adrienne Foreman, R.D., a dietitian at Weight Watchers International. "Instead, try fun activities such as biking, hiking, tennis, canoeing, swimming, and walking tours."

Don't leave your routine at home. If you belong to a health club, find out if they offer reciprocal arrangements with other clubs. You may be able to use a facility near your vacation spot. Or find a hotel that has a pool or exercise room.

ACTIVITY TODAY MAKES DIETING PAY

If the thought of exercise conjures up images of expensive health clubs populated by gorgeous young things in shimmering leotards, you're likely to think of yourself as an exercise misfit. You're more likely to take up exercise if you trade in that thought for a more conservative one. Picture a slender person taking the dog for a long walk. Couldn't *that* person be you? Here are some additional hints to get you up and moving.

Watch the clock. You don't have to shed a lot of sweat to lose weight. You just have to move your body on a sustained basis—ideally 15 minutes at a time—for a total of 30 minutes to an hour each day. Walk, climb stairs, swim, or choose another activity you like.

Burn your fat. The effectiveness of exercise in fat burning depends not on how hard you move, but how steadily. If someone wants to weigh about 10 percent less, they're going to have to move their body an average of 200 minutes a week, and many people will have to move 400 minutes a week. What do those minutes of movement do? They encourage the fat to leave the adipose tissue where it is stored, to go into the bloodstream and then the liver, where it is burned. If you're not active, any fat you lose by dieting will simply recirculate in the blood and return to the adipose tissue.

Pat yourself on the back. "Exercise helps you cope with hassles and promotes a feeling of well-being," Dr. Foreyt says. "And that's important because bad feelings are the major reason people fall off their diets. When people are depressed or stressed, they tend to revert to their childhood and comfort themselves with cookies and candy."

Exercise on empty, burn more calories. Try exercising before a meal. Overweight subjects in a recent study at Mount Sinai Hospital in New York burned significantly more calories when they exercised on an empty stomach than when they exercised after a meal. Lean people burned more when they exercised after they ate.

Chart your progress. A recent study shows that exercisers who monitor their own progress — recording their workouts and progressing regularly or even just discussing it with friends and family — stick to their fitness regimens longer than those who don't.

Skip the elevator. Walking up stairs burns 150 percent more calories than playing tennis and 23 percent more than running, reports a Cleveland Clinic study. Adding two flights of stairs to your daily activity could lead to a weight loss of 10 pounds in a year.

Make cycling easier. Many people ride exercise bicycles with too much resistance, causing unnecessary injuries to muscles and tendons from pedaling too hard. Increase revolutions per minute rather than resistance, and make sure your knees are slightly bent — not fully extended — at the bottom of your stroke.

Garden your weight away. A garden can help you weed your extra weight away. It keeps you outside in the sunshine, instead of inside in front of the television. Plus you get a wonderful sense of accomplishment when you see the success of your little vegetable patch. Another benefit: Fresh, homegrown vegetables taste better than the store-bought varieties.

Squeeze in exercise. Can't find time to squeeze just a half hour of exercise into your busy schedule? Try these suggestions.

- Get rid of a labor-saving device. That wonderful appliance that makes your life easy also robs you of the chance to burn off calories. The automatic dishwasher, for example, can add an extra 2 pounds a year. Having two or more cars for running family errands can add 10 pounds a year. So do a favor for your weight and the environment — burn calories instead of burning electricity and gas.

- Walk to work. If you're not close enough, park your car ½-mile away and walk.
- When you drive to the mall, park your car far from the entrance instead of circling around like a vulture, looking for the closest spot.
- Clear the table one dish at a time. You'll walk a little more as you clear the table.
- If you use fewer wastebaskets, you'll be forced to walk more to fill them up and then empty them.

Find a buddy. If going out to eat is a major social activity, why don't you find an exercise buddy instead? Cold winter weather may be a deterrent against exercise, but warm friends may give you the encouragement and enjoyment needed to stay active. Find a friend who's also watching his or her weight, and arrange to meet regularly for fun and fitness.

Spousercise. You'll follow your exercise program better when working out with your spouse, says a study from St. Francis Medical Center in Peoria. Nearly 50 percent of men who exercised alone quit their program after one year. Two-thirds of those exercising with their wives stuck with it.

MAINTAIN YOUR LOSS WHILE STANDING STILL

If you're determined to lose more than just a few pounds, you're in for the long haul. And after a few months, you may find that no matter how hard you diet, your weight remains about the same. Don't panic—you don't have to starve! You simply need a new strategy.

Know when to stop. Have you reached a plateau and can't seem to budge the dial on the scale? Maintain your weight for at least three to six months, then, if you need to, try to lose weight again. This avoids burnout and gives your metabolism time to readjust gradually, making changes more likely to stick.

Recruit help. Most maintainers have strong support from their families and friends. If you don't have a cheering section, see if you can recruit some help. Make a public commitment to weight loss. Exercise with others. Join a support group. Ask your friends to help you out.

Keep tabs on yourself. "Sometimes people get cocky

when they've lost weight," Dr. Foreyt says. "They try to see how much they can get away with."

If you catch yourself slipping back into your old ways, review what habits kept you fat and which habits made you thin, says Dr. Foreyt. Decide how you're going to cope with tempting situations. "Maintainers rated self-monitoring strategies as one of the most useful ways to keep weight off," Dr. Foreyt says.

Reward yourself without food. Back in the good old days, you were rewarded with candy and cookies and cake. Not anymore. Instead, make a list of nonfood rewards. Reward yourself for sticking to a low-fat diet, for exercising, for finishing a report, or for whatever you want.

The following is a list of rewards from *The Fat-to-Muscle Diet,* co-written by obesity physician, Peter D. Vash, M.D.

- Buy a Walkman for your walking program.
- Order a balloongram to be sent to you.
- Make something with your hands.
- Plan an imaginary vacation to a faraway place. Check out brochures. Put a map of the world on your wall and plan a new vacation a week.
- Send your laundry out this week.
- Treat yourself to a body massage.
- Go dancing.
- Sit on a park bench and people-watch.
- Make a pep-talk tape to play back to yourself.

Picture your perfect weight loss. An instant photo has a powerful impact on your diet. If you deny your true size and shape, a photo can help you face reality. A "before" shot can work as an incentive because it reminds you of the body you want to leave behind. When taken at regular intervals, photos work as a "visual progress report."

LAST-MINUTE HELP WHEN YOU'RE TEMPTED MOST

All your friends eat pizza for lunch and you eat salad. Then one day you hear yourself saying those dreaded words, "with pepperoni, please." What to do?

Lasso your diet when it starts to stray. Remind yourself why you decided to change your eating behavior.

Read back over your motivation list. If you lapse and eat too much, don't feel guilty. Remind yourself of how well you have done and figure out what led to your eating — was it your mood, people you were with, a certain time of day?

Make an immediate plan. When you catch yourself straying, stop. Get rid of the rest of the ice cream or whatever fattening food you're eating. Go for a walk. Get out of the house. If necessary, find an alternative means of satisfying yourself.

Ask for help. Call a friend when you need support.

LOOK 10 POUNDS LIGHTER WHILE YOU LOSE

It's an unfortunate fact of life that it takes a little time to lose weight. If you're eager to *look* slimmer right away, try these techniques.

Line up to slim down. You can lose weight — or the appearance of weight — by creating a few optical illusions. Creating the illusion of height, for example, takes attention away from your width. Vertical lines that lead the eye up make you look taller. Outfits consisting of one color can add height. A "V" neckline also leads the eyes up. To look taller or thinner, you might like to try the following ideas: vertically striped fabrics; long diagonal lines; decoration in lengthwise line on center front; narrow panels; long, narrow pointed collars or narrow "V" or "U" necklines; narrow belts to match garment.

Color yourself slim. The three dimensions of color — hue, value, and intensity — can change your appearance.

Hue: Some colors, like red, yellow, and orange, project a feeling of warmth. Warm colors are advancing and will make you appear closer and thus will increase your size. Colors like blue, green, and purple project a cool feeling. They tend to recede and decrease your size.

Value: Light attracts the eye, so lighter-colored garments will cause the wearer to appear larger than will medium to dark shades of a color.

Intensity: When wearing garments of intense colors, the wearer will appear larger. So to appear smaller, choose a cool hue in a medium value and a less intense color. If your favorite color doesn't fit that description, you still have slimming options. If you want to use warm colors, pick a duller intensity. For example, select rust instead of orange; maroon instead of pink. And if you like bright, warm colors, use them as accents at the neckline or in your accessories.

If you like red, select a red blouse that will be worn under a gray or navy suit. The red will keep the focus on your face.

Choose a pound-shedding fabric. Look for fabrics that are medium to lightweight and are crisp but not stiff. Examples include linen, twill, gabardine, most double knits and fine-wale corduroy.

Dull or matte-finish textures absorb light and generally make the figure look smaller. Look for such fabrics as wool crepe, wool flannel, gingham, denim, wool jersey, sailcloth, broadcloth, and chambray.

A smooth texture is slimming and tends to hide figure irregularities. Fabric examples include flannel, percale, crepe, linen, shantung, seersucker, wool challis, and lightweight tweed.

Focus on figures. The affect of patterned fabrics depends on the size, distinctness, and type of pattern. Indistinct outlines in small to medium patterns decrease the apparent size of the figure. Close, overall placement of design will also give the illusion of a decrease in size. Select subdued prints, geometrics, and plaids. The size of the design should be in proportion to your height. For instance, a tall individual can wear a large print better than a shorter person can.

Select adjustable clothes. A 10- to 15-pound weight loss is necessary to bring about a change in clothing size. Select designs that can be worn while losing weight,

. . . .

AVOID HOLIDAY WEIGHT GAIN

Are you one of the many people who add 10 to 15 extra pounds during the six-week holiday season—and then struggle for months to lose them? This is so common it's almost an American tradition. But it doesn't have to happen. By establishing new holiday traditions, you can weigh the same on January 2 as on November 2. You can maintain health, happiness, and your normal weight throughout the year. Here are some suggestions.

Find something else to talk about. Spend less time cooking, baking, poring over cookbooks, or shopping for delicacies. Try to talk less about dieting, recipes, food, and how delicious it all tastes. The more you do these things, the more excited you get about food, and the more you eat and stimulate eating in others. Focus more on the meaning of the holidays and the joy of spending time with family and friends.

Cut back on fat and sugar. Serve lighter meals, fewer desserts, or no desserts. Forget to buy candy and snack foods. If you must bake holiday goodies, cut down, and try cutting back by one-third or one-half on fat and sugar in favorite recipes. They'll probably taste the same—or even better.

Serve it up smaller. Learn to be content with one serving. One cookie tastes just like a handful; one serving of turkey and stuffing tastes just like the second and third. Put less food on the table. Serve smaller desserts by cutting a pie into eight or ten pieces.

Eat less often. Do you really need those food-filled coffee breaks? Enjoy friends over a cup of coffee or soft drink.

Keep temptation out of sight. Clear away food immediately after meals and put snack foods away. Try getting along without those dishes of candy and nuts—fill the pretty dishes with sparkling Christmas balls and a sprig of evergreen instead.

Relax—it's all right to eat a big meal now and then. Sometimes it happens. Don't worry. One meal will not sabotage your weight. Your body can adjust and handle it. But you need to remember a big traditional meal is just that—one meal. It's not a six-week eating marathon. Return quickly to moderation.

Exercise daily—even on those big-meal days. With all the food and sitting around, physical activity is a welcome change. It reduces stress and gives us renewed vigor and enthusiasm.

If you gain weight, get it off quickly. Eat less and exercise more until that extra weight is gone. It's much easier if you adjust back to normal weight between big meal days. Don't wait until the holidays are over.

SOURCE: Adapted from *Obesity and Health* (November 1989, p. 85). Copyright © 1989 by *Obesity and Health,* Healthy Living Institute, 402 South 14th Street, Hettinger, ND 58639. Reprinted with permission.

· ·

including separates, an ideal choice when your weight loss isn't evenly distributed, or less expensive items such as a new blouse, scarf, or jewelry. Sweaters, vests, or jackets can be worn open over several different sizes. Also consider clothing with elastic waistlines, wrap dresses, or skirts.

Add a sweater. "A sweater is a wonderful thing for a heavy man to wear—it covers the pot belly," says Lois Fenton, an image consultant in Mamaroneck, New York, and the author of *Dress for Excellence*. "Just make sure it is not too short or too tight."

Details count. Men should think vertically when choosing accessories, for instance, wearing long neckties and avoiding bow ties. Wear suspenders.

Padded shoulders are slimming, because they accentuate the inverse triangle of the classic male form. If you don't want to accentuate your rear assets, get that wallet out of your back pocket.

WOMEN'S HEALTH

. . . .

S ugar and spice and everything nice. Well, maybe not *everything*.

Roughly 40 percent of premenopausal women in North America suffer from premenstrual breast discomfort. One in 15 women of reproductive age suffer from endometriosis. Annually 2.5 million U.S. women fall prey to a parasite that causes vaginal infections.

Luckily, there are plenty of smart, sensible, and time-saving measures you can take to help ease yourself over the not-so-nice. In fact:

- In just 30 seconds, you can begin to stop premenstrual breast pain caused by nerve fibers stretched to the max.
- In just 3 minutes, you can banish premenstrual cramps.
- In just 5 minutes a day, you can help counter a uterine prolapse.
- In just 10 minutes, you can defend yourself against the night sweats of menopause.

Here's how.

MAKE MENSTRUAL DISCOMFORT A THING OF THE PAST

Menstrual or premenstrual discomfort is one of the ways your body lets you know what it's up to, beginning on day 1 of your cycle with the onset of your period.

The symptoms fall into four basic subgroups, says Guy Abraham, M.D., a researcher who has conducted extensive research into premenstrual syndrome (PMS) and menstrual discomfort. Some women suffer from water retention, breast tenderness, and gas. Others tire easily and crave sweets. Still other women are most troubled by anxiety and irritability and are prone to bad cramps. The fourth group suffers depression, confusion, feelings of withdrawal.

"The hormones that control menstruation are estrogen and progesterone, and when they begin to amass, they affect the central nervous system," Dr. Abraham says. "Normally, they work in tandem. But estrogen levels may soar, leaving a woman feeling anxious and irritable. Or maybe progesterone predominates, dragging her into depression and fatigue."

So how do you fight back fast? Here's what Dr. Abraham and other experts suggest.

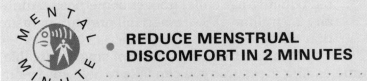

REDUCE MENSTRUAL DISCOMFORT IN 2 MINUTES

Just 1 or 2 minutes a day spent in creating "waking dreams" may significantly lessen your menstrual or premenstrual discomfort.

Here's an exercise to try. It is taken from *Healing Visualizations: Creating Health through Imagery* by psychiatrist Gerald Epstein, M.D.

Dr. Epstein calls this particular visualization The Desert Sand. He recommends that you practice it for 1 to 2 minutes, three or four times a day. Begin the visualization at the first sign of premenstrual discomfort and continue to practice it each day until your period ends.

Close your eyes and breathe in and out three times. See yourself in a desert. Cover your body with sand. Have the sun bake it into your skin. *Sense* the sand soaking up your internal water and the sun drying up the sand. Then open your eyes.

As simple as it may seem, many women find that making simple changes in their diet works wonders. In fact, Dr. Abraham's primary therapy is nutrition. Try these tips for your menstrual tribulations.

Cut out the caffeine. If you get anxious or irritable during your premenstrual period, entirely eliminating caffeine may stop that problem fast, Dr. Abraham says. If you have the caffeine habit, don't go cold turkey during the two weeks prior to your period—you may feel *really* edgy. Instead, start your withdrawal during a week *in your cycle* that you usually feel good.

Munch on magnesium. Whole-grain breakfast cereals and vegetables are high in magnesium, a mineral that can help smooth out contractions of the uterine muscle, the cause of menstrual cramps. Ask your doctor whether magnesium supplements could help, too. Dr. Abraham recommends that you first get off caffeine. If that doesn't help, he prescribes 500 to 1,000 milligrams of magnesium for women whose periods bring on cramps. (Magnesium also helps with irritability, bloating, swelling of the face, breast tenderness, and gas, he says.) You can begin this regimen at any time during your cycle. Expect to see some results within a few days, but know that you'll need to stick with it for three months before the maximum benefits are evident.

Try vitamin B₆. Dr. Abraham's recommended regimen includes vitamin B₆, which he says works along with the magnesium to combat the problems described above. "I usually recommend between 100 and 300 milligrams of B₆ daily. Do not exceed 300 milligrams a day to avoid B₆ toxicity," he says.

You can begin the B₆ at any point in your cycle. Again, expect results within a few days but give the supplement program at least three months before you judge how helpful it is. (Since large doses of B₆ have been associated with nerve damage, this regimen should only be used with the approval and regular supervision of your doctor.)

Consider calcium supplements. Researchers at New York Medical College gave PMS sufferers 1,000 milligrams of calcium carbonate daily. The preliminary but encouraging results: Seventy-two percent of the women reported significant relief within three months of beginning the calcium. The women had less pain, water retention, and mood swings during ovulation, and they had less pain during the actual time of their menstruation.

The researchers say that women suffering from PMS should discuss calcium supplementation with their doctors.

Chicken out on eggs and animal fats. Arachidonic acid, a fatty acid plentiful in animal fats, can stimulate your body to produce a substance that causes cramping, says Dr. Abraham.

Lay off spicy and greasy foods ten days before your period. That's the time when your progesterone levels are highest in your body, Dr. Abraham says. Progesterone is a hormone that, among other things, helps relax smooth muscles in the body, so your digestive organs may not be working their best then.

GETTING PHYSICAL WITH PAIN

During your premenstrual and menstrual phases, your body is the source of pain, tension, and aggravation. But you also can make your body the source of relief, with simple breathing techniques and exercise.

Breathe deeply. Practice inhaling and exhaling slowly and deeply. Shallow breathing, which many of us do unconsciously, decreases your energy level and leaves you feeling tense, making menstrual pain even worse.

Sink into a yoga stretch. Kneel on the floor and sit on your heels. Bring your forehead to the floor and hold your arms against your body along the floor. Close your eyes. Hold this position for as long as it feels comfortable. About 3 minutes should take care of those cramps.

Work out the pain. Walk at a fast pace in fresh air, swim, jog, take up ballet or karate—do something physical you enjoy on a daily basis. Moderate exercise helps your blood circulate, relaxes your muscles, fights fluid retention, and increases your brain's production of pain-blocking endorphins. Dr. Abraham believes that a 20-minute walk each day is the best form of exercise.

More intensive exercise can also help. Studies have shown that 5 to 30 minutes of running can help decrease mental anxiety, and 30 to 40 minutes of running four days a week can bring relief from breast tenderness and fluid retention within four months of starting the running program. Swimming, skiing, and running have proven helpful in relieving premenstrual tension and headaches.

You may have to push yourself in the beginning if you're experiencing menstrual discomfort, but you're likely to find that making the effort on the bad days makes you feel a whole lot better. Over time, the "bad days" may dwindle down to nothing.

Take a mineral bath. Add 1 cup of salt and 1 cup of baking soda to a warm bath. Soak for 20 minutes. The added minerals make the water kinder to your skin, while the warmth increases your blood flow and relaxes your muscles, relieving cramps.

MEDICINE THAT CAN HELP

Sometimes, despite your best efforts with diet and exercise, menstrual symptoms persist. Medication may provide (we're sure you've heard this before) fast relief.

Take ibuprofen for cramps and indigestion. Non-prescription ibuprofen (Advil, Nuprin) may help relieve your cramping uterus and aching legs, back, and head. Prostaglandins, hormonelike substances, are naturally high when you begin your period because their primary job is to help your uterus contract and expel menstrual fluid. However, women with cramps and aching legs, back, and head have abnormally high levels of these hormones, causing the uterus to contract harder and longer than normal and creating the pain. Ibuprofen and other prescription antiprostaglandin drugs help limit the production of prostaglandins.

Menstrual-related diarrhea, nausea, and vomiting may also be brought on by high levels of prostaglandins, says Penny Wise Budoff, M.D., of the Women's Medical Center in Bethpage, New York. Her study showed that antiprostaglandin medications may ease these digestive upsets by limiting the manufacture of the culprit prostaglandins.

The dosage of ibuprofen is what you would normally take for pain relief: one or two tablets at the onset of

QUICK TIPS TO RELIEVE BREAST DISCOMFORT

You've heard of self-cleaning ovens, but did you know that your breasts have a similar built-in feature? The "self-cleaning" mechanism turns on automatically just as you finish your menstrual period. Now that your body "knows" that there's no baby on the way, it reabsorbs the fluid and the extra breast cells it created to enlarge the milk ducts.

But in 30 to 40 percent of women, material that should be reabsorbed is retained in the breasts, creating cysts. You'll feel this as lumpiness.

"Lumpiness is diffused over a wide area. You can feel thickening here and there," says Selig Strax, M.D., medical director of the Guttman Breast Diagnostic Center in New York. "That's different than a lump, which is something you can put your finger around. A lump is like a little ball," and that needs a doctor's examination.

Cysts aren't the only problem. If the fluid isn't reabsorbed, or the breasts overprepare for pregnancy, the swelling that results can be downright severe. (Swelling causes the nerve fibers to stretch, which can create significant pain.) Eight percent of American women suffer from monthly breast changes so disabling it disrupts their lives.

Here are some quick ways to alleviate the discomfort of these monthly, benign breast changes.

Switch to sorbet. It has less fat than ice cream. And choose skim milk over whole, skinless poultry over beef, and low-fat salad dressing over the heavy stuff.

In a Canadian study of 21 women who had persistent and severe cyclical breast discomfort, 6 of the 10 who cut their fat calories to 15 percent of total calories (they made up for the lost calories by increasing carbohydrates) found "significant relief" from pain, swelling, and lumpiness within six months. The remaining 11 women in the study did not cut back on fat, and only 2 of them showed any improvement after six months. The body makes different forms of estrogen, and one of them, estradiol, may be a suspected troublemaker, Dr. Strax says. A high-fat diet may cause the ovaries to produce more estradiol than is good for the body, leading to an overproduction of breast cells and thus, lumpiness, he says.

Slip into a support bra. It will take you half a minute to change bras at the first sign of breast pain. The extra support can prevent the breasts from moving around, helping to reduce the stretching of nerve fibers that can produce pain messages.

Can the caffeine. The results of a Duke University study are encouraging: Of 138 women with persistent monthly breast pain, 69 percent of those who made significant cuts in their consumption of caffeine reported a decrease or total absence of breast pain within a year.

Nurse your baby. "Mothers who decide to nurse notice a definite softening of the breasts," Dr. Strax says. "Nursing cleans out the ducts system, so that whatever partial blockages are in the breast are washed out. I've certainly seen a good deal of the lumpiness disappear in women who have breast-fed their babies."

. . . .

symptoms. Take as often as directed until the symptoms go away. The tablets should be taken with milk or food. (People with ulcers or who are aspirin sensitive should not use ibuprofen.) Acetaminophen won't do as good a job because it does not affect prostaglandins.

Check out estrogen therapy for serious menstrual-related depression. Women who suffer from monthly bouts of depression, withdrawal, memory loss, or suicidal feelings may need small doses of estrogen in the last two weeks of their cycles, Dr. Abraham says.

TIMELY CARE FOR UTERINE DISORDERS

The hard knots of uterine muscle fiber called fibroids; the inner uterine tissues that start growing outside the uterus, a condition known as endometriosis; a uterus that literally loses its support structure and collapses, called prolapse: These serious uterine problems account for about 80 percent of the hysterectomies performed. But don't think you are a candidate for uterine surgery just because your doctor has diagnosed you as having one of these problems. "Doctors today are showing a greater interest in more conservative forms of treatment," says Francis L. Hutchins, Jr., M.D., clinical associate professor of obstetrics and gynecology at Hahnemann Hospital in Philadelphia. These include estrogen creams and tablets, special exercises and devices for uterine prolapse, drugs that reduce the pain of endometriosis and shrink fibroids, and problem-specific surgery that removes just the fibroids or the troublesome endometriosis tissue, instead of the entire uterus. Here's what you need to know.

FINISHING OFF FIBROIDS

Uterine fibroids are found in one-third of women over age 35 but often pose little problem. In fact, more than 50 percent of all fibroids don't produce any symptoms, Dr. Hutchins says. You'll feel them as a lump over the bladder or something "rolling around on the inside during intercourse," says Joseph Bellina, M.D., director of the Louisiana-based Omega International Institute, a fertility clinic, and author of *You Can Have a Baby*.

These hard knots of muscle fiber that grow from the muscular wall of the uterus can become large enough, however, to affect the kidney, bladder, or other organs. Fibroids, which may be fueled by excess levels of estrogen, can cause menstrual problems, iron deficiency anemia, pelvic discomfort, constipation, infertility, and miscarriage. The symptoms range from mild to moderate to severe. If you have progressive abnormal bleeding, or the fibroid(s) partially obstruct your urinary or gastrointestinal tract, you probably will require surgery.

If you've had fibroid pain that's disappeared, chances are the fibroid has grown so big that it has escaped the bounds of the pelvic area. "This is a sign that you need to do something about it," Dr. Bellina says. Here are some suggestions.

Anticipate menopause. Watchful waiting may be your best course of action if you're approaching that time of life. Fibroids are sustained by estrogen, which dwindles after menopause, notes gynecologist Ruth Schwartz, M.D., clinical professor at the University of Rochester School of Medicine in Rochester, New York. If you and your doctor determine that the fibroid isn't causing you problems and you're soon to reach menopause, waiting may be the thing to do.

Ask about the new, faster-healing alternatives to a hysterectomy. If you need to have fibroids removed, you don't necessarily need a hysterectomy. "A lot of pelvic surgery that formerly required opening the abdomen now can be done through a hysteroscope, or more rarely through a laparoscope, to remove fibroids," Dr. Hutchins says. But not all surgeons are familiar with these relatively quick, lower-risk techniques—that's why you should be sure to ask.

A hysteroscope is a telescope-like instrument that's inserted through the vagina into the uterus and is used to cut off small fibroids. Since the surgeon doesn't have to cut into the body to insert the hysteroscope, your body doesn't have to go through the trauma of major surgery.

The laparoscope, which is inserted through a small incision in the abdomen, may be used to detect and remove fibroids on the outside of the uterus. Because the incision is so small, healing time is days rather than weeks. Usually, though, fibroids small enough to be removed by laparoscopy are too small to be causing problems.

Consider Lupron to make fibroid surgery easier. Lupron is a synethetic hormone that essentially stops a woman from making estrogen. The drop in estrogen starves the fibroids, and they shrink. The average woman can expect a 35 percent reduction in the size of her fibroids after 6 to 12 weeks of daily treatment with Lupron, Dr. Bellina says. Since the drug causes the body to mimic menopause, it can cause menopausal symptoms like vaginal dryness and, more significantly, may result in a loss of bone mass. "Women on Lupron have to be monitored very carefully for loss of bone mass," says Dr. Bellina. "Over a period of time, decalcification may occur."

The other problem with Lupron is that as soon as you stop taking it, "you're right back where you were," he says. "Lupron is best used to reduce the volume of the fibroids so that surgery is more successful."

PUTTING AN END TO ENDOMETRIOSIS

Like fibroids, endometriosis depends on a plentiful supply of estrogen and subsides at menopause. Unlike fibroids, endometriosis is often painful. It occurs when endometrial tissue—the same kind that's normally inside the uterus—instead grows outside it, either on the outer wall of the uterus or on other body organs like the ovaries, bowels, bladder, or appendix. As it grows, it anchors itself to internal tissue with small weblike scars. The condition affects up to 7 percent of women in the United States.

With menstruation, this extra endometrial tissue swells

and bleeds, too. Since this blood can't exit the body via the normal route, it causes swelling and inflammation. For women who suffer from the condition, the inflammation may create pain during bowel movements or intercourse, or intense cramps during the menstrual period. Women who have endometrial tissue in their fallopian tubes may also have difficulty getting pregnant.

Again, as with fibroids, there are ways to manage endometriosis before you resort to a hysterectomy.

Take ibuprofen. The hormone prostaglandin stimulates the uterine muscles to contract, expelling menstrual fluid during your period. These contractions can cause painful cramping even if you don't have endometriosis. But the disease can greatly magnify the pain. And again it's ibuprofen to the rescue, helping to limit the production of prostaglandins in your body. Consult your doctor about the recommended dose.

Cut back on caffeine. Instead, opt for fruit juice or herbal tea. If you reduce the caffeine level in your diet, you may find that the severity of your symptoms decreases. "Caffeine is a stimulant," Dr. Bellina says. "When you take a stimulant, any problem gets worse. It makes the whole system go into a hyper mode."

Give careful consideration to danazol. The leading medical treatment for endometriosis, danazol, inhibits your body's ability to produce the hormones that fuel the growth of endometriosis tissue. Danazol is available by prescription only. You may see some results in a month, but it could take six months for the drug to take full effect.

As with any drug, there can be side effects from danazol. One drug comparison trial showed that women in the danazol group had more complaints about weight gain, muscle pain, and depression than the women using a new drug called nafarelin. There were also some problems with liver enzymes and cholesterol counts.

Spray Synarel. Nafarelin is available in a new nasal spray called Synarel. It seems to control endometriosis without the weight gain, muscle aches, or cholesterol changes seen with danazol. It can, however, induce hot flashes and nasal irritation and is more likely to cause vaginal dryness than danazol.

This drug also is available by prescription only. The

VIDEO AND LASERS: LIGHT-SPEED ATTACK ON ENDOMETRIOSIS

While it sounds like something you'd find in a video arcade, video-laseroscopy is actually a brand-new surgical technique that can slice days off your recovery from endometriosis and ovarian cyst surgery.

True to its name, the technique pairs a surgical laser with a tiny video camera and telescopic lens. Surgeons make a small incision in the abdomen, insert a tiny TV camera attached to a long, thin tube called a laparoscope, and study the image projected on a video screen. They use a laser to remove the offending tissue.

Videolaseroscopy offers several advantages over the more traditional hysterectomy surgery for endometriosis, says Farr Nezhat, M.D., who developed the technique with his brother Camran Nezhat, M.D. (The doctors head the Fertility and Endocrinology Center and Endoscopy Laser Institute in Atlanta, Georgia.)

With videolaseroscopy, you can have the surgery, return home from the hospital that day, and be back at work within a few days, Dr. Nezhat says. The procedure is less traumatic than major surgery and you'll lose far less blood. Traditional surgery requires a hospital stay of several days and a recovery period of several weeks. The shorter hospital stay means a lower bill, too.

This procedure also leaves a much smaller scar. Surgeons have to make only a tiny incision, because the video camera and screen allow them to see inside without making a major cut in your stomach.

The technique seems especially effective for endometriosis sufferers who wish to become pregnant. In couples where endometriosis is the sole reason for infertility, the pregnancy success following this operation is about 60 to 75 percent, Dr. Nezhat says.

This technique could be successfully used for treatment of ovarian cysts or when the fallopian tubes are blocked by scar tissue at the ends or near the ovaries.

The only drawback is that you may have to search to find a competent surgeon. The Nezhats continue to train surgeons across the country, but think it may take ten years before the procedure is widely available.

Dr. Francis Hutchins of Hahnemann Hospital warns—and Dr. Nezhat agrees—that it is better to trust a skilled surgeon performing a standard hysterectomy than an inexperienced, ill-qualified surgeon wielding a laser. And to find the best qualified surgeon, ask your doctor or local medical society for a referral. Don't rely on advertisements. Or you can write to Dr. Nezhat at the Fertility and Endocrinology Center, 5555 Peachtree Dunwoody Road, Suite 276, Atlanta, GA, 30342.

twice-daily treatment usually begins during the first four days of the menstrual period. It is used daily until therapy is complete, usually three to six months. According to researchers, it works by temporarily stopping the body's production of hormones that plump up the uterine tissue before menses. In studies, it has brought about partial or total relief from pain of endometriosis within six months, although some results may be apparent within one month.

PROPPING UP A PROLAPSED UTERUS

Like fibroids and endometriosis, uterine prolapse doesn't always require you to have a hysterectomy. Prolapse results when the muscles and ligaments that support the uterus become weak, usually as a consequence of carrying and bearing children. Gravity takes over, the uterus drops and, in extreme cases, "falls" outside the vagina. (The hormonal changes during menopause also contribute to the laxity in the muscles and ligaments supporting the vagina, uterus, and bladder.)

One warning sign of prolapse is that your vagina feels loose during intercourse. Lower back pain, or the feeling of "a knob in the vagina" also point to prolapse.

Here are some alternatives to hysterectomy.

Take a Kegel break. Dr. Hutchins prescribes Kegel exercises in cases of mild prolapse to firm up the region. He says he often sees "substantial improvement," halting the condition.

How do you do a Kegel? Dr. Hutchins tells women that it's best to do them sitting down. "Tighten your pelvic muscles as if you were trying to shut off the flow of urine. Count to 10 and release. Do that ten times, three times a day or as often as you can. You may see results in two months."

Request estrogen tablets or cream. Dr. Hutchins usually prescribes these, along with the Kegel exercises, for women who have mild prolapse. Estrogen is necessary for proper tone of the muscles that support the vagina, uterus, and bladder.

Ask your doctor about a pessary. This ring-shaped device fits inside the vagina, supporting the uterus and vaginal walls. It may be worn full-time or just part-time during unusual stress to the uterus, Dr. Hutchins says. "I had a patient in her forties who was an aerobics instructor. When teaching, she would have symptoms of prolapse, a sensation of pelvic pressure. So we fitted her with an inflatable pessary—you insert it deflated and inflate it to the point of comfort. She can jump around as much as she wants and take it out when she's done."

To prevent inflammation, unpleasant discharge, or ulceration, pessaries must be changed and cleaned frequently, and they must be fitted properly by a doctor.

A stitch in time saves trouble. If you're just beginning to suspect prolapse, do your Kegels first, faithfully. If they—along with estrogen—don't help, you may have no choice but surgery. That's because Kegel exercises and estrogen increase the tone of the underlying muscles but won't help the ligaments that support the uterus, Dr. Bellina says. If your uterus has stretched its ligaments, the sooner you have surgery to shorten them, the better its chance of success. Wait too long and the situation can deteriorate so much you'll need major reconstructive surgery to reposition all your pelvic parts.

Surgery to shorten the ligaments will take about 30 minutes, "and patients are often able to go home the following day," Dr. Bellina says. "You can go back to work in five days, but for three to four weeks you may feel discomfort when you're sitting down. It's a little like having a baby." Of course, if you do have a baby after this kind of surgery, you'll need to have the surgery again.

HAVING A HYSTERECTOMY

You've done what you can to avoid having your uterus removed, but to no avail. You and your doctor agree that a hysterectomy is necessary. What are your options? Well, here is a situation where high-tech may not be the way to go: The scalpel is faster than the laser.

"If you and your doctor have decided that a hysterectomy is absolutely necessary, a skilled surgeon can do the job in 20 to 40 minutes," Dr. Bellina says. "The laser therapy requires 3 to 4 hours to slowly gobble up everything. That's because the particular kind of laser used won't cut through dense tissue as fast as a knife would." The standard operation also carries less risk because it's a shorter operation, he says. However, the laser can be used to remove adhesions, followed by the hysterectomy.

Convalescence time for the standard hysterectomy may also be shorter, says Dr. Bellina, who notes that recovery time is related to the amount of time a person is "under" on the operating table. Another drawback to laser hysterectomy is that it's more expensive and less widely available.

MANAGING MENOPAUSE

The withdrawal of estrogen at menopause sets in motion a process of psychological and physiological change that can last up to ten years after your last period. For many women, these changes begin in their forties. They don't have to be severe. In fact, in a five-year study of nearly 2,500 menopausal women, 85 percent of those asked about symptoms said they are never depressed.

Whether menopause represents a time of ripening into a new phase of your life or just an accursed—and seemingly endless—time of discomfort will depend in part on how well you manage disruptions like hot flashes, night sweats, insomnia, irritability, dry skin, and changes in vaginal tone. Here's how to handle the disquieting manifestations of menopause with dispatch.

COOLING DOWN HOT FLASHES

What's behind those waves of heat that flow through your body like lava, leaving you gasping for cool relief in the daytime and soaking your bedsheets with night sweats? Modern researchers aren't exactly sure, but they do know that estrogen influences the production of neurotransmitters, which carry messages to and from the brain. As estrogen levels drop off, the body's relay system may develop quirks that can temporarily upset your thermostat. Blood vessels may suddenly dilate, bringing on the flush of heat you experience as a "hot flash." These flashes can strike in rapid succession, just 10 to 30 minutes apart. The duration of the attack varies from woman to woman.

Here's how to get the fire inside under control.

Cool off. Slip off your sweater, sip a cool drink, switch on the air conditioner. Anything that helps cool you off on a sultry summer day will also relieve a hormone-triggered heat wave. For the rare occasions when hot flashes are followed by strong chills, just be prepared to rewarm yourself a few minutes later, by putting on a sweater or drinking warm tea.

As a bedtime preventive against night sweats, soak in a tub of tepid water until the water cools (which should take about 10 minutes) or, in winter, lower the thermostat to about 60 degrees when you turn in.

Check out vitamin E. New York University gynecology professor Lila E. Nachtigall, M.D., says 400 international units of vitamin E taken twice a day, with meals, can cut the frequency of hot flashes for some women. It seems to maintain estrogen levels on an even keel, she says. You may see results in as little as 2½ weeks. If you don't see results within 3 weeks, chances are the vitamin E won't work for you.

Check with your physician before beginning vitamin E supplementation. While the vitamin is generally con-

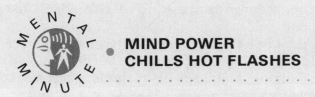

MIND POWER
CHILLS HOT FLASHES

Just because you're going through menopause doesn't mean you've lost all control over your body's internal thermostat. In fact, you can use your mind to reduce the intensity of those hot flashes.

First, relax using the technique outlined in "Progressive Relaxation" on page 376. Close your eyes. Use your imagination to picture a cool mountain stream. Step into it. Experience how cold it feels on your feet. Sense the coolness traveling up through your body and head. See yourself splashing water all over you, as much as you need to feel comfortably cool.

Ahhh. The fire is out.

sidered safe, it can have a blood-thinning effect and may interfere with other medications.

Keep a log and learn to relax. Each time you have a hot flash, note the date, time, intensity, and duration of it. Also record the circumstances preceding it and how you felt emotionally. After you've logged several episodes, try to identify any patterns. You may be able to avoid the triggers that ignited the flash.

De-booze, de-smoke, and decaf yourself. Alcohol, nicotine, and caffeine are all known triggers of hot flashes in some people, as your hot-flash log may reveal.

Take time to relax. In a study of ten menopausal women, psychologist Linda R. Gannon, Ph.D., found that stress increased the frequency, intensity, and duration of hot flashes for five of the women. One good way to beat stress is daily practice of a relaxation technique (see "Progressive Relaxation" on page 376).

BANISHING DRY SKIN

With menopause, your skin naturally becomes thinner and drier. Estrogen levels drop, and estrogen is what helps your body create collagen, a prime component of skin. Sweat glands tend to decrease in size with menopause, too. What to do?

Baby your skin with facial soap. Dermatologist Stephen Schleicher, M.D., codirector of the Dermatology Center in Philadelphia, advises his patients to use a soap meant for sensitive skin on their bodies as well as their faces. "Harsh deodorant soaps only aggravate already dry skin," he says.

Bathe less often and keep the water tepid. Since sweat glands have decreased in size, heavy deodorant soaps and frequent baths may no longer be necessary. "This is important to note, because soaking in a hot tub dehydrates already dry skin," Dr. Schleicher says. "When you do bathe, avoid very hot water and use a moisturizing bath oil to prevent further water loss."

Smooth on a lotion. While your skin is still damp from bathing, apply a moisturizing lotion. It will help seal in the water on your skin.

BRIGHTENING YOUR MOODS

It's true that the hormonal shifts that accompany menopause can affect your emotional well-being. It's also true that you don't have to be a captive to depression. In fact, in a five-year study of nearly 2,500 women who went through menopause, 85 percent of those asked about symptoms said they were never depressed. If you find that you *are* prone to depression, however, here are two quick ways to keep your moods bright.

Schedule fatigue-fighting sessions. If you're irritable because of sleep lost to insomnia or night sweats, take an afternoon nap.

Take a brisk walk to ward off depression. Evidence suggests that regular, energetic exercise may improve your mood by raising levels of endorphins (brain-produced good-humor hormones known to drop during menopause.)

DEFEATING VAGINAL DRYNESS AND LOSS OF TONE

Your vagina fills a crucial and intimate role in your femininity, and it is particularly sensitive to the sweeping changes menopause brings. It needs extra special care during menopause for three important reasons.

- The dwindling levels of estrogen in your system can cause your vaginal walls to become drier and thinner and, consequently, more vulnerable to irritation.
- The hormonal changes also disrupt the delicate alkaline/acid (pH) balance of the vagina. Disruptions in this balance can leave you more open to yeast and bacterial infections and irritation.
- The muscles supporting the bladder, uterus, and vagina may begin to lose their tone.

What can you do? Here's what our experts advise.

Seduce your spouse. Regular sexual activity (once a week or more) helps keep natural moisture flowing and maintains pelvic muscle tone, according to gynecology professor Gloria A. Bachmann, M.D., of Robert Wood Johnson Medical School in New Brunswick, New Jersey.

Take a warm bath to relax before you have sex. This

is a good way to relieve tension arising from menopausal symptoms, Dr. Bachmann advises.

Replace lost lubrication. If you still have a problem with vaginal dryness, you may want to try a brand-new nonprescription lubricant called Replens. It comes in single-dose, tamponlike dispensers, used every three days to provide continuous lubrication. Dr. Bachmann and a colleague tested Replens on 89 menopausal women who said the product stayed in place better than a standard water-soluble lubricant applied with a dispenser.

Another advantage: The lubricant helps normalize vaginal acidity, thus reducing the risk of infections. One note of caution, though: If you have a history of allergic reactions to medications, use this product only under a doctor's care.

Do your Kegels to strengthen pelvic muscles. Specially designed Kegel exercises zero in on crucial muscles: You use the same muscles you would to stop a stream of urine. This contracts the pelvic muscle. Do 10 contractions a day: 5 fast, plus 5 held for 3 to 5 seconds. Build up to a total of 50 or 100 contractions a day.

OVERCOMING CANDIDA ALBICANS

When your body says yes to a yeast infection, you have trouble. Trouble as in vaginal itchiness, burning, and a white, cheesy discharge.

The source of the trouble is the fungus *Candida albicans.*

Normally, the vagina does a fine job keeping itself clean and maintaining just the right alkaline/acid balance to protect against infections. But any number of things can throw that balance off: chemical douches, spermicides, antibiotics, birth control pills, or pregnancy. Once the balance is off, the fungus that causes candida — often present in women who have no symptoms — can go wild, multiplying until you're miserable.

Don't think you can diagnose the nature of your vaginal infection at home. You'll need a doctor to examine your discharge under the microscope and prescribe a specific treatment. Typically, doctors treat yeast infections with antifungal cream, which you insert vaginally every night for a week.

All you can hope to do at home is speed healing and prevent recurrence. Here's what our experts advise.

Skip milk and sugar. Studies show that eating a lot of dairy products, sucrose, or artificial sweeteners—all of which lead to increased urinary sugar—can precipitate and aggravate a yeast infection. Yeast grows rapidly in sugar.

Take a sitz bath. Fill a tub just to hip level with warm water and then add ½ cup of vinegar to help rebalance the vaginal pH, which is usually reduced to less than 4.5 in yeast infection sufferers.

Always wear cotton-crotch panty hose and underwear. They're your best bet against vaginal infections. Cotton "breathes" better than nylon and other synthetic fabrics, allowing moisture to evaporate. Cotton is especially valuable under leotards.

When you exercise while wearing outfits made of nonporous fabric, you cause moisture to pool close to the skin, creating the perfect climate for bacteria and fungus to thrive. The breathability of cotton helps the moisture to evaporate. The more that air can circulate, the less likely you are to develop infection.

Dry thoroughly after bathing. If your crotch area remains damp, the bacteria and fungi normally present in this area could multiply, invade vulnerable vaginal tissue, and initiate an infection. To be safe, use a blow dryer set on cool to remove excess moisture between your legs.

Use a condom. An unribbed, unlubricated condom may prevent you and your partner from passing the infection back and forth.

INDEX

Bacteria
    bad breath from, 146
    cavities and, 136
    traveler's diarrhea from, 491
Bad breath, 145–46
Baldness, 283
Balloon urethroplasty, 359–60
Bandages, 23, 131–32
Basement, asthma and, 4
B-cells, 331
Beans, 66, 306
Bed rest, for back pain, 38
Bedroom, allergens in, 3–4, 6
Bed-wetting, 63–64
Beer, for thicker hair, 284
Bee stings, 415–17
Behavior, Type A, 315–16
Belching, 176–77
Belly button, hemorrhoids and,
    74
Benadryl, 340, 405, 410
Benign prostatic hypertrophy
    (BPH), 358–61
Benzocaine, 127, 148
Benzodiazepines, 200
Benzoyl peroxide, 446–47
Beta-blockers, 34, 200
Beta-carotene
    for emphysema, 119
    immunity and, 327
    muscle damage and, 125
    for night blindness, 222
Beverages. See Liquids
Bicycling
    for immunity, 331
    sex and, 432–33
    stationary, 514
        for osteoporosis, 390–91
Biobrane bandage, 128–29
Biofeedback, for headache, 289,
    292, 294
Birth control pills, high blood
    pressure from, 102
Birthmarks, 445
Bites, tick, 412–15
Blackheads, 446, 447
Bladder and kidney problems, 48
    bed-wetting, 63–64
    incontinence, 48–56
    kidney stones, 59–63
    urinary tract infections,
        56–59
Bleeding, stopping, 121–22
Blemishes, 446–49
Blisters, from sunburn, 405

Blood circulation. See
    Circulation
Blood clots, exercise and, 104
Blood pressure
    checking, 95–96, 506
    high (see High blood
        pressure)
Blow dryer, 276
Bodybuilding, osteoporosis and,
    388, 389–90
Body odor, 464–65
    bad breath, 145–46
    foot odor, 251–52
Boils, 449–50
Bone fractures, 347, 393–94
Bone loss. See Osteoporosis
Bonine, 176
Bowel problems, 65
    celiac disease, 84
    constipation, 70–72
    Crohn's disease, 80–81,
        82–84
    diarrhea, 67–70
    diverticulitis, 79–80
    diverticulosis, 79–80
    flatulence, 65, 66–67
    hemorrhoids, 72–75
    irritable bowel syndrome,
        75–79
    ulcerative colitis, 80–82
BPH, 358–61
Bran
    for constipation, 72
    for heart health, 306
    kidney stones and, 62
Bras
    neck pain and, 298–99
    support, 526–27
Breakfast, weight loss and, 507
Breast discomfort, 526–27
Breasts, neck pain and, 298–99
Breath, bad, 145–46
Breathing
    anger and, 198
    anxiety and, 201
    asthma and, 10, 11, 13
    diaphragmatic, 377, 380
    emphysema and, 120
    for fearful flyers, 501
    gagging and, 488
    for menstrual discomfort,
        524
    panic attacks and, 208–9,
        210
    for stress relief, 377, 380

testing, 316–17
weight loss and, 506
Chromium, 157
Chronic fatigue syndrome
(CFS), 238–44
Cigarette smoking. *See* Smoking
Circadian rhythm, 473, 475,
476
Circulation, 94–96
arterial health and, 96–105
Raynaud's disease, 105–6
Citrus pectin, 307
Climate
allergies and, 2, 4
asthma and, 10–11
bronchitis and, 116–17
colds and, 109–10
cold-weather problems,
417–24
hot-weather problems,
403–17
Raynaud's disease and,
106
seasonal affective disorder
and, 206–7
Cloned skin, for burns, 129–30
Clothing
allergies and, 7–8
chafing and, 451
dandruff and, 280
frostbite and, 421
hypothermia and, 422–23
weight loss and, 517–18,
520
yeast infections and, 539
Clotting, exercise and, 104
Clove (oil), for toothache, 143
Cochlear implant, 192–93
Cockroaches, allergies and, 4–5
Coffee. *See also* Caffeine
habit, 270
heart health and, 307–8
as laxative, 71
peptic ulcers and, 174
Cognitive-behavior therapy, for
depression, 202–4
Cola, 176, 384
Colds, 107–8. *See also* Influenza
fever from, 110–11
prevention of, 108–10
Cold sores, 458–61
Cold treatment
for arthritis, 31
for back pain, 38–39
for bruises, 125
for burns, 126

for eye injuries, 226
for gout, 36
for migraines, 291–92
for pain relief, 22–23, 25–26
for sprains and strains,
123–24
Cold-weather problems, 417–24
Colitis, ulcerative, 80–82
Collagen
in artificial skin, 130
estrogen and, 536
wound healing and, 132,
134
Complexion, 444–46
Computer screens, eyestrain
and, 227–28, 229–30
Condoms, 442, 539
Congestion, 116, 183
Conjunctivitis, 222–23
Constipation, 70–71
fiber for, 71–72
incontinence and, 50
Contact lenses, 221, 225–26
Contraception, urinary tract
infections and, 58
Contraceptives, oral, high blood
pressure from, 102
Cookies, weight loss and, 510
Cooking methods, for dietary
fat reduction, 330
Copper, for insomnia, 468
Corn bran, 306
Corns, 248–49
Coronary artery bypass surgery,
320
Coronary heart disease, 303
Cortaid cream, 405–6
Corticosteroids
for boils, 449
for Crohn's disease, 83
for eczema, 453
for hemorrhoids, 73
for laryngitis, 485–86
for nodules and cysts,
448–49
for ulcerative colitis, 81
Cortisol, 333
Cortisone
for arm and shoulder pain,
28
hemorrhoids and, 73
for sunburn blistering, 405
Cosmetics, insects and, 416
Coughing, from bronchitis,
115
Coughs, 482–84

Cramps
  leg, 339–40
  menstrual, 524, 525
  in summer, 408
Cranberry juice, 57
Cranial electrotherapy stimulation (CES), 289–90
Creativity, 368–70
Crohn's disease, 80–81, 82–84
Crying, depression and, 204
Cryosurgery, for warts, 464
Cumin, body odor from, 465
Curry, body odor from, 465
Cuts. See Wounds
Cyclosporine, 82
Cystitis, 56, 58
Cysts, 448–49, 526

D

Dairy products
  calcium in, 384–85
  lactose intolerance and, 175
  surgery and, 397
  yeast infections and, 539
Danazol, 530
Dander, 4, 6, 7
Dandruff, 5–6, 279–80
Daydreaming, constructive, 369
Deadlines, 211–12
Decongestants, 183
DEET, 414, 415
Dehydration, 409, 492
Dental checkup, 138
Dental problems, 135
  bad breath, 145–46
  bruxism, 151–52
  canker sores, 146–48
  cavities, 135–39
  denture adjustment, 150–51
  discolored teeth, 141–42
  lasers and, 144–45
  periodontal disease, 139–41
  tooth and gum pain, 142–44
  tooth injuries, 148–50
Depression, 202–4
  fatigue from, 236–37
  immunity and, 332
  at menopause, 537
  tinnitus from, 187
  winter, 206–7
Dermatitis, 451–53
DHT, 281
Diabetes, 153–54
  blood sugar monitoring and, 154–55
  diet and, 155–59

exercise and, 159–61
  incontinence and, 54
  stress and, 161
  Type I vs. Type II, 154
  weight control and, 155–56
Diarrhea, 67
  from celiac disease, 84
  from Crohn's disease, 82
  prevention of, 69–70
  traveler's, 491–95
  treatment of, 67–69
Diary
  for alcoholics, 266, 268
  for emotion release, 103
  for hot flashes, 536
  for weight loss, 506
Diet. See also Food(s); Meals; Nutrition
  alcoholism and, 268
  caffeine and, 271
  calcium in, 383–84, 384–85
  cancer prevention and, 90–91
  celiac disease and, 84
  constipation and, 71–72
  cramps and, 409
  Crohn's disease and, 83–84
  depression and, 203–4
  diabetes and, 155–59
  diarrhea and, 68, 69
  diverticula and, 79, 80
  dizziness and, 185
  fatigue and, 242–43
  for fearful flyers, 501
  flatulence and, 66
  gallstones and, 167, 170
  hair problems and, 275
  headache and, 295–96
  heartburn and, 164–66
  heart health and, 305–9
  high blood pressure and, 97–100
  immunity and, 325–29
  incontinence and, 51
  iron in, 17–20
  irritable bowel syndrome and, 77, 78
  itchy ears and, 182
  jet lag and, 497
  kidney stones and, 59–62
  nausea and, 176
  peptic ulcers and, 174
  Pritikin, 311
  quitting smoking and, 263–64

TMD and, 302
vesiculitis and, 355
Dietetic foods, 507
Dieting. *See also* Weight loss
crash, 233–34
Diet pills, 102
Digestive problems, 162
belching, 176–77
dyspepsia (indigestion), 162–64
gallstones, 166–70
heartburn, 164–66
hiccups, 177–78
lactose intolerance, 174–75
nausea and vomiting, 175–76
ulcers, 170–74
Digitalis, 204
Digital-rectal examination, 361
Diuretics, 50, 51
Diverticulitis, 79–80
Diverticulosis, 79–80
Dizziness, 183–86
Doctors, male avoidance of, 353
Dogs, 6, 7, 195
Dramamine, 185, 490, 491
Dressings, wound, 131–32
Drinking
alcohol (*see* Alcohol)
incontinence and, 49–50
Drugs. *See* Medications
Dust, vacuum cleaners and, 2
Dusting, 4
Dust mites, 1, 6
Dyspepsia, 162–64

E

Ear(s)
clogged, from flying, 498
implants in, 192–94
pierced, 180–81
protectors for, 190–91, 192
Ear problems, 179
congestion, 183
dizziness, 183–86
hearing loss, 189–96
infection, 179–81
itching, 182
swimmer's ear, 181–82
tinnitus (ringing), 186–89
wax buildup, 182–83
Echocardiography, 317
Eczema, 451–53
Ejaculation, premature, 437–38
Elbow, tennis, 22, 26

Elbow pain, 22
Elderly. *See* Aging
Electric hair appliances, 276, 278
Electrocautery, for warts, 463–64
Electromagnetic fields, cancer and, 92
Elevators, fear of, 210–11
Emetrol, 176
Emotional problems, 197–98
anger, 198–200
anxiety, 200–202
depression, 202–4
immunity and, 332–37
low self-esteem, 204–6
panic attack, 207–10
perfectionism, 212
phobias, 210–11
procrastination, 211–12
seasonal affective disorder (SAD), 206–7
shyness, 212–13
Emphysema, 118–20
Endometriosis, 527, 529–32
Enemas, 71
Environment
cancer prevention and, 92–93
noise in, 190, 191, 192, 194
Epididymitis, 356
Epstein-Barr virus, 240
ErecAid System, 436
Erection difficulties, 433–37
Erythromycin, 447
Estrogen
collagen and, 536
fibroids and, 528, 529
hot flashes and, 534, 535
menstruation and, 522
for prolapsed uterus, 532, 533
vaginal dryness and, 537
Estrogen replacement therapy (ERT)
for breast discomfort, 527
for heart health, 313
for osteoporosis, 386
sex and, 440
Etidronate, 393
Eustachian tube, 183, 498
Examination(s). *See* Medical examination(s)
Exercise(s). *See also* Walking
alcoholism and, 268
anemia and, 15–16
for anxiety, 201

for irritable bowel syndrome, 77
ulcerative colitis and, 81–82
Fibroids, 527, 528–29
Fibromyalgia, 240
Fish
for heart health, 99–100, 309
immunity and, 330
Fish oil
for arthritis pain relief, 33
diabetes and, 156
immunity and, 327
for psoriasis, 458
for Raynaud's disease, 106
5-ASA, 81
Flatulence, 65, 66–67
Flossing, 137, 140, 142
Flour, gas from, 67
Flu, 112–14
Fluids. See Liquids
Flying problems
altitude sickness, 498–500, 502
clogged ears, 498
fear, 500–501
jet lag, 495–98
Folate
for cold sores, 460
immunity and, 328, 329
restless legs and, 475
Folate deficiency, depression from, 204
Food(s). See also Diet; Meals; Nutrition
additives, cancer and, 91
ethnic
indigestion from, 163–64
weight loss and, 511
irradiated, 91
labels, 506–7
preparation of
diarrhea and, 493–94
for dietary fat reduction, 329–30
shopping list, 507–8
spicy and greasy, progesterone and, 524
for weight loss, 508–11
Foot problems, 245
athlete's foot, 249–50
blisters, 250–51
bunions, 245–46
burning feet, 247
calluses, 247–48

corns, 248–49
heel pain, 252–53
ingrown toenails, 253
metatarsal (ball of foot) pain, 253–54
odor, 251–52
plantar warts, 254
swollen feet, 254–55
tired and aching feet, 255–56
Formaldehyde, 8
Fractures, 347, 393–94
Fragrances, high blood pressure and, 103
Frostbite, 420–21
Fungus
athlete's foot from, 249–50
Candida albicans, 538–39
Furniture
allergies and, 3–4, 7
back pain and, 42, 43

G

Gagging, 487
Gallbladder, 166, 169
Gallstones, 166–67
imagery for, 168
prevention of, 167–70
surgery for, 169
Gardening, 11, 514
Gargling, for sore throat, 482
Garlic, for heart health, 308
Gas
belching, 176–77
flatulence, 65, 66–67
Gastroesophageal reflux, 164, 165
Gastrointestinal problems. See Bowel problems; Digestive problems
Gatorade, 408
Genisphere, 56
Genital herpes, 441–43
Giardiasis, 76
Ginger, 176, 490
Gingivitis, 139–40
Glasses
for computer work, 229, 230
over-the-counter, 225
protective, 226
Glaucoma, 217–18
Glucose, diabetes and, 153, 154–55, 157, 158
Gluten intolerance, 84
Gonorrhea, 442

Hoarseness, 484–87
Hormones. *See also* Estrogen;
   Progesterone; Prostaglandins;
   Testosterone
      menstruation and, 522
      neurohormones, 331, 332
      osteoporosis and, 386–87
Hospital, choice of, 399
Hospital stay, for heart attack,
   320
Hostility, 315
Hot flashes, 534–36
Hot water, sleep and, 470
Hot-weather problems,
   403–17
Humidity
      chapped skin and, 419–20
      colds and, 109–10
      complexion and, 446
      dry eyes and, 220
      hair and, 276–77
      for laryngitis, 485
      pneumonia and, 115
      postnasal drip and, 117
      for sore throat, 483–84
Hydrocortisone, 250, 452
Hypertension. *See* High blood
   pressure
Hyperventilation, in panic
   attacks, 208–9, 210
Hypnosis, for asthma, 13
Hypothermia, 422–24
Hysterectomy, 527, 528, 531,
   533–34
Hysteroscope, 529
Hytrin, 359

IBS. *See* Irritable bowel
   syndrome
Ibuprofen
      for arm and shoulder pain,
         24
      for back pain, 40
      for colds, 110, 111
      for endometriosis, 530
      for epididymitis, 356
      for gout, 35
      for headache, 290, 294
      for insect stings, 416
      for menstrual cramps, 525,
         527
      peptic ulcers and, 174
      for shinsplints, 346
      for sore throat, 482

Ice treatment
      for back pain, 38–39
      for burns, 126
      for cold sores, 459
      for epididymitis, 356
      for gout, 36
      for insect stings, 415–16
      for migraines, 291–92
      for neck pain, 297
      for pain relief, 22–23,
         25–26
      for pimples, 447
      for shinsplints, 346
      for sprains and strains,
         123–24
      for sunburn, 405
      for TMD, 301
IgA, 333
Imagery
      for anger, 199
      for anxiety, 201
      for arthritis, 32
      for asthma, 13
      for eye problems, 228–29
      for gallstones, 168
      for hair growth, 285
      for hot flashes, 535
      for incontinence, 53
      for irritable bowel syn-
         drome, 77
      for kidney stones, 61
      for leg cramps, 340
      for low self-esteem, 206
      for menstrual discomfort,
         522
      for peptic ulcers, 172–73
      in progressive relaxation,
         376–78
      for quitting smoking, 264
      for sleep, 471
      for sore throat, 481
Immunity, 325
      emotions and, 332–37
      exercise for, 331–32
      fat and, 329–30
      genital herpes and, 441–42
      music and, 336–37
      nutrition and, 325–29, 330
      vitamins and, 109
Immunoglobulin A (IgA), 333
Imodium, 68, 492, 493
Implants
      ear, 192–94
      for glaucoma, 218
Impotence, 433–38

for port-wine stain removal,
445
for wound healing, 134
Laughter, 103, 332–34
Laxatives, 71
Learning, 365–68
Leg pain, 338–39
cramps, 339–40
intermittent claudication,
341–43
knee pain, 347–51
shinsplints, 345–47
stress fractures, 347
varicose veins, 343–45
Legs, restless, 474–75
Lemon, for oily hair, 278
Lens, artificial, 216, 217
Lenses, contact, 221, 225–26
Leuprolide acetate, 78
Lidocaine injections, for arm
and shoulder pain, 28
Lifting, back pain and, 43
Ligament sprains, 122–25
Lips, chapped, 418–20
Liquids
for asthma, 10, 12
for bronchitis, 115–16
indigestion and, 163
for influenza, 113
traveler's diarrhea and, 492
vesiculitis and, 355
Lithotripsy, 63, 169
Loperamide, 68
Losec, 165
Love, immunity and, 334
Lower esophageal sphincter,
164, 166
Lozenges, for sore throat, 482
Lubricants, for vaginal dryness,
538
Lupron, 78, 529
Lyme disease, 412–13
Lymphocytes, 332, 333

M
Macrophages, 327
Macular degeneration, 218–19
Magnesium, 387–88, 523
Magnetic fields, cancer and, 92
Male pattern baldness, 280–83
Margarine, weight loss and,
509
Marriage. *See* Spouse
Massage
for headache, 293
for leg cramps, 339

for pain relief, 22, 23
for swollen feet, 255
Mattress, 43, 478
Mayonnaise, hair and, 276
Meals
altitude sickness and, 500
exercise and, 514
jet lag and, 497, 498
mental energy and, 374–75
weight loss and, 511–13
Meats
cured, migraines from,
295
fat in, 507, 509–10
Meat tenderizers, for insect
stings, 416
Medial tibial stress syndrome,
345
Medical examination(s)
for cancer prevention, 88–89
digital-rectal, 361
for testicular cancer, 362
Medications
depression from, 204
fatigue from, 235
impotence from, 434–35
incontinence from, 50
Raynaud's symptoms from,
106
sleep apnea from, 479
sun sensitivity from, 407
Meditation, immunity and, 335
Melanomas, 88
Memory, 371–73
Men
bicycle injury in, 432–33
doctor avoidance by, 353
Men's health problems, 352
baldness, 280–83
epididymitis, 356
hernia, 354–55
impotence, 433–38
prostate problems, 356–61,
363
testicular cancer, 362
vesiculitis, 355–56
Menopause problems, 534
bone loss, 386
depression, 537
dry skin, 536
fibroids, 528, 529
hot flashes, 534–36
vaginal dryness, 537–38
Menstrual discomfort, 521–27
Menstruation, endometriosis
and, 529–30

Nosebleed, 122
Nuprin. *See* Ibuprofen
Nursing, breast discomfort and, 527
Nutraderm, 446
Nutrition
    anemia and, 17–20
    celiac disease and, 84
    Crohn's disease and, 83–84
    immunity and, 325–29, 330
    surgery and, 397, 400–401

O

Oat bran, 306
Oatmeal
    for eczema, 452
    for sunburn pain, 127
Obesity. *See also* Weight control; Weight loss
    cancer and, 89
    gallstones and, 169–70
    heartburn and, 166
Odor, body. *See* Body odor
Odors, motion sickness and, 490
Oil(s)
    aromatic, for sore throat, 483
    food
        cholesterol and, 98
        diabetes and, 157–58
    olive, for heart health, 309
Oily hair, 278–79
Oily skin, moisturizers for, 445–46
Olive oil, 309
Omega-3 fatty acids. *See also* Fish oil
    for heart health, 309
    immunity and, 330
    for Raynaud's disease, 106
Onion, for heart health, 308
Orabase(-B), 148
Oral rehydration therapy (ORT), 68
Orgasm
    Kegel exercises and, 432
    migraines and, 292
ORT, 68
Osteoarthritis, 29
Osteoporosis, 381–82
    calcium and, 383–86, 387
    exercise and, 388–90, 390–91
    hormones and, 386–87
    magnesium and, 387–88

    risk factors for, 382
    treatment of, 390–94
    weight gain and, 388
Overweight. *See* Obesity; Weight control; Weight loss
Oxalate, kidney stones and, 60, 62
Oxygen, altitude sickness and, 498–99

P

Pain
    arm and shoulder, 21–28
    arthritis, 29–36
    back, 37–47
    from gallstones, 167
    head, 287–96, 299–302
    heel, 252–53
    knee, 347–51
    leg, 338–47
    metatarsal (ball of foot), 253–54
    muscle, 24–25
    neck, 287, 296–302
    from TMD, 299–302
    tooth and gum, 142–44
Paint fumes, laryngitis and, 485
Palladium, radioactive, 361
Panic attack, 207–10
Papaverine, 437
Paper cuts, 130
Pectin
    for heart health, 307
    for ulcerative colitis, 81–82
Pelvic muscle tone, 537
Penile prosthesis, 433, 437
Peptic ulcers, 170
    causes of, 171
    imagery for, 172–73
    medications for, 165
    symptoms of, 170–71
    treatment of, 171, 173–74
Pepto-Bismol, 68–69, 492–93, 495
Perfectionism, 212–13
Peridex, 138
Periodontal disease, 139–41
Permanone Tick Repellent, 414–15
Pessary, 532–33
Petroleum jelly, 450, 452
Pets
    allergens from, 6–7
    diarrhea and, 70

Pets (continued)
    high blood pressure and, 102
    ticks and, 415
PET scans, 318
pH balance, of vagina, 537
Phentolamine, 437
Phenylpropanolamine (PPA), 102
Phobias, 210–11
    flying, 500–501
Phosphate, calcium and, 384
Physical therapists, 25
Physicians, male avoidance of, 353
Piles, 72–75
Pillows, 44, 478
Pilocarpine, 217
Pimples, 446–49
Pinkeye, 222–23
Plantar warts, 254–55
Plants, in house, mold from, 9
Plaque (dental), 136–40
Pneumonia, 114–15
Poison ivy, 409–12
Pollen, 7, 8, 9
Polyunsaturated fats, 98
Popcorn, weight loss and, 510
Port-wine stains, 445
Positive attitude
    cancer and, 89–90
    depression and, 203
    immunity and, 337
    for low self-esteem, 205, 206
    for quitting smoking, 258
Positron emission tomography (PET) scans, 318
Postnasal drip, 117–18
Posture
    back pain and, 42, 43, 46
    TMD and, 301–2
Potassium, high blood pressure from, 98–99, 100
Potassium-sodium ratio, 99, 100, 120
PPA, 102
Prednisone, 81, 83, 448
Premature ejaculation, 437–38
Premenstrual discomfort, 521–27
Preparation H, 73, 127
Presbyopia, 225–26
Prescriptives Oil-Free Skin Renewer, 446
Pritikin diet, 311
Pritikin program, for heart health, 310–11

Probe coagulator, infrared, 75
Problem solving, 370–71
Procrastination, 211–12
Progesterone
    hair loss and, 286
    menstruation and, 522, 524
    for osteoporosis, 386, 387
Progressive relaxation, 376–78
Proscar, 359
Prostaglandin E$_1$, 437
Prostaglandin E$_2$, 327–28
Prostaglandins, 525, 530
Prostate problems, 356
    benign prostatic hypertro-phy (BPH), 358–61
    cancer, 360–61, 363
    prostatitis, 357–58
Prostate-specific antigen im-munoassay, 360
Protein
    calcium and, 383
    jet lag and, 497
    kidney stones and, 60
Psoralen baths, 458
Psoriasis, 456–58
Psychotherapy, short-term, 197–98, 201, 442
Psyllium, 72, 307
Ptosis, 231
Public speaking, 214
Pubococcygeus muscles, 432
Purine, gout and, 36
Purpose soap, 452, 454
Pyelonephritis, 56
Pyorrhea, 140

Q

Quinine, 339–40
Q-Vel, 339–40

R

Radiation synovectomy, 34
Radon, 92–93
Rash, from tick bites, 412, 413
Raynaud's disease, 105–6
Reflux, gastroesophageal, 164, 165
Relaxation. See also Anxiety; Stress; Tension
    for fearful flyers, 501
    immunity and, 335
Relaxation exercises. See also Imagery
    for asthma, 12–13
    for back pain, 41
    headache and, 294

T

Tabasco, for sore throat, 483
Tagamet, 165, 171
Talcum powder, 450
Talking, laryngitis and, 485
Tannic acid, as carpet spray, 3
Tannin, for mouth pain, 148,
    150
Tapes, surgery and, 396, 402
T-cells, 328, 331, 332, 333
Tea
    for canker sores, 148
    for foot odor, 252
    for sore throat, 483
Tears, artificial, 220
Teeth
    bleaching of, 142
    brushing of, 136–37, 140,
        142
    desensitization of, 144, 145
    grinding of, 151–52, 301
Teeth problems. See Dental
    problems
Temporomandibular disorder
    (TMD), 188, 299–302
Tendinitis, 22, 24, 124
Tennis elbow, 22, 26
TENS, for headache, 289
Tension. See also Anxiety;
    Relaxation; Stress
    fatigue from, 235–36
    mental performance and,
        379–80
Terazosin, 359
Testicular cancer, 362
Testosterone, 281
TestPack Chlamydia, 443
Tetracycline, 142
Thiamine deficiency, depression
    from, 204
Thinking. See also Learning
    visual, 367
Throat problems, 480
    coughs, 482–84
    gagging, 487
    laryngitis, 484–87
    sore throat, 113–14, 480–82
    tickle, 484
Thrombolysis, 318–20
Ticks, 412–15
Tinactin, 250
Tinnitus, 186–89
Tiredness. See Fatigue
TMD (TMJ), 299–302
Tobacco. See Smoking
Toenails, ingrown, 253

Tongue
    bleeding, 150
    burned, 127
Toothbrush
    cavities and, 137
    cold sores and, 459–60
    electric, 140
    traveler's diarrhea and, 495
Tooth cap, knocked off, 149–50
Toothpaste
    for insect stings, 416
    for whiter teeth, 142
Tooth problems. See Dental
    problems
Toxins, 93
Transcutaneous electrical nerve
    stimulation (TENS), 289
Transrectal needle biopsy, 363
Transurethral resection of the
    prostate (TURP), 359
Travel problems, 489
    altitude sickness, 498–500,
        502
    clogged ears, 498
    jet lag, 495–98
    motion sickness, 489–91
    turista (diarrhea), 491–95
Tretinoin (Retin-A), 447, 454
Trichloroacetic acid, 455
Tricyclic antidepressants, 243–44
Trimethoprim, 57
Turista, 491–95
TURP, 359
Tylenol. See Acetaminophen
Type A behavior, 315–16

U

Ulcerative colitis, 80–82
Ulcers, peptic. See Peptic ulcers
Ultrasound
    echocardiography, 317
    for pain relief, 25
    scan for prostate cancer,
        360–61, 363
Underwear, men's, fertility and,
    427
Urethra damage, 55
Urethritis, 56
Uric acid, gout and, 35, 36
Urinary incontinence. See
    Incontinence
Urinary problems, in men, 355,
    358, 360
Urinary tract infections, 56–59
Urushiol, 410, 411

Walking *(continued)*
    for stress relief, 380
    for varicose veins, 343–44
Warts, 254, 462–64
Water
    diarrhea and, 70
    hot, sleep and, 470
    kidney stones and, 60
    for laryngitis, 485
    quitting smoking and, 263
    salt *(see* Salt water)
    for soaking nails, 456
    for throat tickle, 484
    traveler's diarrhea and, 494
    walking in, for arthritis, 30
    weight loss and, 512
Water irrigation, periodontal disease and, 140
Weakness. *See* Fatigue
Weight control. *See also* Obesity; Weight loss
    cancer prevention and, 89
    diabetes and, 155–56
    fertility and, 426
    for intermittent claudication, 342
    sleep apnea and, 477–78
Weight gain
    during holidays, 518–19
    osteoporosis and, 388
Weight lifting, 26, 160
Weight loss, 503. *See also* Obesity; Weight control
    clothing for illusion of, 517–18, 520
    eating tips for, 511–13
    exercise for, 513–15
    food flavor and, 510–11
    food selection for, 508–10
    holidays and, 518–19
    incontinence and, 51
    mind-set for, 505–6
    plateaus in, 515–16
    preparation for, 503–5
    rewards for, 516
    strategy for, 506–8
    temptation and, 516–17
Wellbutrin, 439
Wheezing, in infants, 12
Whiteheads, 446, 447
Wine, red, headache from, 295
Winter problems, 417–24
Witch hazel, 224

Women's health problems, 521
    acne, 448
    anemia, 15–16
    Candida albicans (yeast infections), 538
    hair loss, 283–86
    incontinence, 52, 55, 56
    menopause changes, 534
        depression, 537
        dry skin, 536
        hot flashes, 534–36
        vaginal dryness, 537–38
    menstrual discomfort, 521–27
    osteoporosis, 381–94
    sexual problems, 438–40
    uterine disorders, 527–28
        endometriosis, 529–32
        fibroids, 528–29
        prolapsed uterus, 532–34
Wool clothing, allergies and, 8
Work, return to, after heart attack, 320
Wounds, 121. *See also* Bruises; Burns
    healing of, 130–35
    stopping bleeding from, 121–22

X

Xylitol, 139

Y

Yawning, 302, 498
Yeast, diarrhea and, 68
Yeast infections, 538–39
Yoga breathing exercises, for asthmatics, 13
Yoga stretches, for menstrual discomfort, 524

Z

Zantac, 171
Zinc
    for acne, 448
    for body odor, 465
    for cold sores, 460–61
    immunity and, 327, 328, 329
    for sore throat, 482
Zovirax, 461, 462